MW00441935

skinnytaste®
Simple

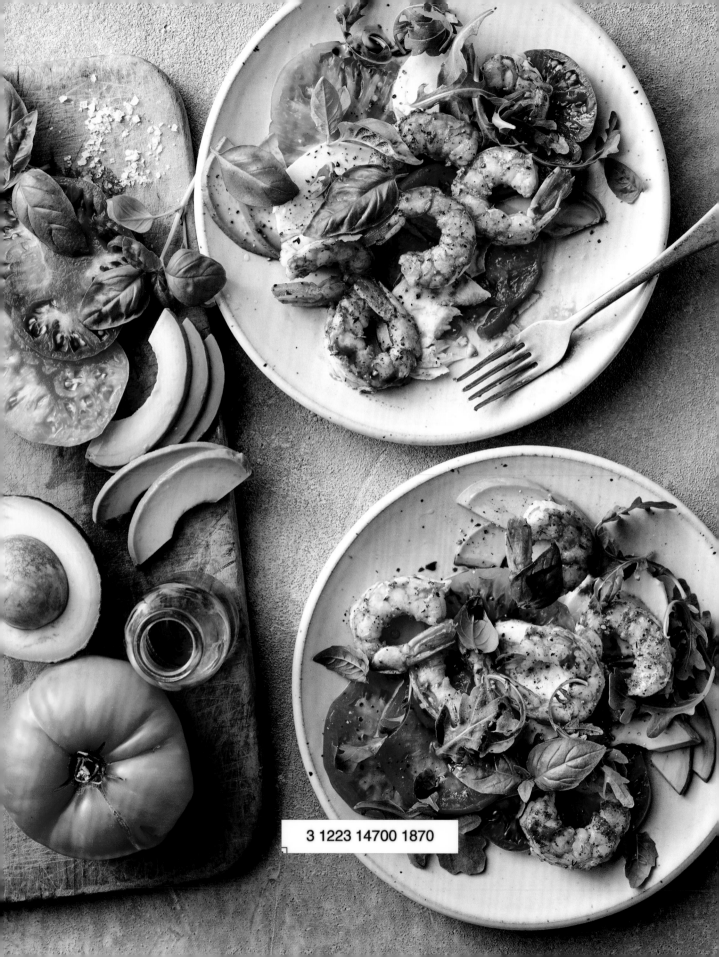

3 1223 14700 1870

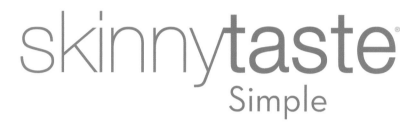

skinnytaste Simple

Easy, Healthy Recipes with 7 Ingredients or Fewer

Gina Homolka

with Heather K. Jones, R.D.

Photographs by Eva Kolenko

Clarkson Potter/Publishers
New York

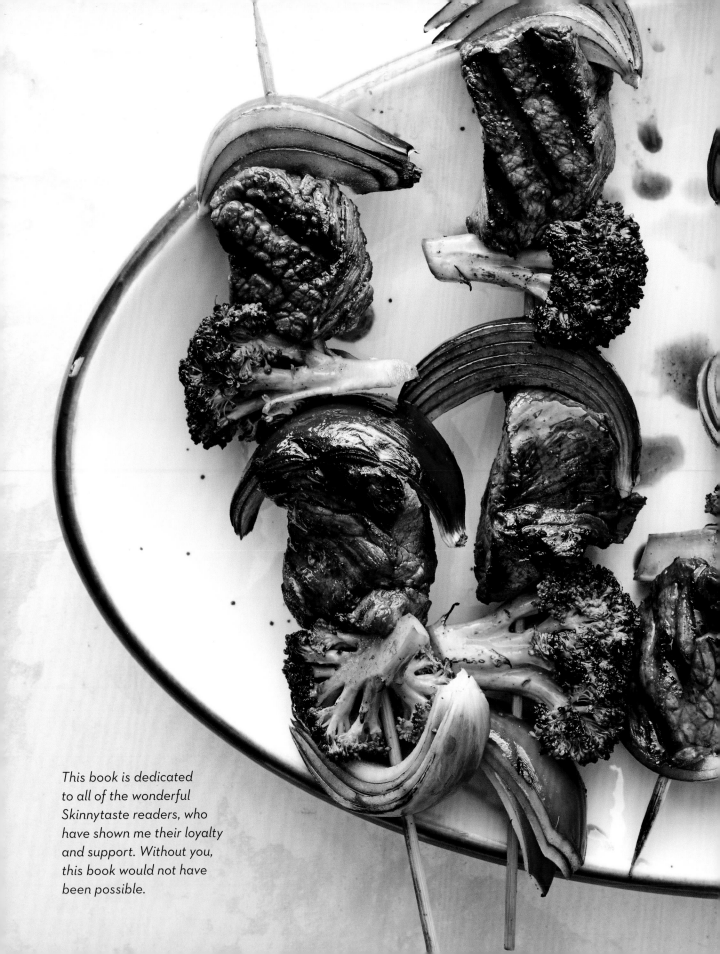

This book is dedicated to all of the wonderful Skinnytaste readers, who have shown me their loyalty and support. Without you, this book would not have been possible.

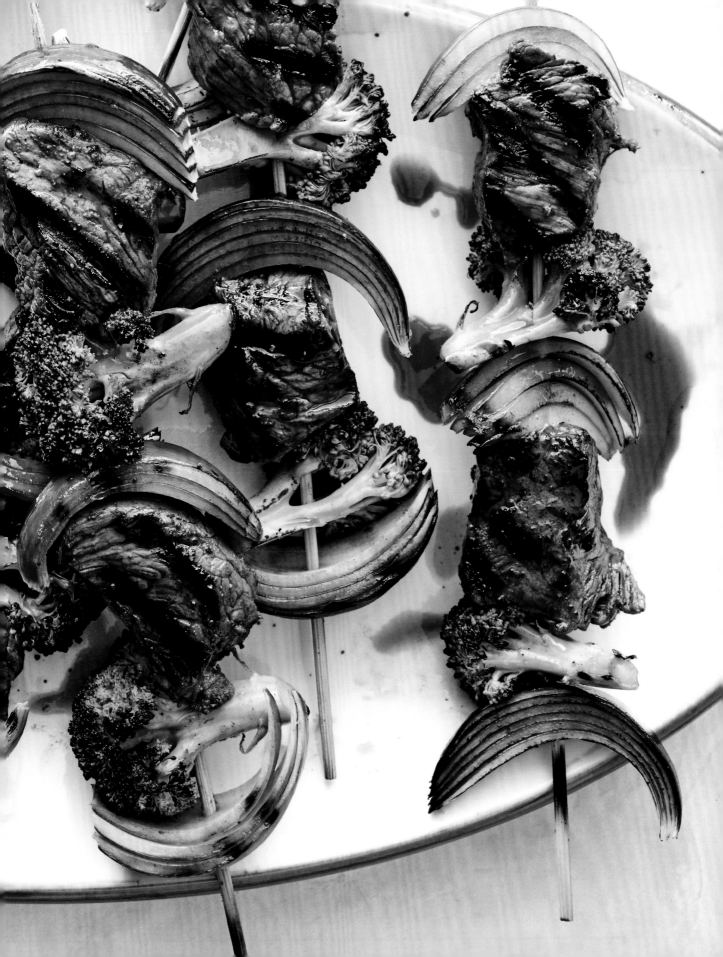

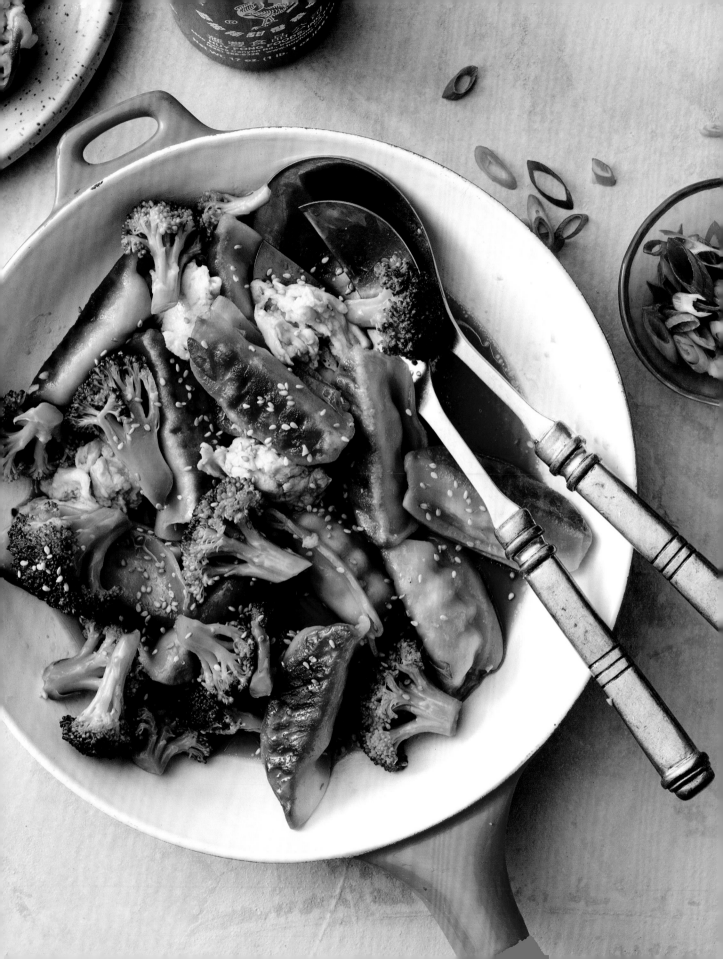

Contents

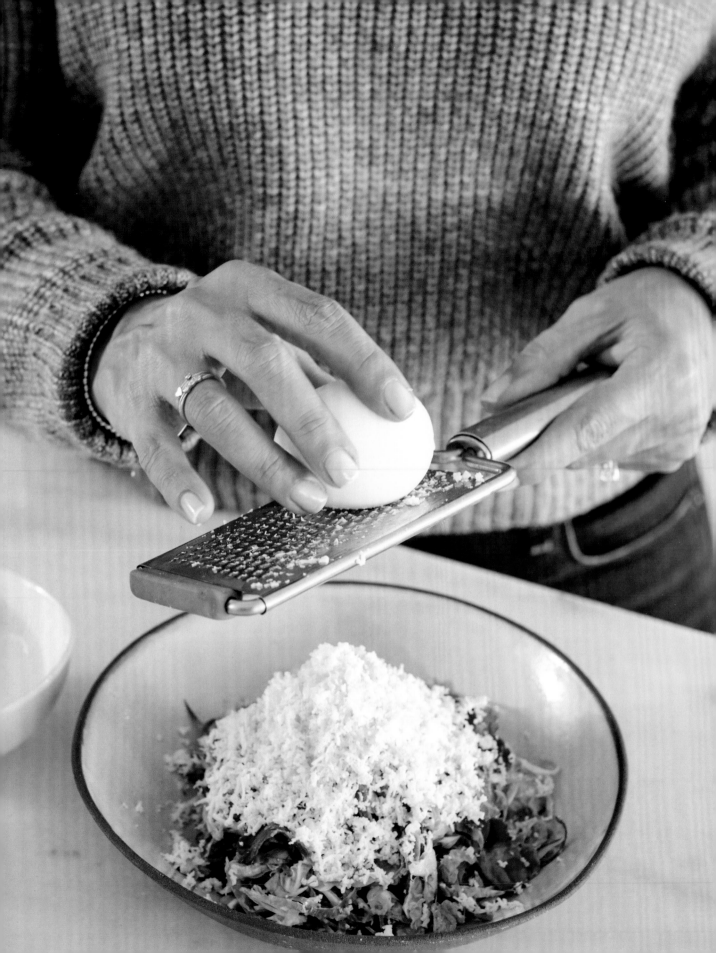

Introduction

Over the years, I've met so many people who have told me they want to eat healthier, but they don't like to cook. Their reasoning is that it's too hard, too much work, or they don't have time. And to be honest, anytime I see a recipe in a cookbook that has a long list of ingredients, I usually avoid it myself! When I have a lot going on, I'm lucky if I get a healthy meal on the table every night, so cooking complicated recipes that require a lot of time is certainly a luxury. Even though I'm often short on time, I love cooking at home and knowing what goes into the food I'm eating.

That's why this cookbook is filled with healthy recipes that use no more than 7 ingredients. I want to make feeding yourself and your family good-for-you meals easier than ever. Whether you're busy, tired, a beginner cook, looking for budget-friendly meals—or all of the above!—this book is for you.

My hope is to get everyone to enjoy cooking their own homemade meals, and with these recipes, there are no excuses. We are all busy but still want to eat well, so this book is both simple to cook from and doesn't require a large shopping list, which also means saving more money at the grocery store.

How do you create flavorful dishes with minimum fuss? I have a few tricks: finding winning flavor and ingredient combinations; using super fresh in-season produce; seasoning with lots of bright herbs, spices, and citrus; and utilizing condiments and sauces that pack a lot of flavor. I've made it as simple as possible to cook nutritious and delicious food, with just 7 ingredients or fewer, any night of the week. The dishes in this book have become recipes I repeat over and over in my home, and I can't wait for you to try them, too.

Not only are the recipes in these pages simple and easy, but they can also help you stick to your wellness goals. I made sure to include plenty of protein in each dish because it's satiating, so you can fill up on simple, tasty foods without going overboard on portion sizes. Many of the recipes are also veggie-packed and include lightened-up versions of your favorite indulgences, like Baked Beef Stew with Butternut Squash (page 218) and Instant Pot Spaghetti Rings with Beef (page 205). Since all of the recipes are short, I focused on the quality of ingredients and flavors over quantity. The result is a book jam-packed with nutritious dishes that couldn't be simpler to make.

There's everything from breakfast items to recipes for sharing with friends to a whole chapter on soups and main-dish salads, to dinner recipes. I've also included desserts like Coconut Rice Pudding with Mango (page 293) and Mini Blueberry Swirl Cheesecakes (page 273) that you can enjoy anytime. To make things even simpler, there are a lot of sheet pan recipes, such as Sheet Pan Tomato Soup with Grilled Cheese Croutons (page 91), as well as one-pot dishes like One-Pot Creamy Gnocchi with Chicken and Leeks (page 185), and even some Instant Pot and air fryer recipes like Instant Pot "Baked" Ziti with Spinach (page 115) and Air Fryer Chicken Drumsticks (page 175).

When I first started exploring this concept, I have to admit I was hesitant—I thought it would be tough. How do you cut back on ingredients without losing flavor? But I love a good challenge, so I had a lot of fun testing these recipes. Even with so few ingredients, these recipes are packed with flavor and turned out to be some of my favorites from any of my cookbooks. And since this is my 7th cookbook, it felt like a 7-ingredient cookbook was meant to be.

I hope you enjoy the simplicity of this cookbook and love it as much as I do! It's sure to become a favorite on your bookshelf, and it's the perfect book to share with friends or family members who love easy, healthy meals as much as you do. If you share a meal from this book on social media, be sure to tag me so I can see what you're cooking and reshare on my social channels. I love seeing everyone's favorite cookbook recipes in action!

The Simple Pantry

I've kept the recipes to 7 ingredients or fewer using easy-to-find vegetables, proteins, herbs, and spices. You'll notice many of the recipes have a handful of ingredients mentioned in the directions, but not in the ingredient list. That's because items like salt, pepper, and oil are so basic that I am certain you always have them on hand, which is why I haven't counted them toward the 7 total ingredients (but I have calculated them in the nutrition information).

1. Salt
The salt I cook with every day is Diamond Crystal kosher salt. Note that different brands and different types of salt vary not only in the amount of sodium per measured amount, but also in taste. When cooking the recipes in the book—both for flavor and for the sodium values listed—you should use Diamond Crystal kosher salt. If you use another type of salt or a different brand of kosher salt, just remember to taste as you go.

2. Black pepper
Just like salt, freshly ground black pepper is a kitchen staple that even most noncooks keep on hand.

3. Cooking oils
The oils I cook with most are extra-virgin olive oil, olive oil (including the spray), and occasionally vegetable oil. I typically cook with extra-virgin olive oil because I love the taste, but when I need an oil with a high smoke point, I will use olive oil, grapeseed oil, or avocado oil. For salad dressing and finishing a dish, I always use extra-virgin olive oil because it gives the dish the best flavor. I also love toasted sesame oil in Asian-inspired dishes.

Recipe Key
Look for these helpful icons throughout the book:

- Ⓠ Quick (ready in 30 minutes or less)
- Ⓥ Vegetarian
- GF Gluten-Free
- DF Dairy-Free
- FF Freezer-Friendly
- AF Air Fryer
- PC Pressure Cooker
- SC Slow Cooker

Weight Watchers Points
For those of you on WW, I've linked all my recipes to the WW recipe builder, which will give you the points conveniently located on my website under the cookbook tab: *skinnytaste.com/cookbook-index*

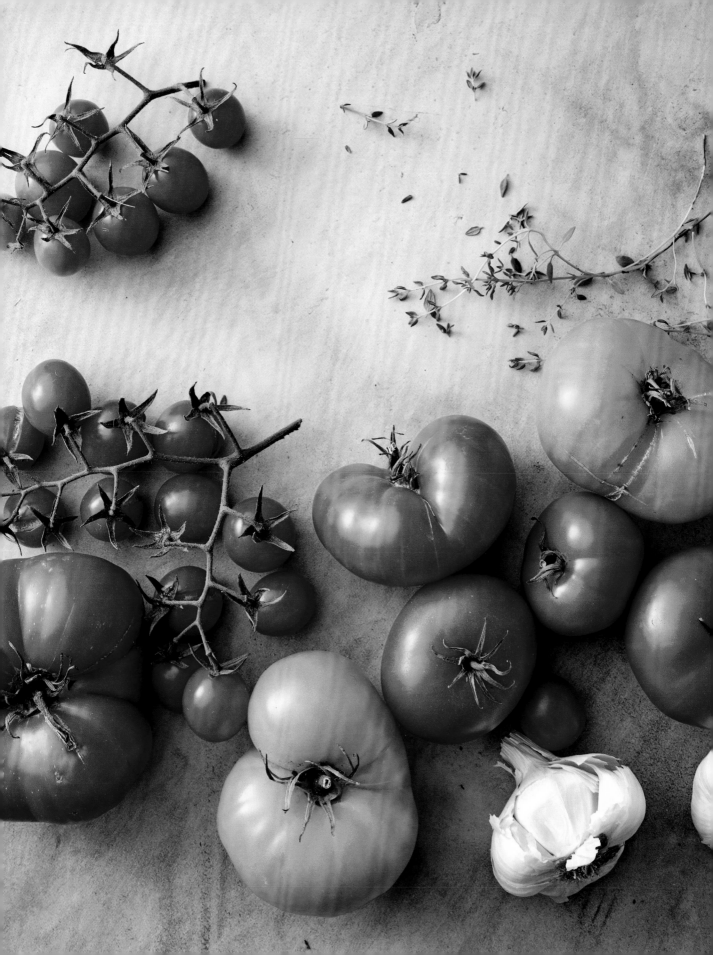

7 Tips for Cooking with 7 Ingredients or Fewer

1. Control the Quality

With limited ingredients, you want to make sure you're using the highest quality ingredients possible. Get to know your local butchers, fishmongers, farmers, and bakers. I buy ethically sourced and humanely raised meat, poultry, dairy, and eggs, as well as sustainable seafood, whenever I can. Shop at farmers' markets and buy in-season produce (see more on this below, in number 2). Always sample different brands of cheese, dairy, broths, grains, condiments, and spices, then choose discriminatingly. I think finding the best and freshest ingredients for my recipes is half the fun! My local suppliers know me by name, and I consider them friends.

2. Cook Seasonally

In-season fruits and vegetables have the best flavor because they're picked when ripe and aren't stored for long periods of time before making it to your table. There's nothing worse than a mealy winter tomato from the grocery store or a rock-hard peach when they're out of season. Shopping for in-season produce (and freezing extra summer produce for the winter) gets you the most flavor bang for your buck, which is important when that produce is one of 7 or fewer ingredients in a recipe. Whenever possible, I like to buy produce from my local farmers' market or the displays of local in-season produce at my grocery store to make sure I'm getting the freshest fruits and veggies available.

3. Embrace Color

I like to use a variety of colors in every dish I make to help me "eat the rainbow." Eating a range of colors increases your intake of various nutrients that are beneficial to your health. We also eat with our eyes, so making dishes visually appealing is always a priority for me. I make dishes more exciting by adding color from ingredients like multicolor peppers and fresh herbs, and using a variety of vegetables in salads, sides, and crudité platters.

4. Take Advantage of Prepared Foods

Cooking with fewer ingredients means you have to find ways to get creative while still making sure you're eating unprocessed foods. Foods like rotisserie chicken, pizza dough, and good-quality jarred sauces make meals simpler without adding a ton of unwanted processed ingredients. These prepared foods make a great starting point for entirely new dishes and cut down on your prep time and ingredient list.

5. The Freezer Is Your Friend

Aside from a short ingredient list, I wanted these recipes to be quick and simple because we're all busy. I keep my freezer stocked with lots of convenient whole foods to help make whipping up a meal fast: Frozen brown rice, empanada wrappers, pizza dough, frozen pot stickers, veggies, berries, etc., are all great items to keep on hand for shortcut meals. I also always have a stock of frozen proteins to use when I need to whip up a last-minute meal: Shrimp, fish, ground beef or turkey, chicken breast, tofu, and edamame are all great options to keep in your freezer to make mealtime even easier.

6. Get Creative with Condiments and Sauces

Condiments and sauces are the secret weapons in recipes with minimal ingredients. They last a long time in the fridge, so once you buy them to use in a recipe, you'll be set for quite a while. I keep all sorts of high-quality condiments and seasoning sauces on hand to level up my simplest meals. Using Sriracha, toasted sesame oil, hoisin sauce, BBQ sauce, vinegars, and more can transform a plain dish into an extraordinary one without any extra effort. As you cook through the recipes in this book, your pantry will expand naturally to include a variety of condiments, vinegars, oils, and sauces that will easily transform your meals.

7. Spice It Up

Whether you cook every night or just occasionally, you don't need to worry about having every single spice and herb on hand. Your seasoning pantry will grow gradually as you continue to experiment with new recipes, but there are some staples I always keep on hand. I use these seasonings often and recommend starting with them if you're building your pantry for the first time: kosher salt, black pepper, garlic powder, cumin, paprika, cinnamon, and dried oregano, just to name a few.

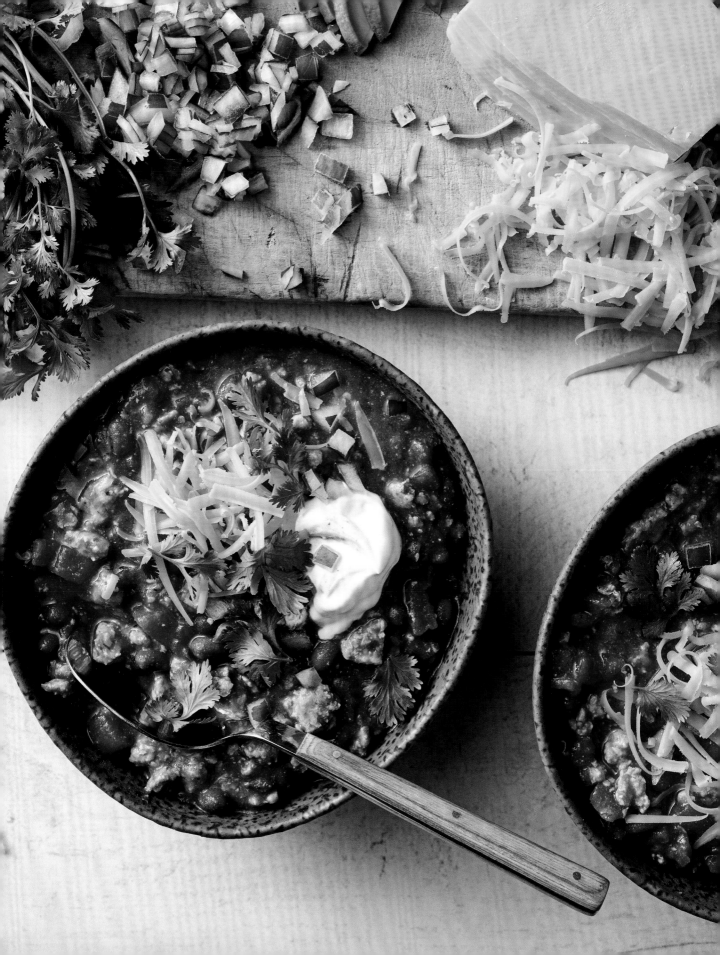

Morning Meals

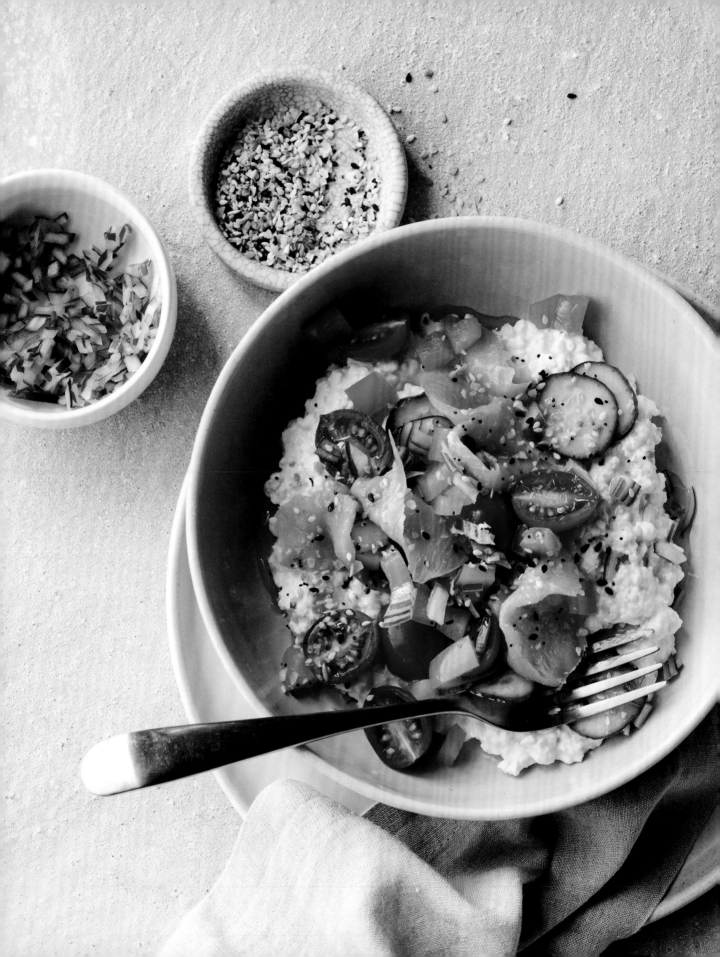

Everything but the Bagel Cottage Cheese and Lox Bowl

SERVES 1

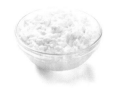

I love cottage cheese: It's loaded with protein and makes the perfect base for this savory bowl that's inspired by all the toppings I love on a bagel (minus the bread!). Perfect for breakfast or a snack, these bowls are an easy way to get more nutrient-rich foods into your day. If you're not a fan of cottage cheese, you can use plain yogurt instead.

¾ cup low-fat (2%) cottage cheese (I like Good Culture)

1 ounce Nova lox, chopped

½ cup sliced Persian (mini) cucumbers

½ medium orange or yellow bell pepper, chopped

10 grape tomatoes, halved

1 thin slice red onion, chopped

1 teaspoon salt-free everything bagel seasoning

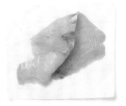

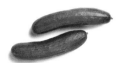

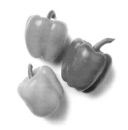

Place the cottage cheese in a small bowl. Layer the lox, cucumbers, bell pepper, and tomatoes on top of the cottage cheese. Garnish with the red onion, drizzle with 1 teaspoon extra-virgin olive oil, and sprinkle with the everything bagel seasoning.

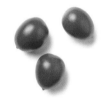

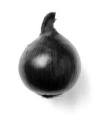

Per Serving (1 bowl) ● Calories 252 ● Fat 10 g ● Saturated Fat 3 g ● Cholesterol 29 mg
Carbohydrate 17 g ● Fiber 4 g ● Protein 29 g ● Sugars 13 g ● Sodium 745 mg

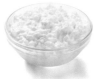
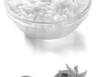

Maple Pecan Cottage Cheese

SERVES 1

I always have cottage cheese in my fridge, and depending on my mood, I enjoy it sweet or savory. This is my go-to when I want something sweet. The maple syrup gives it that salty-sweet combo that really works, and you can use your favorite ripe fruit that's in season.

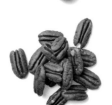

¾ cup low-fat (2%) cottage cheese (I like Good Culture)
½ cup diced fruit, such as berries, apples, peaches, or pears
8 pecan halves, coarsely chopped
1 tablespoon pure maple syrup

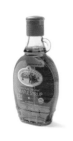

Place the cottage cheese in a small bowl. Top with the fruit and pecans and drizzle with maple syrup.

Sweet + Savory Cottage Cheese Bowls

Cottage cheese bowls are a delicious and healthy way to start the day! See page 19 for my Everything but the Bagel Cottage Cheese and Lox Bowl, and here are a few more toppings to try:

• Chopped apples + walnuts + maple syrup + cinnamon
• Sliced cucumbers + avocado + grape tomatoes + salt and freshly ground black pepper
• Sliced mango + banana + shredded coconut
• Raspberries + blueberries + pistachios + honey
• Chopped hard-boiled eggs + bell peppers + chives + salt and freshly ground black pepper
• Chopped pineapples + macadamia nuts
• Burst cherry tomatoes (cooked with EVOO in a pan until they burst) + chopped basil + balsamic vinegar + salt and freshly ground black pepper

Per Serving (1 bowl) ● Calories 285 ● Fat 12 g ● Saturated Fat 3 g ● Cholesterol 23 mg
Carbohydrate 28 g ● Fiber 2 g ● Protein 22 g ● Sugars 23 g ● Sodium 512 mg

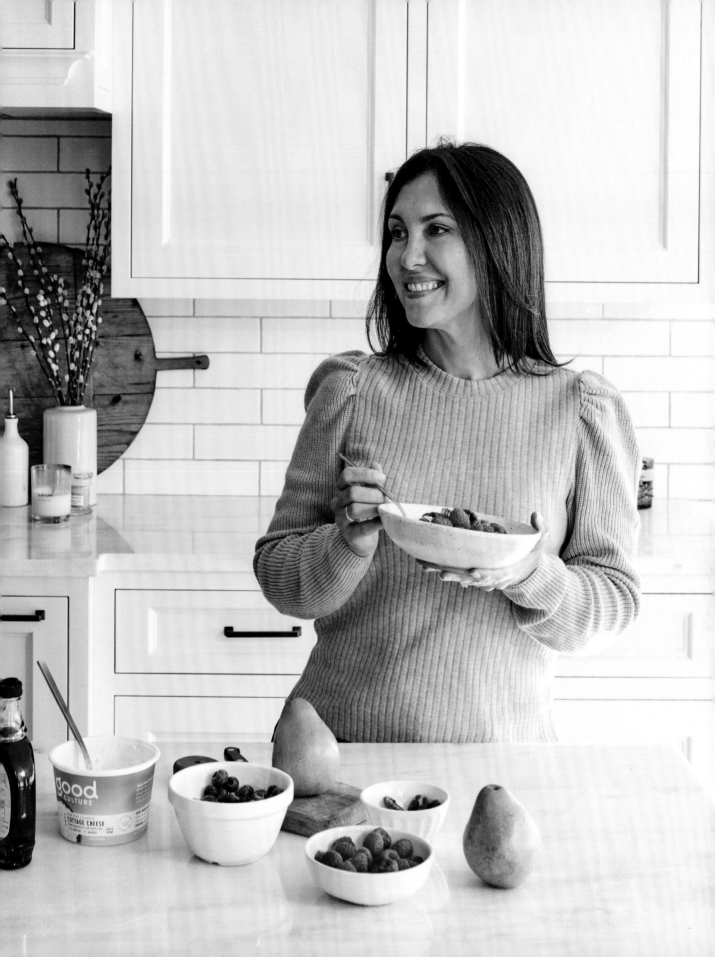

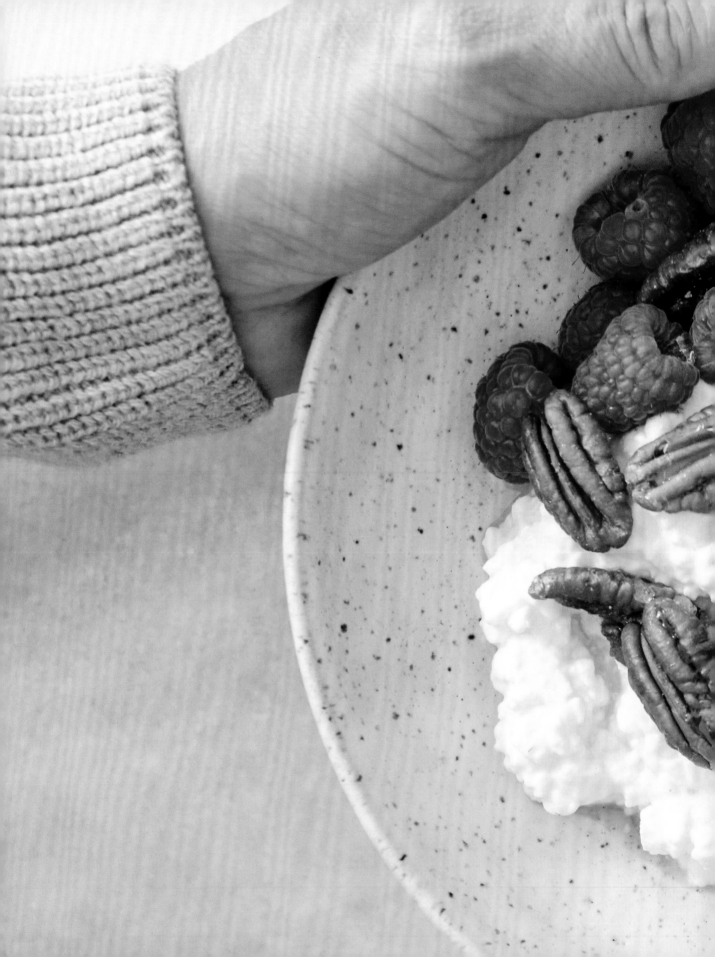

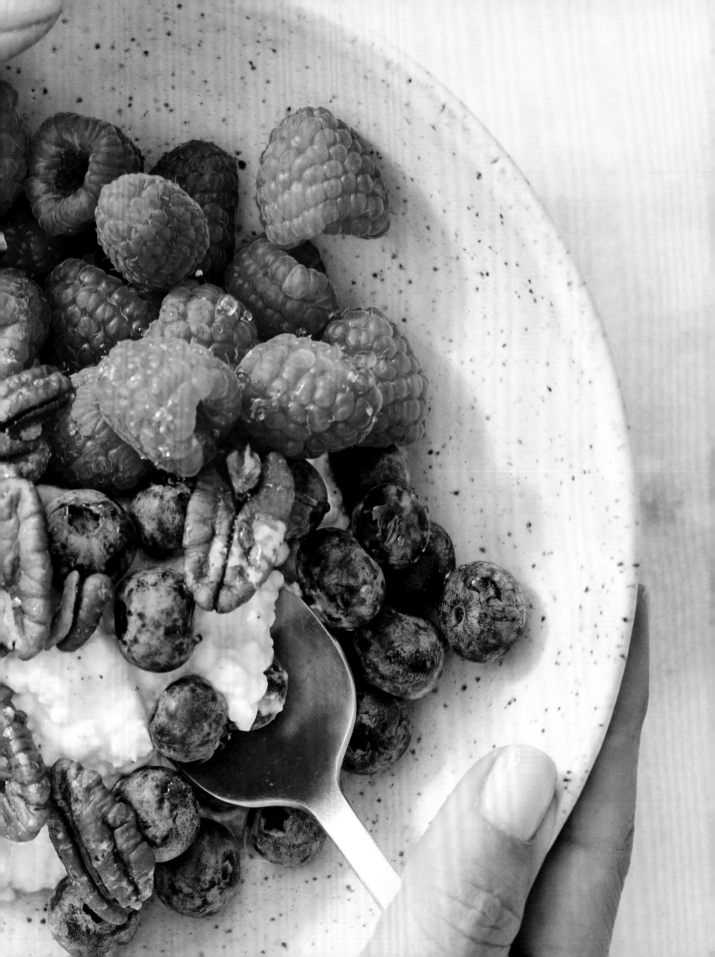

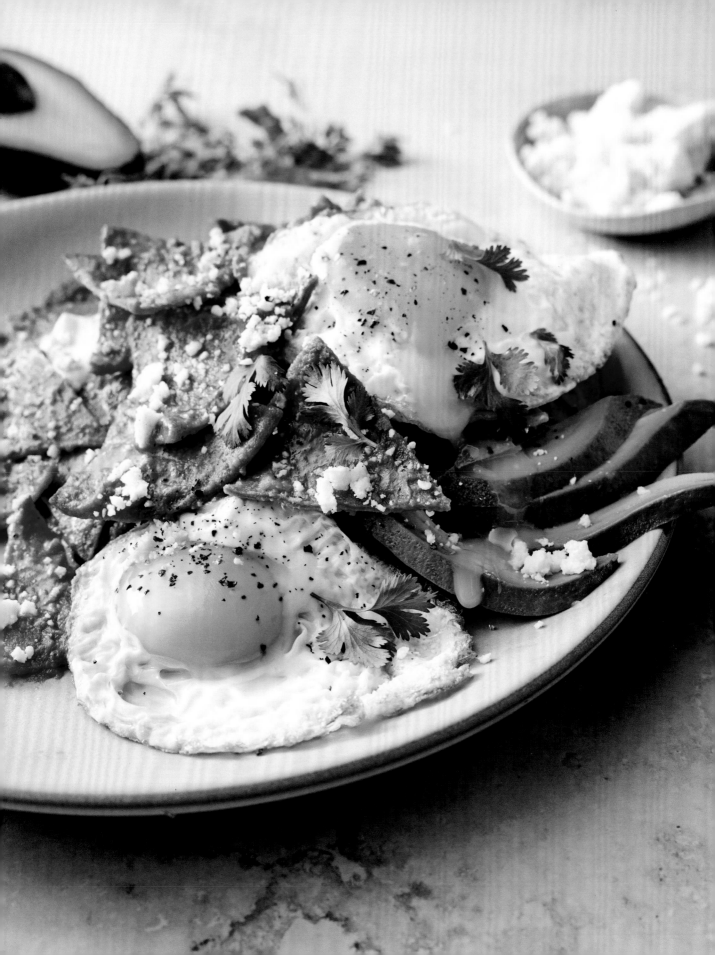

Red Chilaquiles with Fried Eggs

SERVES 4

Chips for breakfast? Yes, please! Chilaquiles, a traditional Mexican breakfast made with tortillas simmered in tomato or tomatillo sauce and topped with cheese, are a nacho lover's dream. But unlike nachos, chilaquiles are a meal to be eaten with a fork. This dish is also an amazing way to have breakfast for dinner. Fried chips are typically used in chilaquiles, but here they're made lighter by baking them. Top with fresh cilantro, avocado, or sour cream, if you have them!

12 (6-inch) corn tortillas (I like Guerrero)

½ medium yellow onion, diced

2 garlic cloves, minced

1½ cups canned tomato sauce (about 12 ounces)

1 tablespoon diced canned chipotle peppers in adobo sauce

8 large eggs

4 tablespoons crumbled Cotija cheese or feta cheese

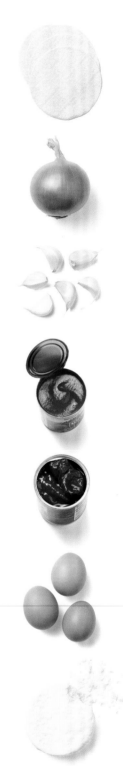

Preheat the oven to 425°F.

Stack the tortillas on top of each other and cut into 8 wedges. Spray two sheet pans with extra-virgin olive oil and arrange the wedges in an even layer on both sheet pans. Lightly spray the wedges with olive oil and sprinkle with ¼ teaspoon kosher salt. Bake for 4 minutes, then remove the sheet pans from the oven to carefully flip the chips, and continue to bake for 4 minutes more, or until the chips are golden and crisp all over. Set aside to cool.

Heat a medium skillet over medium heat and add 2 teaspoons extra-virgin olive oil. Add the onion and sauté, stirring occasionally, until softened and translucent, about 5 minutes. Add the garlic and sauté for 30 seconds more until fragrant. Remove the skillet from the heat and pour the mixture into a high-powered blender or food processor. Add the tomato sauce, chipotle peppers, ⅓ cup water, and ½ teaspoon kosher salt and process on high until smooth.

(recipe continues)

Per Serving (1 cup chilaquiles + 2 eggs + 1 tablespoon cheese) ● Calories 380 ● Fat 17 g Saturated Fat 5 g ● Cholesterol 380 mg ● Carbohydrate 40 g ● Fiber 6.5 g ● Protein 20 g Sugars 5 g ● Sodium 973 mg

Pour the sauce into the skillet. Set over medium heat and cook until the sauce has slightly reduced and the flavors have melded, 4 to 5 minutes.

Meanwhile, to make the eggs, heat a large skillet over medium-low heat and spray with olive oil. Working in batches if needed, carefully crack the eggs into the skillet. Cover and cook until the whites turn opaque, 3 to 5 minutes. Sprinkle the eggs with a pinch of kosher salt and freshly ground black pepper to taste.

Add the chips to the skillet with the sauce and toss to evenly coat. Divide the mixture equally among four plates (about 1 cup each). Top each serving with 2 eggs and sprinkle each with 1 tablespoon of Cotija cheese. Serve immediately.

High-Protein Oat Waffles

SERVES 5

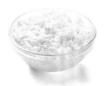

I'm obsessed with these high-protein waffles! I top mine with nut butter plus whatever fruit I have on hand, usually banana and some strawberries, but you can top yours with any type you wish (or syrup, too!). Protein-packed oats, cottage cheese, and eggs are what make these crisp and fluffy waffles keepers.

SKINNY SCOOP: If you don't have oat flour on hand, simply process 1 cup plus 2 tablespoons rolled oats in a blender until finely ground. Also, you may omit the sugar or use your favorite sweetener instead.

2/3 cup small curd whole-milk (4%) cottage cheese

2 large eggs, separated

1 teaspoon vanilla extract

1 tablespoon sugar (optional)

1 cup oat flour* (see Skinny Scoop)

½ teaspoon baking powder

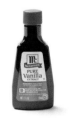

*Read the label to be sure this product is gluten-free.

In a blender, combine the cottage cheese, egg yolks, vanilla, and sugar (if using). Add 6 tablespoons water, the oat flour, baking powder, and ¼ teaspoon kosher salt and blend until the mixture has the consistency of a smooth batter. Transfer to a medium bowl, using a spatula to scrape all the batter out.

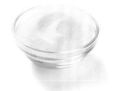

In a medium bowl, with an electric mixer, beat the egg whites to soft peaks, then gently fold them into the batter.

Preheat a waffle iron according to the manufacturer's instructions. Spray the hot iron with olive oil. Pour about ¼ cup of the batter into the iron and cook until the waffle is golden brown and steam is no longer being released. Repeat with the remaining batter (you'll have 10 waffles total) and serve.

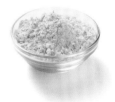

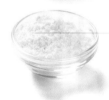

Per Serving (2 waffles/¼ cup batter each) ● Calories 156 ● Fat 5 g ● Saturated Fat 1.5 g Cholesterol 79 mg ● Carbohydrate 19 g ● Fiber 2.5 g ● Protein 9 g ● Sugars 0.5 g Sodium 246 mg

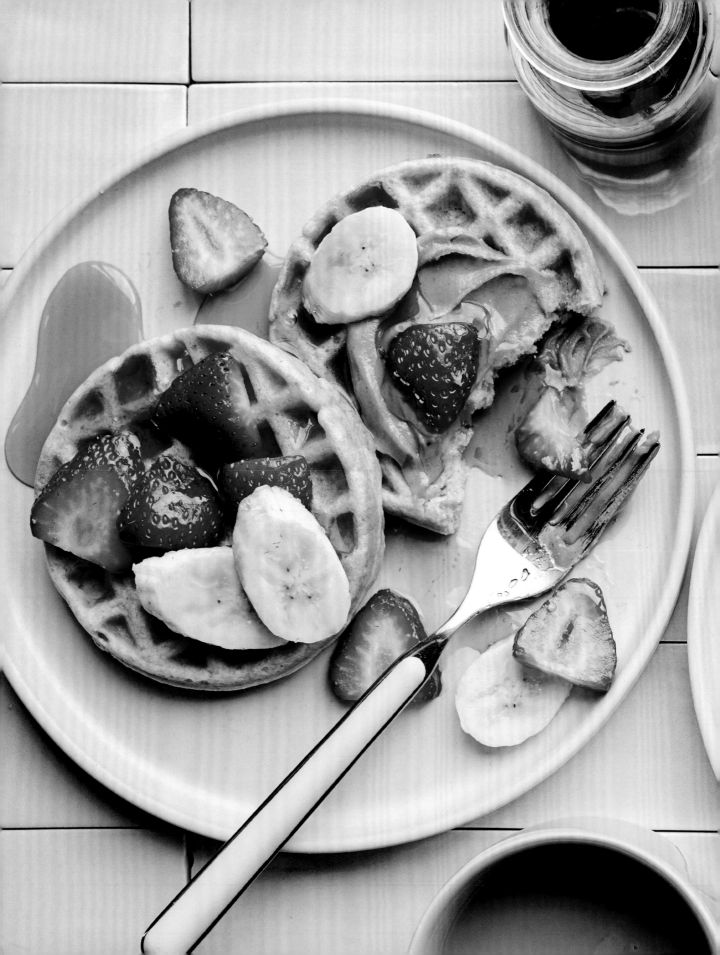

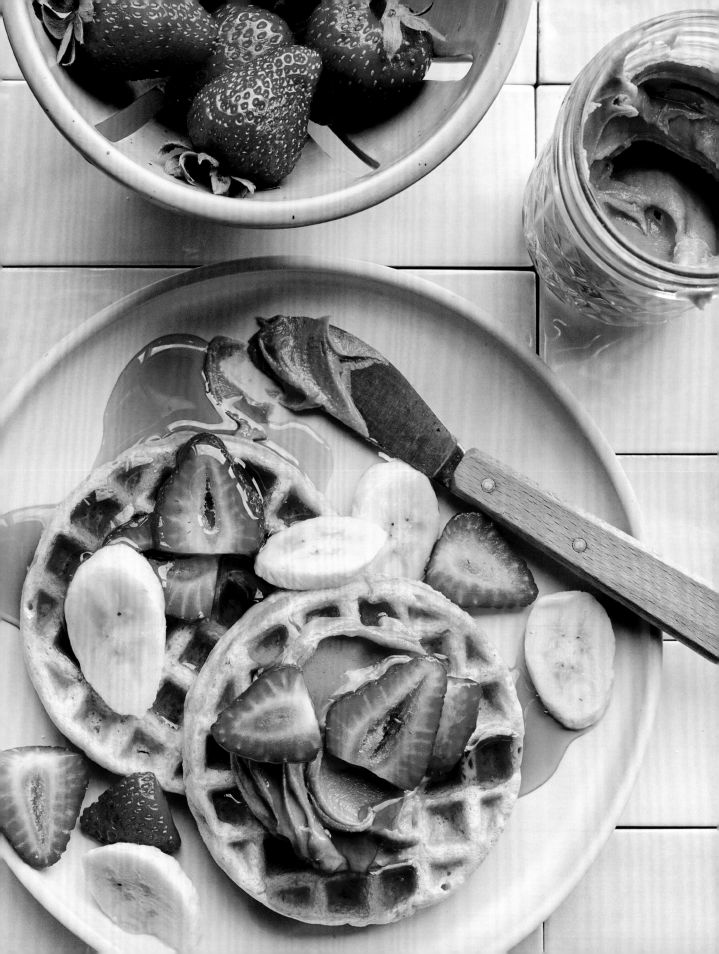

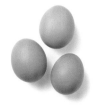

Ham and Swiss Omelet Wrap

SERVES 1

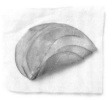

I love this hack for making quick breakfast wraps: Cook the egg right onto the tortilla. It's an omelet and a wrap all in one, and it's seriously delish! This dish was inspired by a recipe from Nadiya Hussain, but I've seen the same technique done with an Indian kati roll, only using a roti instead. This recipe is so versatile, you can switch it up with whatever you prefer in your omelet. If you want to make it dairy-free, skip the cheese, or swap the Swiss for any cheese you like. If you want to make it vegetarian, just omit the ham and add more veggies.

2 large eggs
1 ounce thinly sliced low-sodium ham, chopped (scant ⅓ cup)
1 ounce light Swiss or nondairy cheese, chopped (scant ⅓ cup)
¼ cup loosely packed baby spinach or baby kale, chopped
1 (8- or 9-inch) low-carb whole wheat or gluten-free tortilla
Hot sauce (optional), for serving

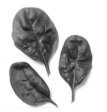

In a medium bowl, beat the eggs, then add the ham, cheese, spinach, and ⅛ teaspoon kosher salt.

Spray a nonstick medium skillet with the olive oil and heat over medium-low heat. Pour the egg mixture into the pan and swirl the pan to create a round omelet to match the size of your tortilla. Place the tortilla on top of the egg mixture and press gently with your hands (the uncooked eggs will act as a sort of glue that sticks to the tortilla).

Let the bottom of the eggs cook until set and no longer runny, 1 to 2 minutes, then run a flat spatula along the outside of the omelet, carefully releasing the outer edges to prepare for flipping. Flip the omelet and cook, tortilla side down, for about 1 minute more, or until the tortilla is browned and begins to crisp.

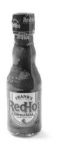

Transfer the omelet/tortilla to a plate and carefully roll it up. Place seam side down and cut in half. Serve with hot sauce, if desired.

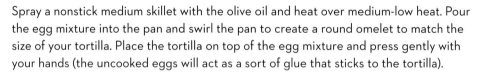

Per Serving (1 wrap) ● Calories 301 ● Fat 15 g ● Saturated Fat 5.5 g ● Cholesterol 400 mg
Carbohydrate 20 g ● Fiber 12 g ● Protein 31 g ● Sugars 1 g ● Sodium 872 mg

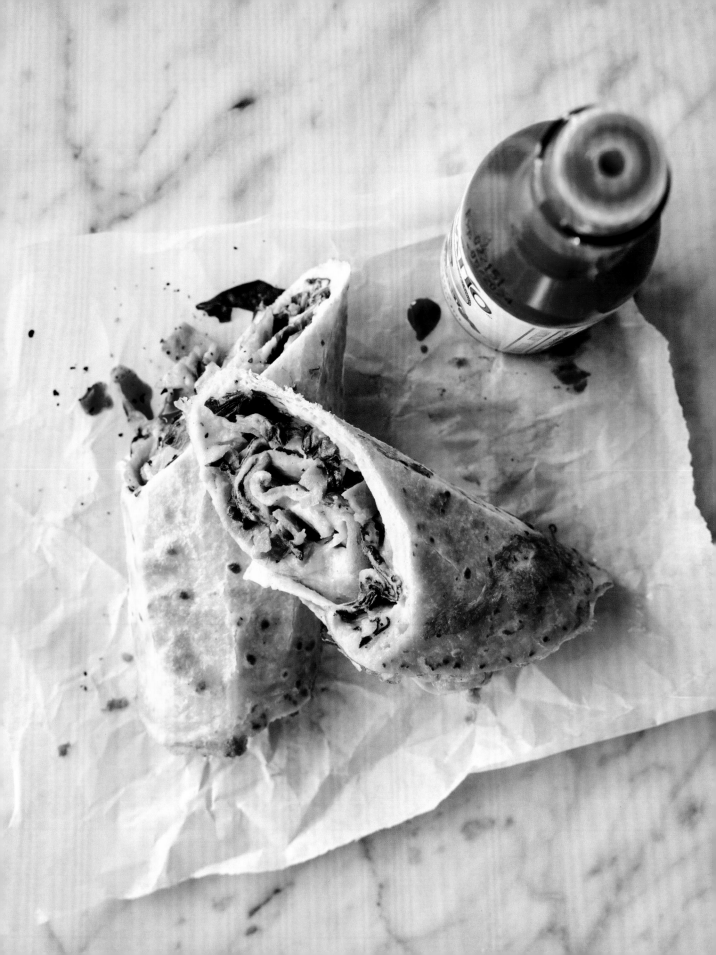

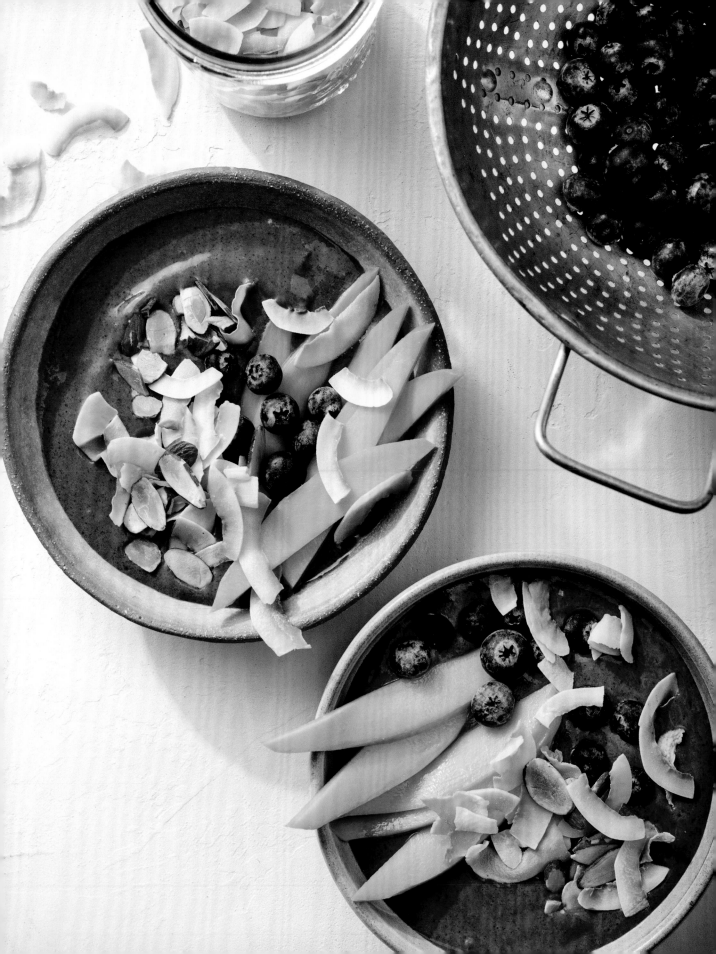

Açai Berry Bowls

SERVES 2

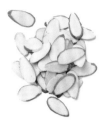

Açai bowls are what healthy breakfast dreams are made of! The only problem is they're often loaded with added sugar, but this one is lightly sweetened with a ripe banana and has yogurt for extra protein. Since açai bowls are all about the toppings, feel free to load them up with all your favorites! I love sliced strawberries, banana, chia seeds, and granola, too, but here I opted for toasted coconut and almonds for crunch and fresh mango for a tropical vibe.

SKINNY SCOOP: Açai berry puree is usually sold near the frozen fruit in most natural foods stores, supermarkets, or even Trader Joe's. Before blending, you may need to put the packet in warm water to soften it slightly.

2 tablespoons sliced almonds (½ ounce)

2 tablespoons unsweetened coconut chips or shredded coconut (½ ounce)

1 cup frozen blueberries

1 (3.53-ounce) packet frozen unsweetened açai berry puree (I used Sambazon; see Skinny Scoop)

1 ripe medium banana, sliced then frozen

½ cup plain 0% Greek yogurt or nondairy yogurt

1 cup sliced fresh mango

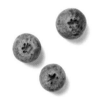

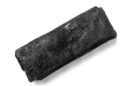

Heat a small skillet over medium-low heat. Add the almonds and coconut and toast, stirring frequently, until the coconut becomes golden and the almonds begin to slightly brown, about 3 minutes. Remove from the heat and set aside.

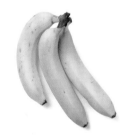

Put ¼ cup of the blueberries into each of two bowls. Add the remaining ½ cup blueberries to a blender and add the açai, frozen banana, and yogurt. Blend until smooth.

Pour the puree (about ¾ cup each) into the bowls over the blueberries and mix. Top each with the mango and almond/coconut mixture. Serve immediately.

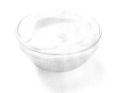

(To meal prep, make the fruit puree, place in a freezer-safe container, and freeze. Store the almonds and coconut in an airtight container or zip-top plastic bag. When ready to eat, thaw the puree slightly in the microwave for about 45 seconds to 1 minute and top with the almond/coconut mixture and fresh mango.)

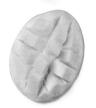

Per Serving (1 bowl) ● Calories 292 ● Fat 11 g ● Saturated Fat 5 g ● Cholesterol 3 mg Carbohydrate 44 g ● Fiber 8.5 g ● Protein 10 g ● Sugars 28 g ● Sodium 34 mg

Cajun-Spiced Shakshuka

SERVES 3

Shakshuka, a classic North African and Middle Eastern dish with eggs poached in a sauce of tomatoes, gets a Cajun twist! This egg dish can be eaten for breakfast or any meal of the day. Serve it with some crusty bread on the side to soak up all the delicious sauce and runny yolks, and garnish with chopped parsley if you have it on hand.

¾ cup chopped onion

2 garlic cloves, minced

2½ cups chopped tomatoes (about 3 vine tomatoes)

¾ cup diced green bell pepper

1 tablespoon Cajun seasoning*

6 large eggs

3 slices crusty bread or gluten-free bread (1 ounce each), toasted

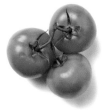

*Read the label to be sure this product is gluten-free.

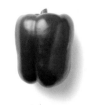

Heat a large deep skillet over medium heat and add 1 teaspoon extra-virgin olive oil. Add the onion and garlic and cook, stirring occasionally, until soft, 3 to 4 minutes.

Stir in the tomatoes, bell pepper, and Cajun seasoning. Cover and cook over medium-low heat until the flavors meld and the tomatoes soften, about 10 minutes.

Reduce the heat to low. Uncover the skillet, make 6 small divots around the sauce for the eggs to be cracked into, and add the eggs. Cover again and cook until the egg whites are opaque and the yolks are cooked to your liking, 6 to 8 minutes. Serve with crusty bread.

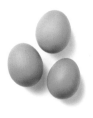

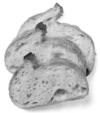

Per Serving (2 large eggs + ½ cup veggies + 1 ounce bread) ● Calories 292 ● Fat 12 g Saturated Fat 3.5 g ● Cholesterol 372 mg ● Carbohydrate 29 g ● Fiber 4 g ● Protein 18 g Sugars 8 g ● Sodium 657 mg

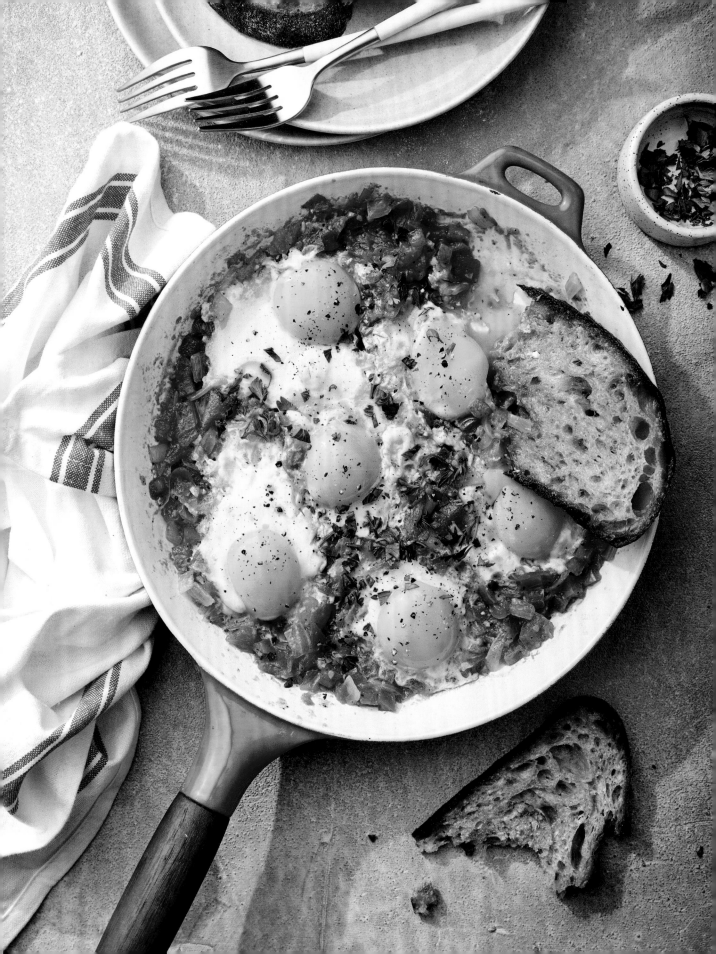

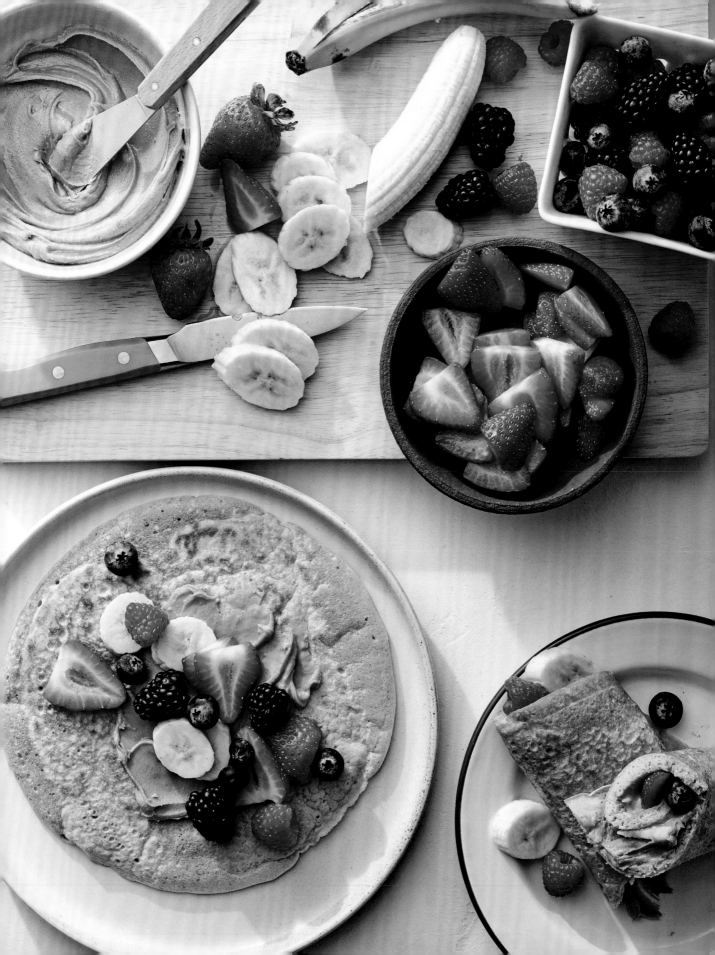

Peanut Butter-Banana-Berry Pancake Roll-Ups

SERVES 2

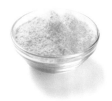

Pancakes you can eat with your hands! This glorified peanut butter and jelly wrap uses a protein-packed pancake to keep the ingredients together and mess-free. It's the perfect way to start the day and easy to eat on the run.

¾ cup whole-grain protein pancake mix (I like Kodiak Power Cakes or Birch Benders)

½ teaspoon vanilla extract

Pinch of ground cinnamon

2 tablespoons peanut butter or your favorite nut butter

1 medium banana, sliced

⅔ cup mixed berries (sliced, if large)

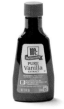

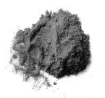

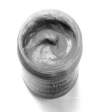

In a medium bowl, combine the pancake mix and 1 cup water and whisk until smooth (you want the batter to be on the thin side, more like a crepe batter than a thick pancake batter). Add the vanilla and cinnamon and whisk again until just incorporated.

Meanwhile, spray a nonstick medium skillet or griddle with olive oil and heat over medium heat.

Add half of the batter to the skillet, spreading with a spatula, if needed, to form a 7-inch pancake. Cook until bubbles form on the top side, 2 to 3 minutes. Flip and cook about 1 minute more or until the pancake is fully cooked and browned on both sides. Transfer the pancake to a plate and repeat with the remaining batter.

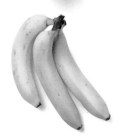

Set the pancakes on a plate or cutting board, and spread 1 tablespoon of the peanut butter evenly over each. Divide the banana and the berries between the pancakes, placing the fruit in the center, and roll the pancake tightly. Slice each roll in half and serve.

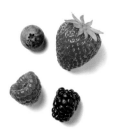

Per Serving (1 roll-up) ● Calories 316 ● Fat 10 g ● Saturated Fat 1.5 g ● Cholesterol 8 mg
Carbohydrate 45 g ● Fiber 7 g ● Protein 15 g ● Sugars 15 g ● Sodium 354 mg

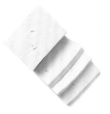

Vegan Scrambled Tofu

SERVES 2

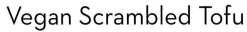

Q V GF DF

It's kind of crazy how much this tofu dish looks and tastes like scrambled eggs. Don't get me wrong, I love eggs, but when I am trying to get more plant-based protein, this recipe hits the spot. Hot sauce or Sriracha is a must for me when I eat this scramble, but if you prefer yours milder, just skip the hot sauce and add a pinch more salt. This is great alone or served with home fries, on toast, or in a breakfast burrito.

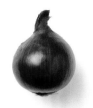

1 (16-ounce) package extra-firm tofu, drained

¼ cup diced red onion

¼ cup chopped red, yellow, or orange bell pepper

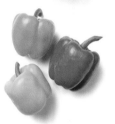

¼ cup diced seeded jalapeños

½ teaspoon ground turmeric

¼ teaspoon sweet paprika

A few dashes hot sauce or Sriracha (optional)

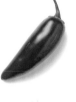

Cut the tofu into 4 blocks. Use a paper towel to soak up some of the liquid from the tofu. Using your hands, squeeze the tofu through your fingers until it resembles the texture of scrambled eggs.

Heat a medium skillet over medium-low heat and add 1 tablespoon extra-virgin olive oil, the onion, bell pepper, and jalapeños and cook until softened, 3 to 4 minutes. Add the tofu and season with ¾ teaspoon kosher salt, the turmeric, paprika, and freshly ground black pepper to taste. Cook, stirring well so that the seasoning evenly coats the tofu, until the tofu is heated through, 3 to 4 minutes.

Divide the scramble between two plates and serve topped with hot sauce or Sriracha, if desired.

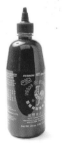

Per Serving (1 generous cup) ● Calories 320 ● Fat 19 g ● Saturated Fat 2.5 g ● Cholesterol 0 mg Carbohydrate 12 g ● Fiber 4 g ● Protein 25 g ● Sugars 5 g ● Sodium 436 mg

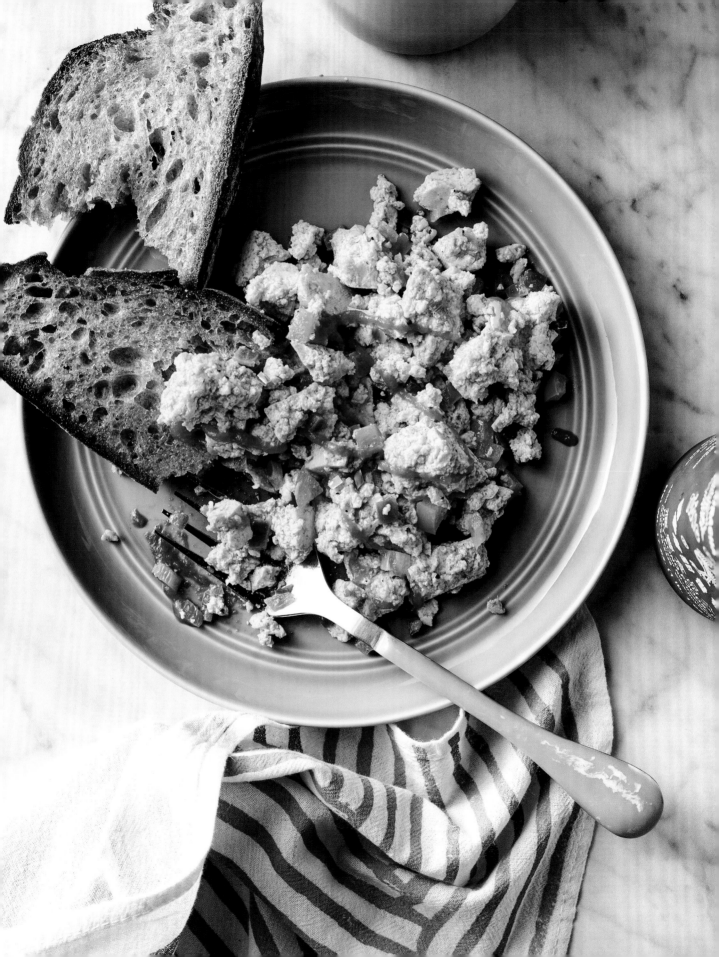

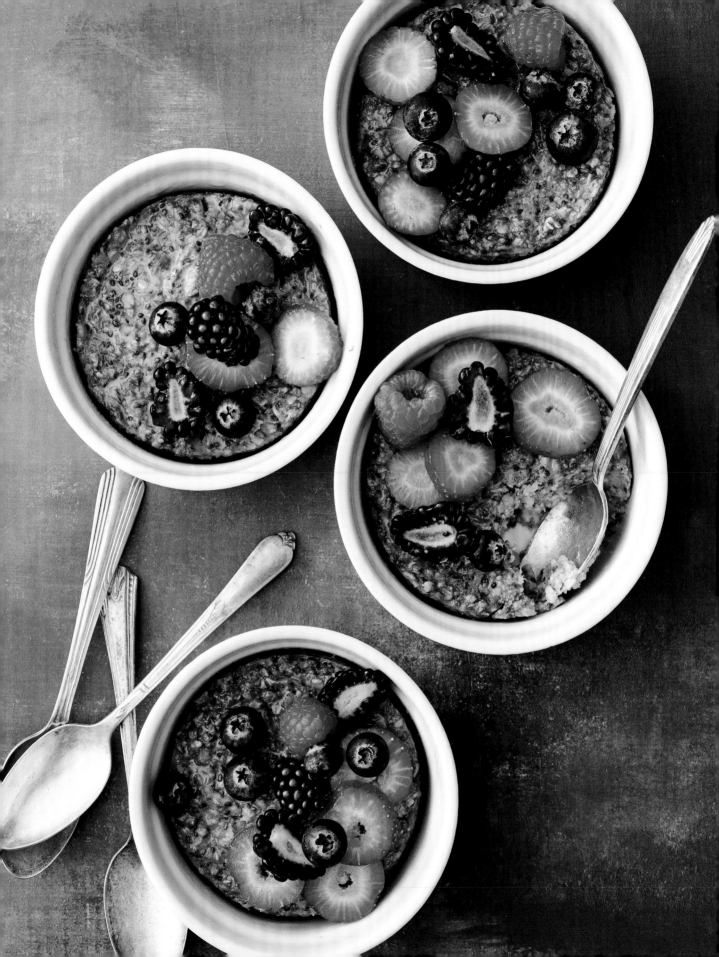

Heart-Smart Baked Oatmeal

SERVES 4

These creamy baked oats are not just delicious but also combine lots of high fiber and nutritious foods that naturally lower your cholesterol. I use mashed banana to sweeten the oatmeal naturally. That way you don't have to add too much sugar. I also love that I can meal prep this for an easy breakfast so I can eat it throughout the week (just pop it in the microwave to reheat). For added fiber and to include a rainbow of fruits in my day, I usually serve this topped with some fresh berries.

SKINNY SCOOP: If you have only rolled oats, pulse them in a food processor 5 to 8 times until finely ground (they will be similar in consistency to quick-cooking oats with a few bigger pieces).

1¹⁄₃ cups quick-cooking oats* (see Skinny Scoop)

1 cup unsweetened nut milk or other milk of choice

2 ripe medium bananas, mashed

2 tablespoons chia seeds or ground flaxseeds

4 teaspoons vanilla extract

1 tablespoon monk fruit sweetener, raw sugar, or maple syrup

⅛ teaspoon baking powder

*Read the label to be sure this product is gluten-free.

Preheat the oven to 350°F. Spray four 1- to 1½-cup ramekins or ovenproof Pyrex bowls with oil.

In a large bowl, combine the oats, milk, bananas, chia seeds, and vanilla and mix thoroughly. Set aside to allow the oats to absorb some of the milk, about 5 minutes.

In a small bowl, combine the sweetener of your choice, baking powder, and ⅛ teaspoon kosher salt. Add the mixture to the oats and stir until combined. Divide the oat mixture among the prepared ramekins and place them on a baking sheet.

Bake until the oats are just set, yet still creamy, 20 to 24 minutes. Allow to cool for a few minutes before eating.

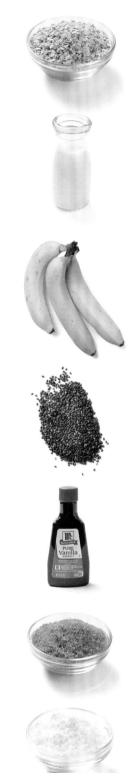

Per Serving (1 bowl) ● Calories 203 ● Fat 4 g ● Saturated Fat 0.5 g ● Cholesterol 0 mg
Carbohydrate 35 g ● Fiber 6.5 g ● Protein 5 g ● Sugars 8 g ● Sodium 83 mg

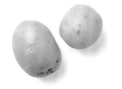

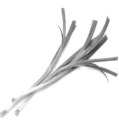

Loaded Waffled Hash Browns

SERVES 4

GF

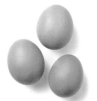

Once you make hash browns in a waffle iron, you'll never want to make them any other way! The waffle iron gives you so much surface area for crisp golden edges without needing a ton of oil. Topping them with runny eggs and cheese takes them to the next level! To simplify this more, you can use 8 cups frozen hash browns in place of the potatoes.

2 pounds Yukon Gold potatoes (about 4 potatoes)

4 scallions, thinly sliced, plus extra for garnish

4 large eggs

4 tablespoons shredded cheddar cheese

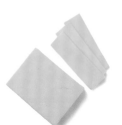

Preheat the oven to 200°F. Preheat a standard 7-inch round waffle maker on the highest setting.

Peel the potatoes and shred them on the large holes of a box grater into a large bowl. Transfer to a clean cloth and squeeze to extract as much liquid as possible (discard the liquid). Place the potatoes in the bowl and add the scallions, 1¼ teaspoons kosher salt, and freshly ground black pepper to taste and stir to combine.

Spray both sides of the waffle iron generously with olive oil. Scoop a generous ½ cup of the potato mixture onto the bottom and spread in an even layer. Close the iron tightly and cook until the potatoes are browned on the edges and cooked through in the center, 8 to 10 minutes. Transfer to the oven to keep warm and repeat with the remaining ingredients to make 7 more hash brown waffles.

Meanwhile, heat a griddle or skillet over medium-low heat. When hot, spray with oil and carefully add the eggs. Top each egg with 1 tablespoon cheddar, cover, and cook until the eggs set but are still runny, about 2 minutes.

To serve, place 2 hash browns on each plate and top with an egg, scallions, a pinch of kosher salt, and freshly ground black pepper to taste.

NO WAFFLE IRON? NO PROBLEM! You can cook them in batches in a hot cast-iron skillet over medium-high heat until the bottom is browned, carefully flipping with a spatula, 8 to 10 minutes on each side.

Per Serving (2 hash browns + 1 egg + 1 tablespoon cheese) ● Calories 281 ● Fat 7 g
Saturated Fat 3 g ● Cholesterol 193 mg ● Carbohydrate 42 g ● Fiber 5 g ● Protein 13 g
Sugars 3 g ● Sodium 501 mg

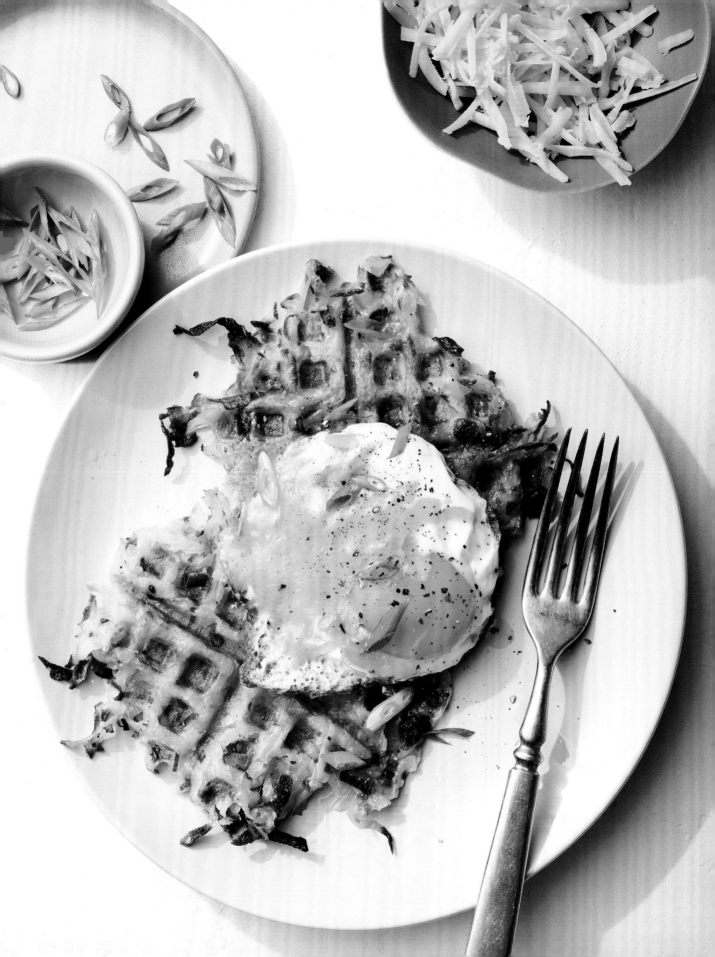

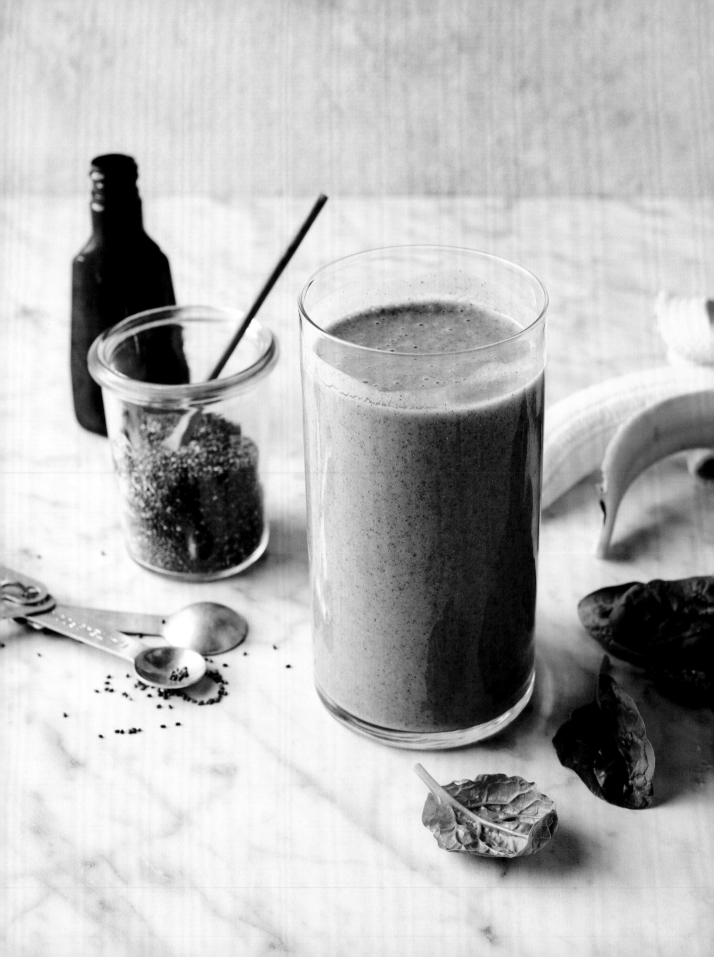

Banilla Protein Smoothie

SERVES 1

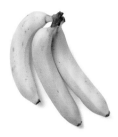

I love the convenience of this easy and delicious protein-rich shake that's perfect for a post-workout boost. I created this recipe because I really hated the artificial flavors in the premade protein shakes I've tried—and trust me, I've tried a ton of them! In this real-food shake, I use a ripe banana and vanilla extract to sweeten it naturally, unflavored pea protein powder (you can also use whey), and a handful of spinach. Chia seeds are a great source of fiber, and adding them to a smoothie is easy! For variations I add nut butter, berries, or collagen powder for an even more nutrient-rich smoothie.

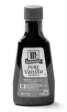

1 ripe medium banana

1 teaspoon vanilla extract

¼ cup unflavored organic pure pea protein or whey protein powder

2 tablespoons chia seeds

1 cup ice

A small handful of baby spinach

Stevia or monk fruit sweetener (optional)

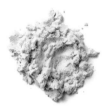

In a blender, combine the banana, vanilla, protein powder, chia seeds, 1 cup water, the ice, and spinach and blend until smooth. If you want it sweeter, add Stevia or monk fruit sweetener, to taste. Serve immediately.

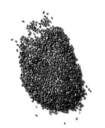

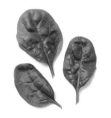

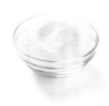

Per Serving (1 smoothie) ● Calories 357 ● Fat 10 g ● Saturated Fat 1 g ● Cholesterol 0 mg
Carbohydrate 38 g ● Fiber 11.5 g ● Protein 28 g ● Sugars 15 g ● Sodium 45 mg

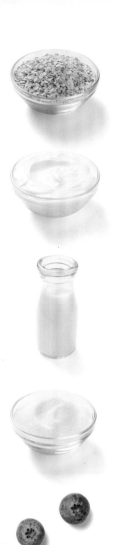

Creamy Overnight Oats
with Blueberries and Pistachios

SERVES 1

 V GF DF

These overnight oats make my heart and belly happy! What really makes these oats special is swirling in the warm burst of blueberries, then topping them with pistachios for crunch. I use whole-milk yogurt, which adds protein and an ultracreamy texture, but any yogurt will work in this recipe. I've also used coconut yogurt for a dairy-free option, and it comes out just as delicious. Double or triple the recipe for meal prep—your future self will thank you!

½ cup quick-cooking oats,* preferably organic

⅓ cup plain whole-milk Greek or coconut yogurt

⅓ cup unsweetened milk of choice

4 teaspoons monk fruit sweetener or sugar

⅓ cup blueberries

2 tablespoons pistachios

Granola (optional), for topping

*Read the label to be sure this product is gluten-free.

In a small bowl, combine the oats, yogurt, milk, and 1 teaspoon sweetener of choice. Cover and refrigerate overnight.

In a small saucepan, combine the blueberries, remaining 3 teaspoons sweetener, and 1 tablespoon water. Cook over medium-low heat, stirring occasionally, until the berries release their juices and burst, 6 to 8 minutes. (You can make this ahead, then reheat in the microwave with a little water before using.)

In the morning, remove the oats from the fridge and pour them into a large shallow bowl. Swirl in the blueberry mixture, top with pistachios and granola (if using), and serve.

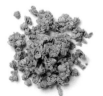

Per Serving (1 bowl) ● Calories 365 ● Fat 14 g ● Saturated Fat 4 g ● Cholesterol 15 mg
Carbohydrate 77 g ● Fiber 7 g ● Protein 18 g ● Sugars 13 g ● Sodium 63 mg

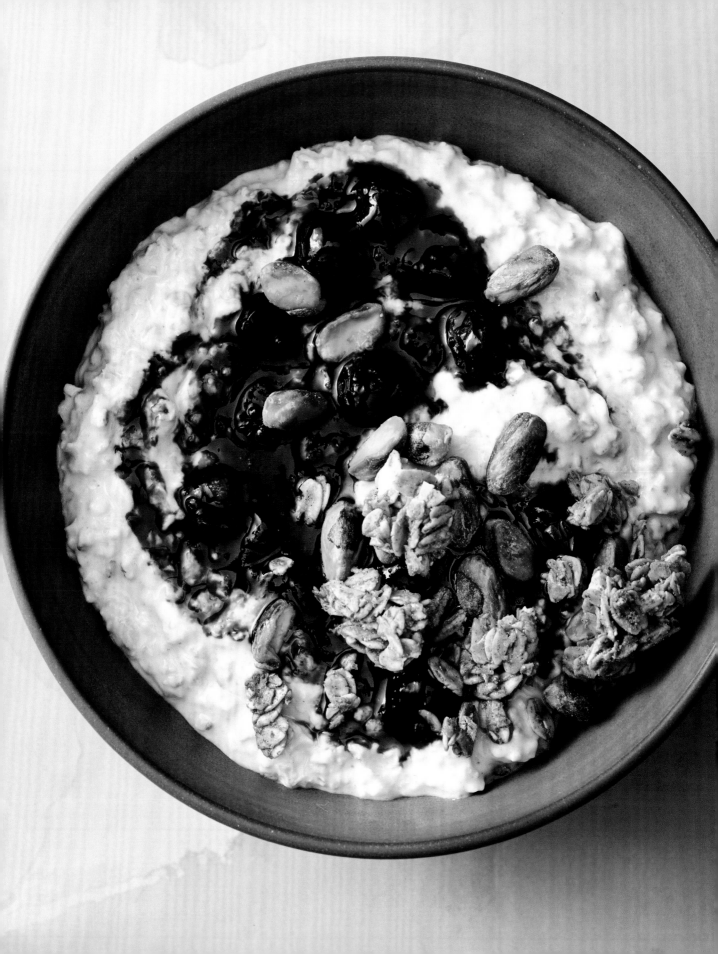

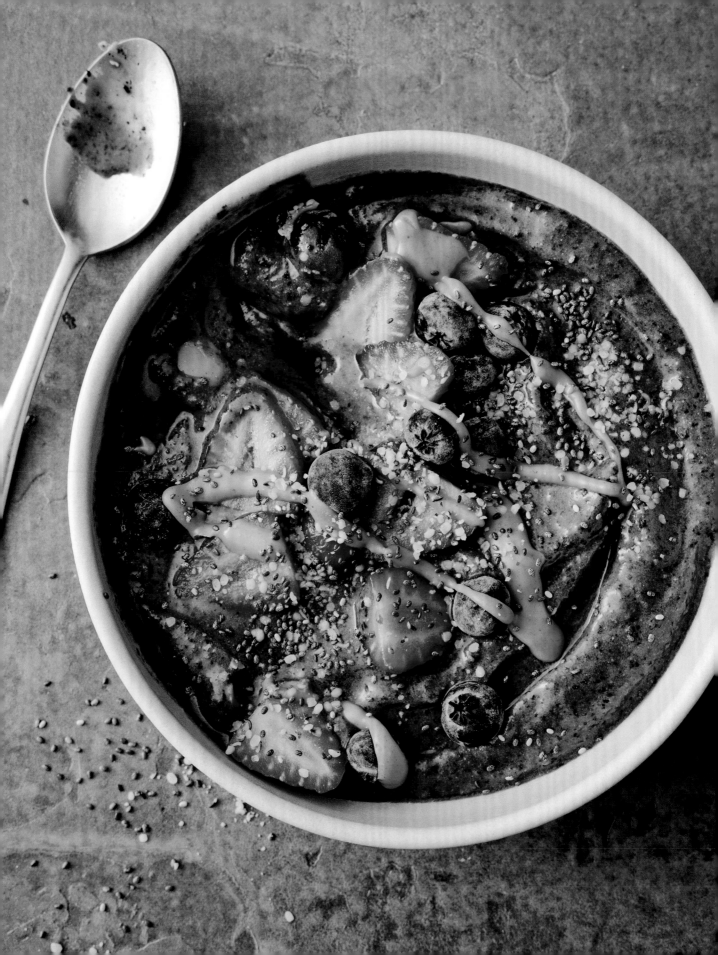

PB & J Smoothie Bowl

SERVES 1

This is the ultimate smoothie bowl—it tastes JUST like peanut butter and jelly. Packed with protein, it's the perfect start to your day!

SKINNY SCOOP: I always buy fresh blueberries and keep some in my freezer for smoothies and smoothie bowls. This way, nothing gets tossed because it has spoiled.

¼ cup nondairy milk of your choice, such as almond or oat

⅔ cup frozen blueberries, plus 2 tablespoons fresh for topping (see Skinny Scoop)

⅔ cup sliced frozen strawberries, plus 2 tablespoons fresh for topping

1 scoop (about 23 grams) grass-fed or dairy-free vanilla protein powder*

2 tablespoons smooth peanut butter

1 tablespoon chia and/or hemp seeds, for topping

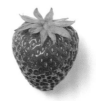

*Read the label to be sure this product is gluten-free or dairy-free, if needed.

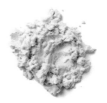

In a blender, combine the milk, frozen blueberries, frozen strawberries, protein powder, and 1 tablespoon of the peanut butter and blend until smooth. Pour the mixture into a bowl and top with fresh blueberries and fresh sliced strawberries.

In a small microwave-safe bowl, microwave the remaining 1 tablespoon peanut butter until melted, 30 to 45 seconds. Drizzle over the bowl. Top with chia and/or hemp seeds. Eat right away with a spoon!

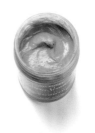

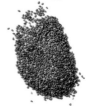

Per Serving (1 bowl) ● Calories 440 ● Fat 24 g ● Saturated Fat 4 g ● Cholesterol 0 mg
Carbohydrate 47 g ● Fiber 11 g ● Protein 22 g ● Sugars 21 g ● Sodium 305 mg

For

Sharing

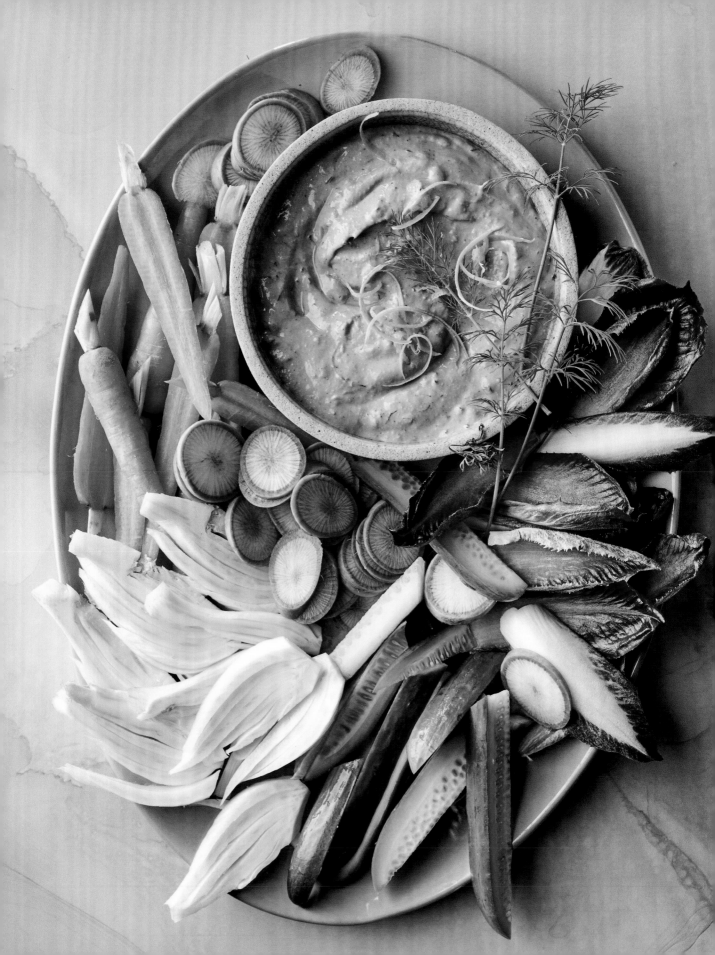

Greek Goddess Dip

SERVES 6

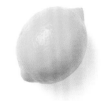

This Greek-inspired Green Goddess dip is loaded with herbs and bright flavors and gets its creaminess from avocado and yogurt, but adding feta makes it over-the-top delicious! For maximum effect, I include 2 whole cups of herbs and you can experiment with different combinations. Personally, I like to make this with equal parts basil, parsley, and dill, but to keep it to 7 ingredients, choose your favorites. This dip practically begs for crudités of any kind: sliced fennel, cauliflower or broccoli florets, baby carrots, and endive, just to name a few.

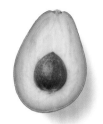

Zest and juice of 1 lemon

4 ounces peeled and pitted avocado (from 1 small)

1/2 cup plain 2% Greek yogurt

1/2 cup crumbled feta cheese

2 garlic cloves, smashed with the side of a knife

**2 cups loosely packed fresh herbs in any combination,
  such as parsley, basil, dill, and/or tarragon**

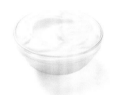

In a blender, combine the lemon juice, avocado, yogurt, feta, garlic, 1 tablespoon extra-virgin olive oil, and 1 teaspoon kosher salt. Puree until smooth, adding 2 to 4 tablespoons water if necessary to get the motor going.

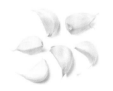

Add 1 cup of the herbs and pulse until they are very finely chopped. Add the remaining 1 cup herbs and repeat. (Pulsing the herbs in batches ensures the final dip has some texture.)

Transfer to a serving bowl and serve at room temperature or chilled, garnished with the lemon zest. It will keep in the fridge for up to 1 week.

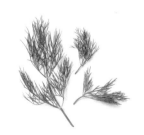

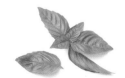

Per Serving (1/4 cup) ● Calories 105 ● Fat 8 g ● Saturated Fat 3 g ● Cholesterol 13 mg
Carbohydrate 4 g ● Fiber 2 g ● Protein 5 g ● Sugars 2 g ● Sodium 315 mg

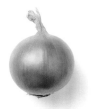

French Onion Greek Yogurt Dip

SERVES 6

Classic for a reason, this perfect caramelized onion dip has the sweetness of slowly cooked onions balanced with the bright tanginess of creamy yogurt. Worcestershire sauce is the secret ingredient that gives the dip a pop of flavor. Here, Greek yogurt takes the place of the cream cheese, sour cream, or mayo typically used in onion dip recipes; I used full-fat for a richer flavor and creamier texture.

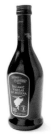

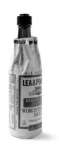

2 medium yellow onions, diced

1 tablespoon balsamic vinegar

1 teaspoon Worcestershire sauce*

2 cups plain whole-milk Greek yogurt

1 teaspoon dried parsley

*Read the label to be sure this product is gluten-free.

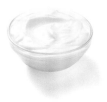

In a large heavy skillet, heat 2 tablespoons extra-virgin olive oil over medium heat. Add the onions, reduce the heat to medium-low, and cook, stirring occasionally, until they are evenly caramelized and soft, 25 to 30 minutes.

Add the vinegar and Worcestershire sauce and stir, scraping up any bits from the bottom of the pan. Remove from the heat and let cool for at least 10 minutes (so it doesn't melt the yogurt in the next step).

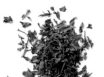

Stir in the yogurt, dried parsley, 1½ teaspoons kosher salt, and ¼ teaspoon freshly ground black pepper until thoroughly incorporated.

Serve at room temperature or chilled; it will keep in the fridge for up to 1 week.

Per Serving (½ cup) ● Calories 150 ● Fat 9 g ● Saturated Fat 3.5 g ● Cholesterol 13 mg
Carbohydrate 11 g ● Fiber 1 g ● Protein 8 g ● Sugars 8 g ● Sodium 326 mg

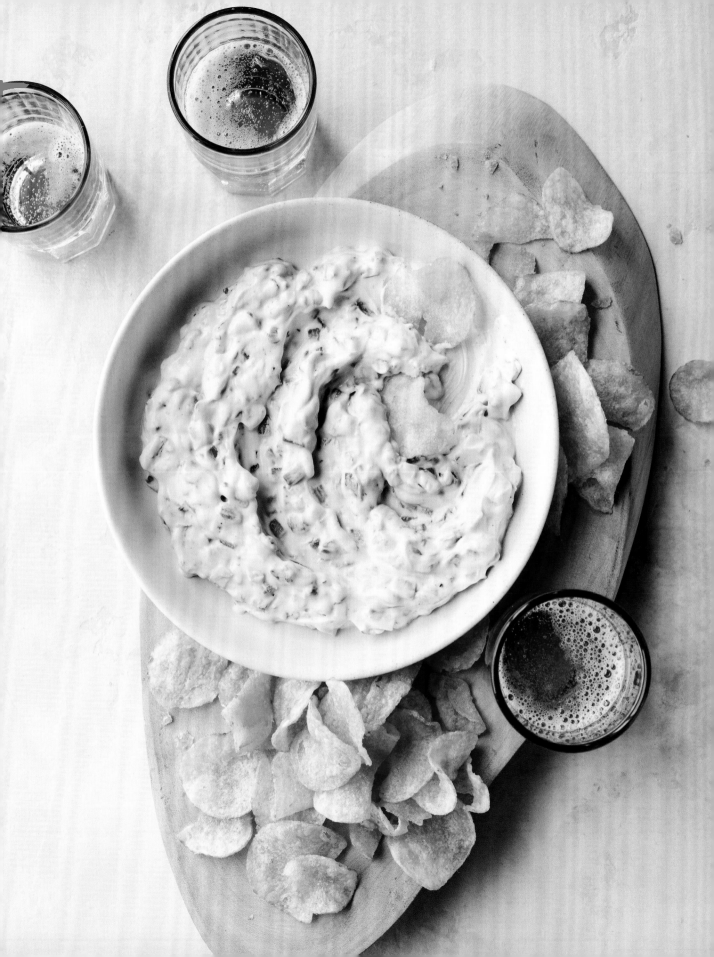

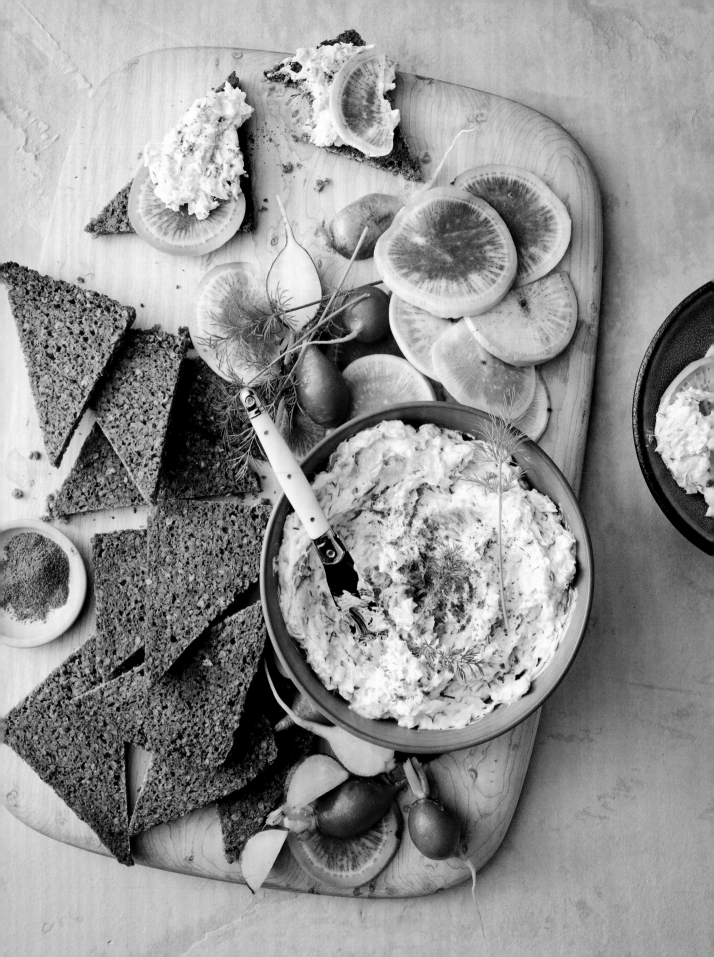

Smoked Fish Dip

SERVES 8

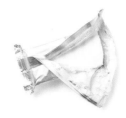

This Florida fish shack classic is elegant enough for a party but also perfect for a casual beach picnic. I was first introduced to smoked fish dip (aka pâté) at The Ordinary in Charleston, one of my favorite seafood restaurants. Theirs is made with amberjack, but any smoked, flaky fish works great in this dip (just avoid cold-smoked fish like lox). Look for smoked fish at the supermarket, usually by the lox and herring. Serve with sliced colorful crudités, such as watermelon radish, rainbow carrots, and cucumbers as well as pumpernickel toast points or crackers.

8 ounces ⅓-less-fat cream cheese, at room temperature

Grated zest and juice of 1 lemon

2 shallots, finely diced

1 large celery stalk, finely diced, plus the leaves for garnish

2 tablespoons chopped fresh dill, plus more for garnish

¼ teaspoon cayenne pepper, or more to taste (optional)

8 ounces smoked fish, such as trout

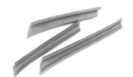

In a medium bowl, use a fork to combine the cream cheese with the lemon juice and 1 teaspoon kosher salt, whipping until it's smooth.

Add the shallots, celery, dill, cayenne (if using), and lemon zest and stir until incorporated.

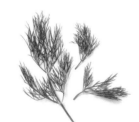

Remove the skin from the smoked fish and use your fingers to flake it into the bowl as you would lump crabmeat, removing any small pin bones but being careful not to mash it to a paste. Fold the fish into the dip.

Serve at room temperature or chilled, topped with a dash of cayenne pepper, dill, and celery leaves, for garnish. It will keep in the fridge for up to 1 week.

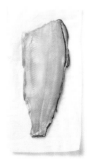

Per Serving (⅓ cup) ● Calories 156 ● Fat 9 g ● Saturated Fat 4.5 g ● Cholesterol 50 mg
Carbohydrate 2 g ● Fiber 0.5 g ● Protein 13 g ● Sugars 1 g ● Sodium 394 mg

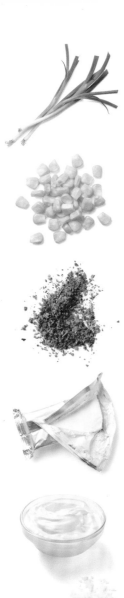

Baked Elote Dip

SERVES 10

This cheesy skillet dip will have everyone crowding around the snack table. It takes its inspiration from Mexican elote, grilled ears of corn coated with a blend of crema, mayonnaise, salty Cotija cheese, and smoky, tangy chili powder. This version swaps the mayo for cream cheese and turns it into an ooey-gooey dip with a toasty brown top, perfect for your favorite baked chip.

6 scallions, thinly sliced, dark green portion kept separate

16 ounces frozen corn kernels or 3 cups fresh

1 teaspoon Tajín or Trader Joe's Everything but the Elote Seasoning Blend

4 ounces ⅓-less-fat cream cheese

¼ cup light sour cream

7 ounces Cotija cheese, grated (1¾ cups)

Chopped fresh cilantro, for garnish

Adjust an oven rack in the center and another 6 inches from the broiler and preheat to 350°F.

In a 10-inch ovenproof skillet or cast-iron skillet, heat 1 teaspoon extra-virgin olive oil over medium heat. Set aside 2 tablespoons of the scallion greens for garnish. Add the white and light-green parts to the skillet along with ¼ teaspoon kosher salt and cook until softened, 2 to 3 minutes.

Add the corn and Tajín seasoning. Continue to sauté until the corn starts to soften, 3 to 5 minutes. Add the cream cheese and stir until it is fully incorporated.

Remove the pan from the heat and fold in the sour cream along with ¾ cup of the Cotija. Transfer to the oven and bake until the edges start to bubble and brown, 10 to 12 minutes.

Carefully remove the pan from the oven and preheat the broiler. Sprinkle the remaining 1 cup cheese over the top and transfer to the rack under the broiler. Broil until browned (watch carefully so it doesn't burn), 2 to 3 minutes.

Remove the pan from the oven and sprinkle the reserved scallion greens and some cilantro over the top. Serve immediately.

Per Serving (⅓ cup) ● Calories 156 ● Fat 10 g ● Saturated Fat 5.5 g ● Cholesterol 30 mg Carbohydrate 11 g ● Fiber 1 g ● Protein 7 g ● Sugars 1 g ● Sodium 438 mg

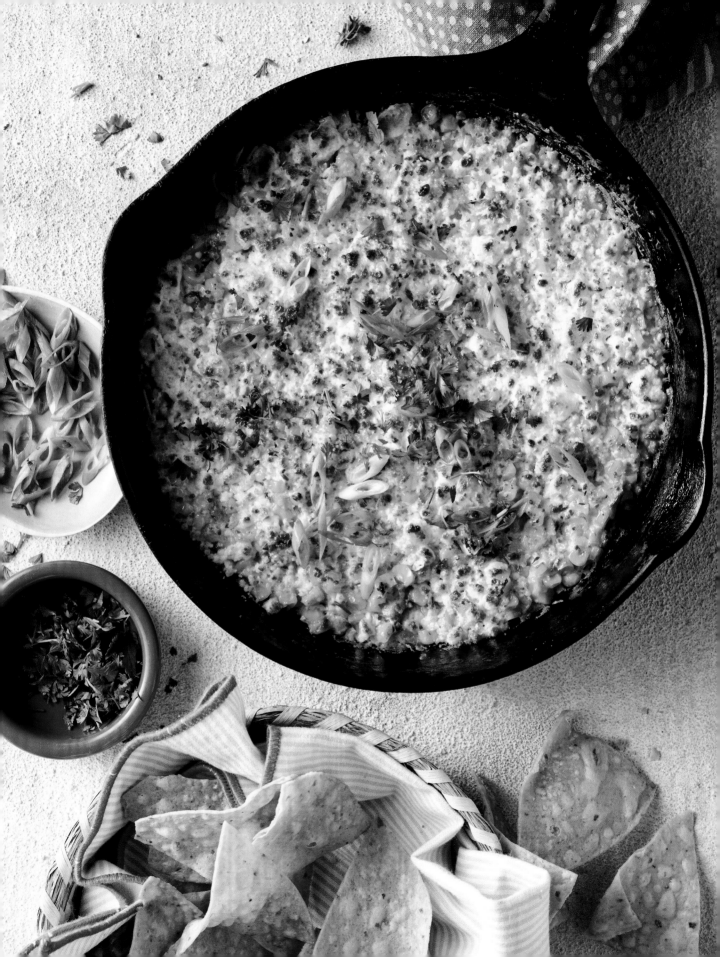

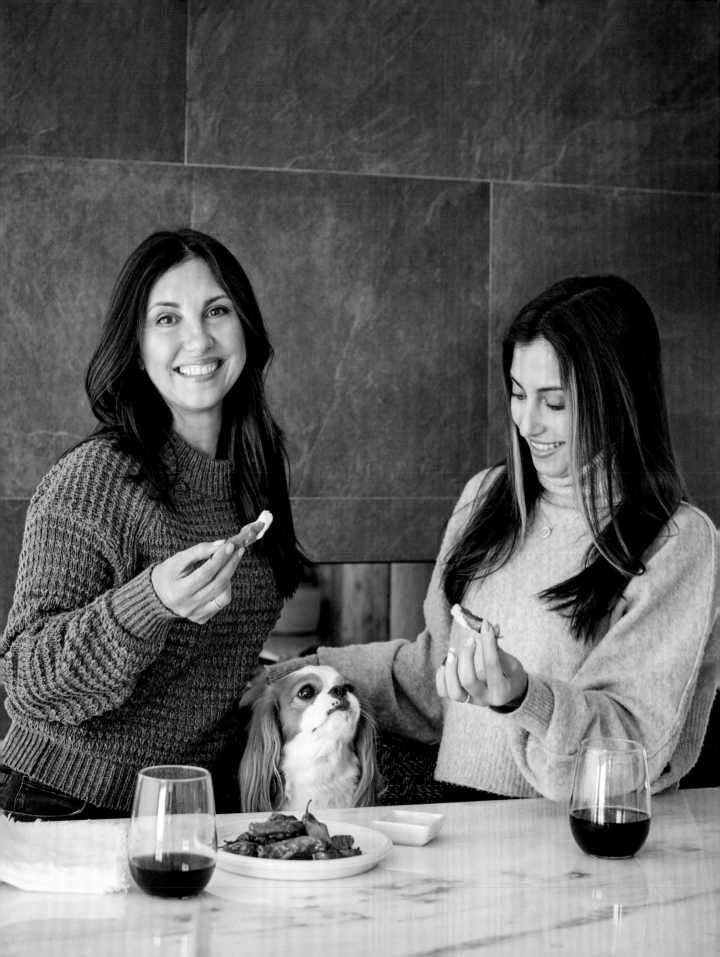

Air-Fried Blistered Shishitos with Smoked Paprika Aioli

SERVES 2

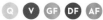

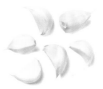

Shishito peppers are one of my favorite snacks! I always order them—instead of fries!—when I see them on a menu, but making them at home is so simple. You can use the air fryer or broiler here. Shishito peppers can be found at farmers' markets, some grocery stores, and Trader Joe's.

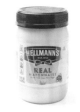

½ garlic clove

3½ tablespoons mayonnaise

2 tablespoons fresh lemon juice

¼ teaspoon smoked paprika

8 ounces shishito peppers

To make the aioli, use a Microplane to grate the garlic into a small bowl (or use a garlic press). Add the mayonnaise, 1 tablespoon of the lemon juice, the smoked paprika, and ¼ teaspoon kosher salt and stir to combine. Refrigerate the smoked paprika aioli until ready to use.

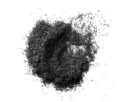

Spray the shishito peppers all over with olive oil. Transfer them to an air fryer basket in one batch and cook at 400°F for 6 to 8 minutes, shaking halfway through, until the peppers are soft and slightly charred and blistered.

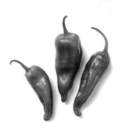

To serve, transfer the shishitos to a large plate and sprinkle with ¼ teaspoon kosher salt and toss with the remaining 1 tablespoon lemon juice. Serve the aioli alongside for dipping.

NO AIR FRYER? NO PROBLEM! Place the peppers on a sheet pan 6 inches from the heating element and broil for 6 minutes, flipping halfway.

Per Serving (4 ounces shishitos + 2 tablespoons aioli) • Calories 205 • Fat 18 g • Saturated Fat 2 g Cholesterol 18 mg • Carbohydrate 5 g • Fiber 0 g • Protein 0 g • Sugars 0 g • Sodium 447 mg

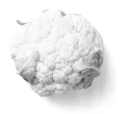

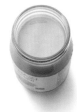

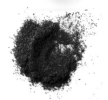

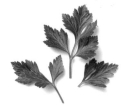

Roasted Garlic and Cauliflower Hummus

SERVES 8

In this hummus-inspired dip, roasted cauliflower takes the place of chickpeas, making it a low-carb, full-flavored spread. A whole head of garlic roasts along with the cauliflower, and the result adds an irresistible caramelized sweetness to the spread. As with any hummus, use good tahini, since it rounds out all of the delicious flavors, and serve with toasted pita wedges or assorted crudités.

1 medium head cauliflower (about 20 ounces of florets), cored and cut into 2-inch florets

1 head garlic

⅓ cup tahini

3 tablespoons fresh lemon juice

½ teaspoon smoked or sweet paprika

Chopped fresh parsley, for garnish

Preheat the oven to 400°F.

Scatter the cauliflower on a sheet pan. Drizzle on 1 tablespoon extra-virgin olive oil, sprinkle with 1 teaspoon kosher salt, and toss to coat.

Remove the papery outer layers of the whole head of garlic and cut the top ¼ inch or so off the head, exposing the cloves but leaving them intact. Place in a sheet of foil and coat with ½ tablespoon extra-virgin olive oil. Tightly wrap the garlic in the foil and add it to the baking sheet with the cauliflower.

Roast the cauliflower and garlic, flipping the cauliflower halfway through, until browned in some parts but not all over, 20 to 25 minutes. Use a knife or fork to prick the garlic through the foil; if it isn't easy to pierce, transfer the foil-wrapped garlic to a different baking sheet and continue cooking for another 15 minutes. Let cool.

Measure out ⅓ cup roasted cauliflower and set aside for garnish. Add the remaining cauliflower to a food processor. Squeeze the roasted garlic cloves into the food processor, discarding the papery skin. Add the tahini, lemon juice, ½ tablespoon extra-virgin olive oil, and ¼ teaspoon kosher salt. Process, pausing occasionally to scrape down the sides, until it's creamy and airy, about 5 minutes. Add 3 to 4 tablespoons cold water as needed to help it become creamy.

To serve, transfer to a wide, shallow bowl. Top with the reserved ⅓ cup cauliflower, sprinkle with paprika and parsley, and finish with a drizzle of extra-virgin olive oil. Serve immediately. (The hummus can be stored in the refrigerator for up to 4 days.)

Per Serving (¼ cup) ● Calories 120 ● Fat 9 g ● Saturated Fat 1.5 g ● Cholesterol 0 mg
Carbohydrate 8 g ● Fiber 3 g ● Protein 3 g ● Sugars 2 g ● Sodium 209 mg

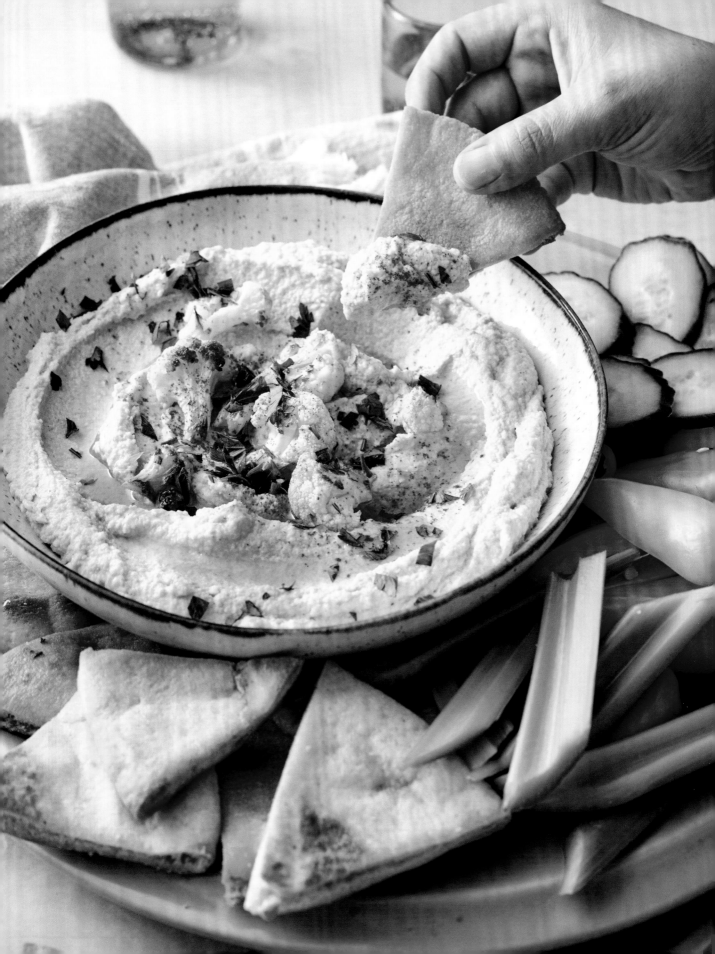

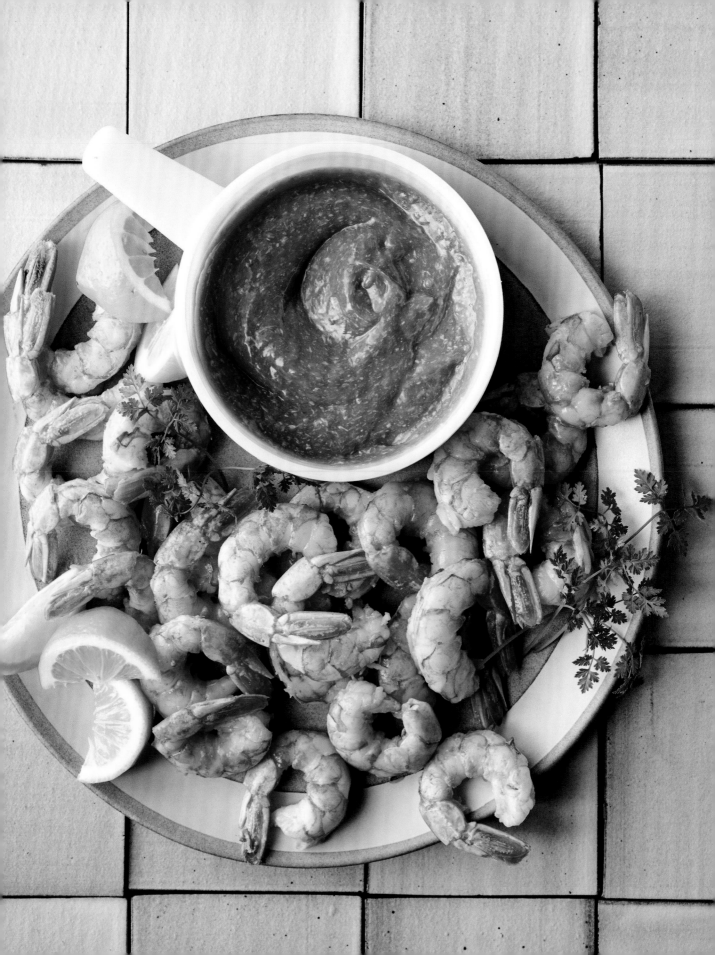

Roasted Shrimp Cocktail

SERVES 6

When I go to parties on the weekend, I like to bring a light, high-protein appetizer, like shrimp cocktail, because it is always such a crowd pleaser! Since there are so few ingredients in this shrimp cocktail, two things are key: Cook the shrimp yourself for maximum freshness and whip up this homemade cocktail sauce. It's too easy not to! One of the simplest ways to prepare shrimp is to roast them in the oven: It's hands off and foolproof. If you like it spicy, add a few dashes of your favorite hot sauce to the cocktail sauce.

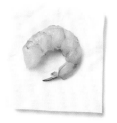

36 extra-jumbo (16/20 count) tail-on peeled and deveined shrimp (2½ pounds total)

2 lemons, 1 halved, 1 sliced into wedges for serving

1 cup ketchup

½ cup prepared horseradish

1 teaspoon Worcestershire sauce*

*Read the label to be sure this product is gluten-free.

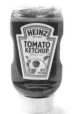

Preheat the oven to 400°F. Spray two large sheet pans with olive oil.

Combine the shrimp and 2 tablespoons extra-virgin olive oil on one of the sheet pans and toss to combine. Transfer half to the second sheet pan and spread all the shrimp in a single layer.

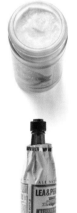

Roast until the shrimp turn pink and firm and are cooked through, 6 to 8 minutes. Remove from the oven and squeeze one of the lemon halves over the shrimp. Transfer to a large bowl and refrigerate to chill.

In a small bowl, combine the ketchup, the juice from the remaining lemon half, the horseradish, and Worcestershire sauce and refrigerate the cocktail sauce until ready to eat.

Serve the shrimp with the cocktail sauce and lemon wedges.

Per Serving (6 shrimp + ¼ cup cocktail sauce) ● Calories 293 ● Fat 8 g ● Saturated Fat 2.5 g Cholesterol 279 mg ● Carbohydrate 14 g ● Fiber 1 g ● Protein 40 g ● Sugars 11 g Sodium 756 mg

Spicy Vegan Cashew Queso

SERVES 8

Cashews are a vegan's best friend: Soaking and blending them with just a few ingredients creates such a creamy, spicy, flavorful dip that even nonvegans will be crowding around the bowl! No presoaking is needed, as the nuts will soften in hot water in the time it takes for you to cook the onion and tomatoes. Pickled jalapeño brings the heat, and nutritional yeast adds that signature cheesy flavor. It's a rich, comforting dip perfect with tortilla chips or raw vegetables or on top of nachos.

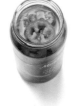

1 cup raw cashews

4 tablespoons chopped pickled jalapeños, plus 2 tablespoons brine from the jar

1 medium yellow onion, diced

1 (10-ounce) can Ro-Tel diced tomatoes and green chilies, drained

2 garlic cloves, minced

1½ tablespoons taco seasoning

⅓ cup nutritional yeast

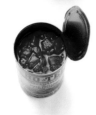

Place the cashews, ⅔ cup boiling water, and the 2 tablespoons jalapeño brine in a blender but do not process yet. Let the nuts soak and soften while you cook the vegetables.

In a medium skillet, heat 1 tablespoon extra-virgin olive oil over medium heat. Add the onion and 1 teaspoon kosher salt and sauté, stirring occasionally, until translucent and starting to brown on the edges, 7 to 10 minutes.

Add the drained tomatoes and chilies, garlic, and taco seasoning. Cook, stirring occasionally, until very fragrant, 2 to 3 minutes. Remove from the heat. Measure out 1 tablespoon of the tomato mixture and set aside for garnish.

Blend the soaked cashews on high until very smooth. Add the nutritional yeast and the tomato mixture from the skillet and blend again on high speed until very smooth.

Transfer the queso to a large serving bowl and stir in 2 tablespoons of the chopped pickled jalapeños. Garnish with the reserved tomato mixture and remaining 2 tablespoons pickled jalapeños.

Per Serving (scant ⅓ cup) • Calories 147 • Fat 9 g • Saturated Fat 1.5 g • Cholesterol 0 mg
Carbohydrate 12 g • Fiber 2.5 g • Protein 5 g • Sugars 4 g • Sodium 405 mg

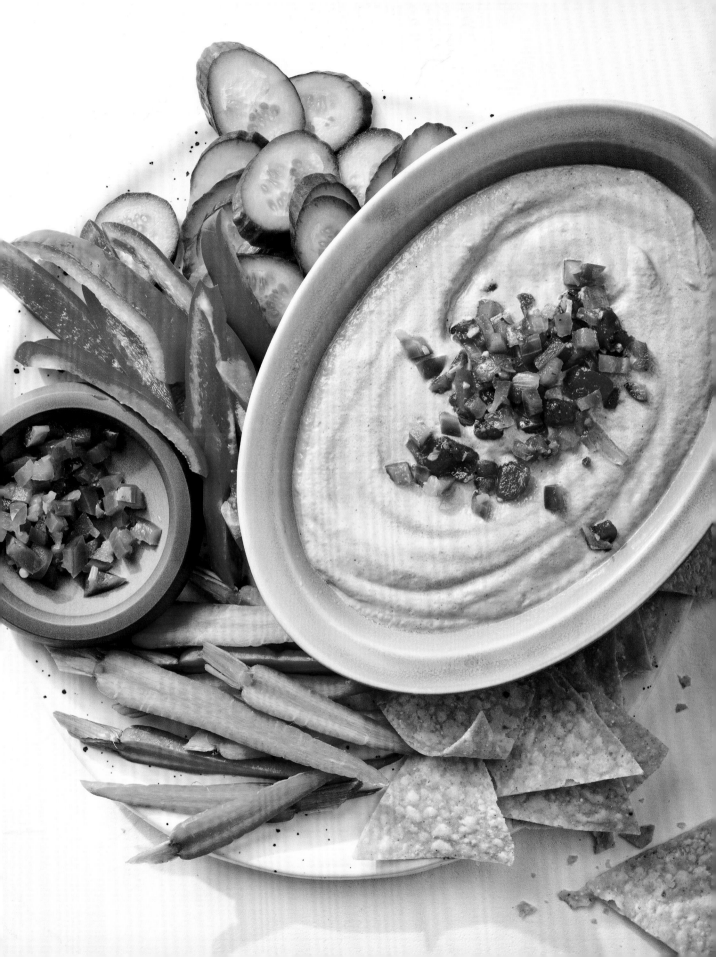

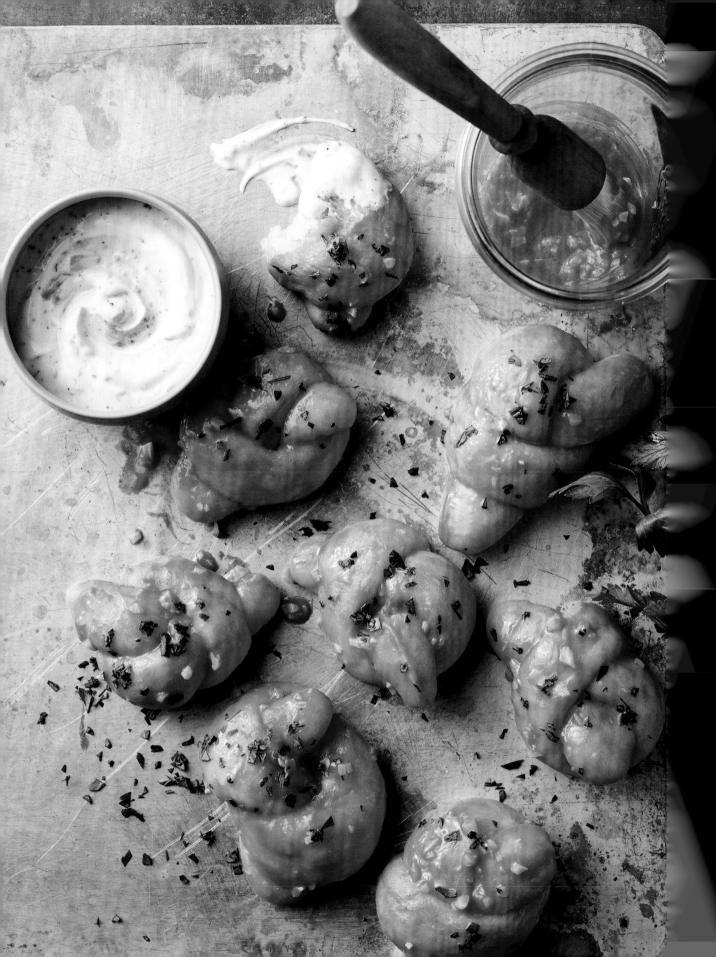

Buffalo Garlic Knots

MAKES 8

I've "Buffalo-ed" everything from chicken strips to cauliflower, classic dips, and even chickpeas. So it was only a matter of time before I took garlic knots and smothered them in Buffalo sauce, too! And, boy, am I glad I did: Once you start, it's hard to stop eating them, and they make the perfect appetizer or party snack. They're delicious on their own, or you can serve with ranch or blue cheese dressing on the side for the classic combo.

SKINNY SCOOP: A thick Greek yogurt, such as Fage or Stonyfield, is a must here. Some brands are not as thick and will result in sticky dough.

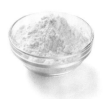

1 cup all-purpose or white whole wheat flour, plus more for dusting

2 teaspoons baking powder

1 cup plain 0% Greek yogurt, drained of any excess liquid (see Skinny Scoop)

1 tablespoon unsalted butter

3 garlic cloves, chopped

¼ cup Frank's RedHot sauce

1 tablespoon finely chopped fresh parsley

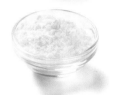

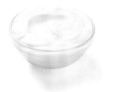

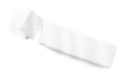

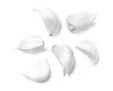

Adjust an oven rack to the top third of the oven and preheat the oven to 375°F. Line a sheet pan with parchment paper or a silicone baking mat.

In a large bowl, combine the flour, baking powder, and ¾ teaspoon kosher salt and whisk well. Add the yogurt and mix with a spoon until incorporated. Use your dry hands to knead the mixture about 15 times until the dough is smooth. If it's too sticky you can add a little more flour. Shape into a ball.

Dust a clean work surface with flour. Divide the dough into 8 equal portions, then roll each portion into a 9-inch-long rope. Tie each rope into a knot-like ball and transfer to the prepared baking sheet. Spray the tops with olive oil.

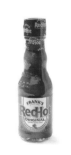

Bake until golden, about 18 minutes. Let them cool for 5 minutes.

Meanwhile, in a small nonstick skillet, melt the butter over medium-low heat. Add the garlic and cook until golden, about 2 minutes. Add the hot sauce and remove the Buffalo garlic sauce from the heat.

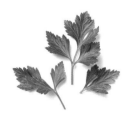

Brush the knots all over with the Buffalo garlic sauce and sprinkle with chopped parsley. Serve immediately.

Per Serving (1 garlic knot) ● Calories 87 ● Fat 2 g ● Saturated Fat 1 g ● Cholesterol 5 mg
Carbohydrate 14 g ● Fiber 0.5 g ● Protein 5 g ● Sugars 1 g ● Sodium 524 mg

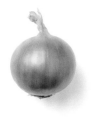

Spinach Empanadas

SERVES 12

In South America, there's lots of different vegetable fillings for empanadas (mushrooms, pumpkin, beans, peppers, corn, you name it), but spinach empanadas are always my favorite. In addition to making a great appetizer, they can also be enjoyed for lunch, and any leftovers will heat up well the next day. Serving with hot sauce is a must for me!

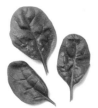

1½ cups diced onion (about 1 large)

3 garlic cloves, chopped

11 ounces baby spinach

2 large eggs

⅓ cup part-skim ricotta cheese, drained

¼ cup grated Parmesan cheese

12 frozen empanada dough rounds, for baking, thawed

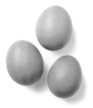

Preheat the oven to 375°F. Spray a sheet pan with olive oil.

In a large deep skillet, heat ½ tablespoon extra-virgin olive oil over medium heat. Add the onion and cook until softened, about 5 minutes. Add the garlic and cook until fragrant, about 2 minutes. Add the spinach, 1¼ teaspoons kosher salt, and ¼ teaspoon freshly ground black pepper. Cook, stirring frequently, until the spinach is wilted, 3 to 4 minutes. Transfer to a colander for a few minutes to cool and drain.

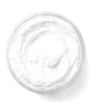

In a large bowl, beat one of the eggs. Add the ricotta, Parmesan, and cooled spinach filling and mix well.

In a small bowl, beat the remaining egg and set aside. Place an empanada round on your work surface and roll it out to 4 inches in diameter. Take about 3 tablespoons of the spinach mixture and place in the center of the round. Moisten the edges with the beaten egg and fold in half to form a half-moon shape. Gently press down the edges and twist to crimp or use a fork to seal the edges; transfer to the prepared sheet pan. Repeat with the remaining filling to make 12 empanadas. Brush the empanada tops with the beaten egg.

Bake the empanadas until they are puffed and golden brown and the filling is hot, 20 to 25 minutes, rotating the pan front to back after 10 minutes for even browning.

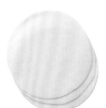

Transfer the empanadas to a wire rack. Serve warm or at room temperature.

Per Serving (1 empanada) ● Calories 151 ● Fat 6 g ● Saturated Fat 2 g ● Cholesterol 35 mg Carbohydrate 17 g ● Fiber 1 g ● Protein 5 g ● Sugars 1 g ● Sodium 345 mg

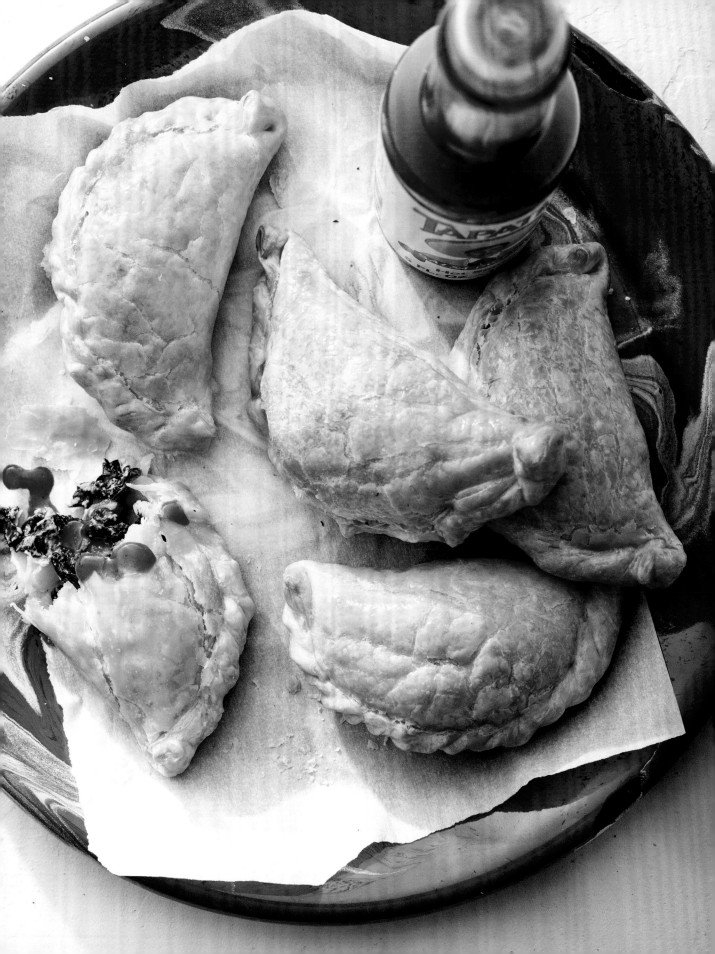

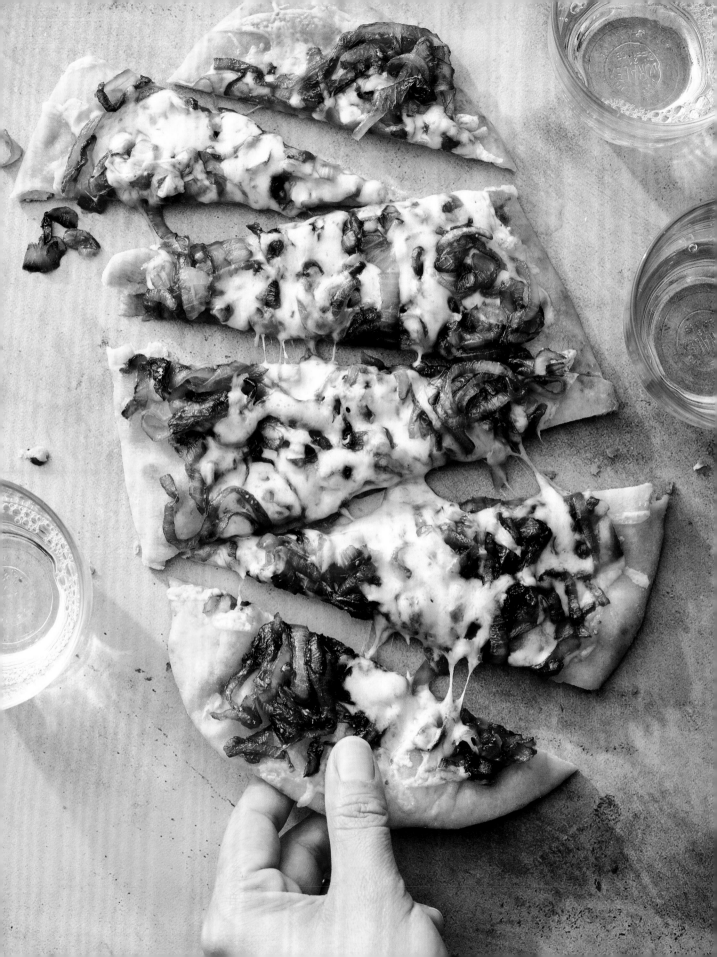

Caramelized Onion and Fig Flatbread

SERVES 6

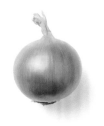

When I'm having friends over for dinner I like to the keep the appetizers as simple as possible. I usually make a cheese board, some dips (like the Greek Goddess Dip, page 53), along with crudités and something hot, like these delicious flatbreads, which Tommy just devours! Using store-bought naan as the base for these flatbreads does the trick. The caramelized onions can be made a day ahead, then you can assemble and bake right before your guests arrive.

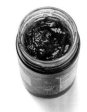

2 medium onions, thinly sliced

1 tablespoon fig jam

3 ounces fontina cheese, shredded (¾ cup)

2 naan flatbreads, such as Stonefire Original

1 teaspoon balsamic glaze, for drizzling

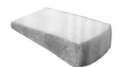

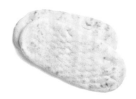

Heat a small heavy-bottomed pot over low heat and add 2 teaspoons olive oil, the onions, and ⅛ teaspoon kosher salt. Cook until the onions are caramelized and golden, 30 to 35 minutes, stirring every 5 minutes—after 25 minutes, you may need to stir every minute. If the onions dry out, add a tablespoon of water as needed. Set the onions aside. Stir in the fig jam.

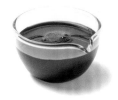

Preheat the oven to 400°F. Spray a sheet pan with oil.

Place flatbreads on the sheet pan and sprinkle half the cheese over both. Dividing evenly, top with the caramelized onions and then the remaining cheese. Bake until the cheese is melted, 6 to 7 minutes.

Drizzle each with some balsamic glaze. Slice into strips and eat right away.

Per Serving (⅓ flatbread) ● Calories 244 ● Fat 9 g ● Saturated Fat 3.5 g ● Cholesterol 21 mg Carbohydrate 31 g ● Fiber 2 g ● Protein 9 g ● Sugars 11 g ● Sodium 466 mg

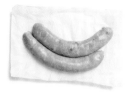

Air Fryer Mini Arancini Bites

SERVES 10

Arancini is always made with leftover risotto, but we never have risotto lying around the fridge. The solution? Making them with frozen brown rice, which I always have on hand! Instead of stuffing them like typical arancini recipes, all of the ingredients get mixed together and then rolled into bite-size balls, perfect for sharing. The air fryer does a great job of giving them a golden crust. Serve with warmed marinara (or even more pesto) on the side for dipping.

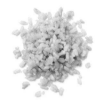

5½ ounces Italian chicken or turkey sausage links,* casings removed

2 cups frozen or leftover cooked brown rice, heated

2/3 cup shredded mozzarella cheese

½ cup prepared pesto

1 cup marinara sauce

2 large eggs plus 2 large egg whites

1 cup seasoned bread crumbs, regular or gluten-free

*Read the label to be sure this product is gluten-free.

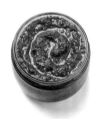

In a medium skillet, cook the sausage over medium heat, breaking it up as you go, until cooked through, about 5 minutes. Set aside to cool, then place in a small food processor and process until minced. (Alternatively, finely mince with a knife.)

In a medium bowl, combine the minced sausage, rice, mozzarella, pesto, and ¼ cup of the marinara sauce and mix well. Add the 2 egg whites and mix again, until fully incorporated.

Roll into 30 balls (a heaping tablespoon each) and transfer to a sheet pan. Freeze for 15 minutes to firm or refrigerate for up to 24 hours.

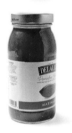

When ready, in a medium bowl, beat the 2 whole eggs. Place the bread crumbs in another medium bowl. Dip an arancini ball in the egg, then the bread crumbs, shaking off any excess. Transfer to a platter. Repeat with the remaining rice mixture.

Spray the air fryer basket with oil. Working in batches, add the balls in a single layer. Spray the tops generously with more olive oil. Air-fry at 400°F for 8 to 10 minutes, flipping halfway, until they are golden brown. Warm the remaining ¾ cup marinara sauce and serve on the side for dipping the hot arancini.

NO AIR FRYER? NO PROBLEM! Bake on a sheet pan in a 400°F oven for 8 to 10 minutes per side.

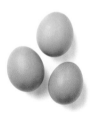

Per Serving (3 arancini bites) ● Calories 191 ● Fat 11 g ● Saturated Fat 3 g ● Cholesterol 57 mg Carbohydrate 15 g ● Fiber 1 g ● Protein 9 g ● Sugars 2 g ● Sodium 454 mg

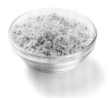

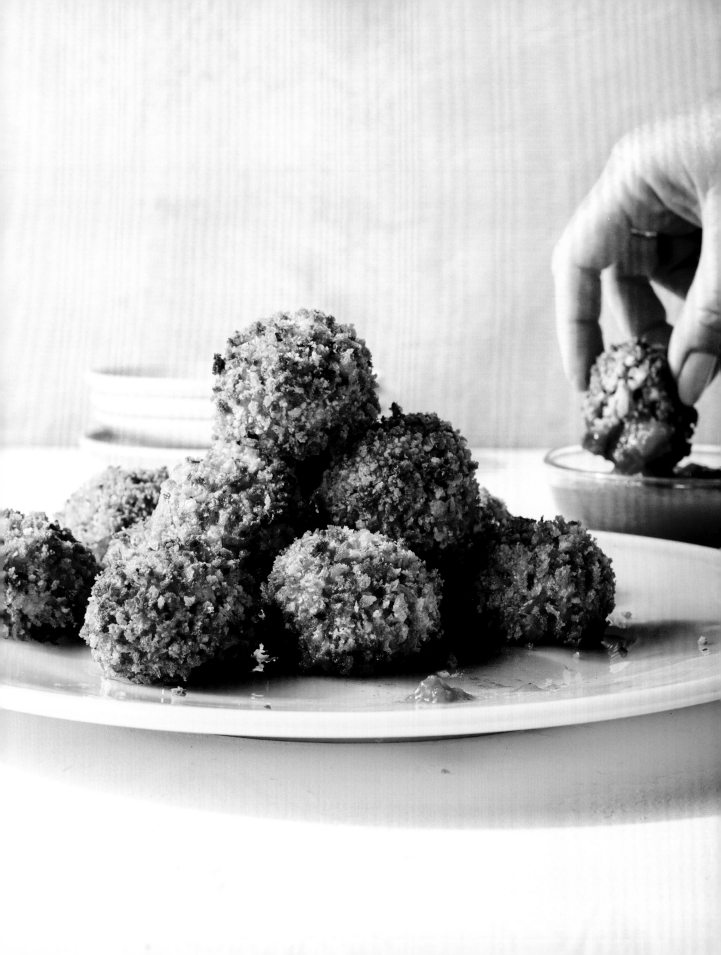

Hearty Soups and Big Salads

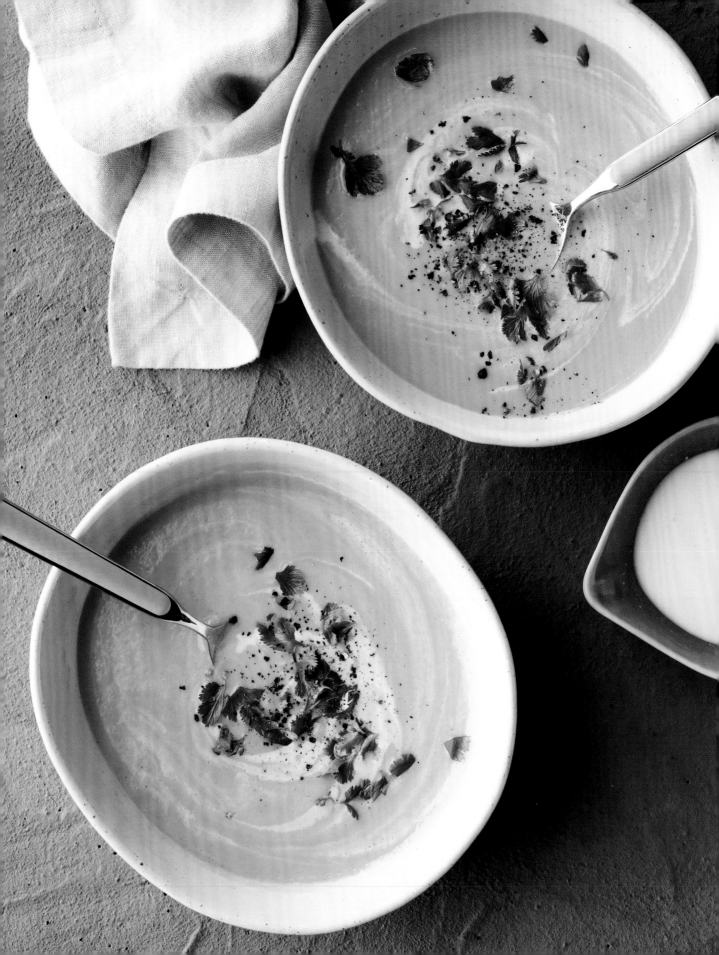

Creamy Coconut Curry Soup with Summer Squash

SERVES 6

 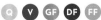

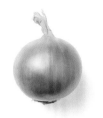

Although the ingredients in this creamy soup are simple, the flavors are rich. Make it vegan with vegetable broth if you desire, and if you want to level it up, add some chopped cilantro just before serving. This is the perfect soup to enjoy as a first course, or to eat alongside a sandwich or salad to make it a meal. Enjoy it hot or chilled, depending on your mood (and the weather!).

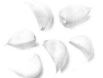

1 medium onion, chopped

2 garlic cloves, minced

1 tablespoon grated fresh ginger

2 teaspoons yellow curry powder*

1½ pounds yellow summer squash (3 to 4 medium), cut into large chunks

1 (32-ounce) carton chicken or vegetable broth*

¼ cup canned full-fat coconut milk, plus more (optional) for garnish

*Read the label to be sure this product is gluten-free.

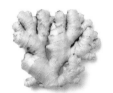

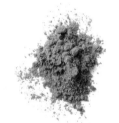

Heat a large pot over medium heat and add 1 tablespoon extra-virgin olive oil, the onion, garlic, and ginger. Season with the curry powder and ½ teaspoon kosher salt and sauté until the onion is golden, 4 to 5 minutes.

Add the squash and broth and bring to a boil over high heat. Reduce the heat to low, cover, and simmer until the squash is tender, 18 to 20 minutes.

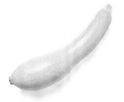

Remove from the heat, and working in batches if necessary, transfer the mixture to a blender (filling it only halfway full each time) and puree until smooth. (Alternatively, use an immersion blender in the pot.) Return the soup to the pot, add the coconut milk, and simmer over medium heat until heated through, 2 to 3 minutes.

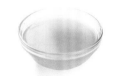

Drizzle each serving with additional coconut milk, if desired, and serve.

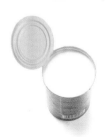

Per Serving (1 generous cup) ● Calories 91 ● Fat 5 g ● Saturated Fat 2 g ● Cholesterol 0 mg
Carbohydrate 11 g ● Fiber 3.5 g ● Protein 3 g ● Sugars 5 g ● Sodium 854 mg

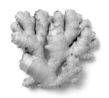

Shortcut Shrimp Ramen

SERVES 4

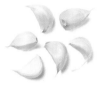

Madison loves ramen, and she gave this recipe an enthusiastic two thumbs up! It's a quick and easy way to take packaged instant ramen noodles and turn them into a delicious meal, complete with protein and veggies! You can switch up the protein and use leftover chicken breast, tofu, crispy chicken thighs, or soft-boiled eggs. Or swap the mushrooms for other veggies like bok choy, spinach, or corn. She often tops her soup with furikake or sesame seeds, but I always reach for Sriracha or an extra drizzle of soy sauce and toasted sesame oil for mine.

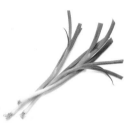

1 teaspoon grated fresh ginger

3 garlic cloves, minced

3 large scallions, chopped, plus more for garnish

12 ounces peeled medium shrimp, halved lengthwise

7 cups reduced-sodium vegetable or chicken broth

1²/₃ cups (5 ounces) thinly sliced fresh shiitake mushrooms

2 (3-ounce) packages instant ramen noodles, flavor packet discarded

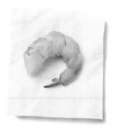

In a large pot, heat 1 teaspoon olive oil (or toasted sesame oil) over medium-high heat. Add the ginger, garlic, and scallions and sauté until fragrant, about 30 seconds. Add the shrimp and sauté until the shrimp are almost cooked through, 1 to 2 minutes maximum (they will finish cooking in the soup later). Transfer to a plate.

Add the broth and mushrooms to the pot and bring to a boil. Reduce the heat to medium-low, cover, and cook until the mushrooms have softened, 5 to 6 minutes.

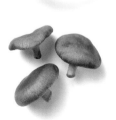

Stir in the ramen noodles and cook until tender, 2 to 3 minutes. Taste and adjust the salt as needed (you can add a splash of soy sauce if you have it on hand). Return the shrimp to the pot. Remove from the heat and serve right away, garnished with chopped scallions.

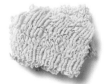

Per Serving (about 2 cups) ● Calories 338 ● Fat 10 g ● Saturated Fat 4 g ● Cholesterol 126 mg
Carbohydrate 32 g ● Fiber 2.5 g ● Protein 27 g ● Sugars 3 g ● Sodium 1,212 mg

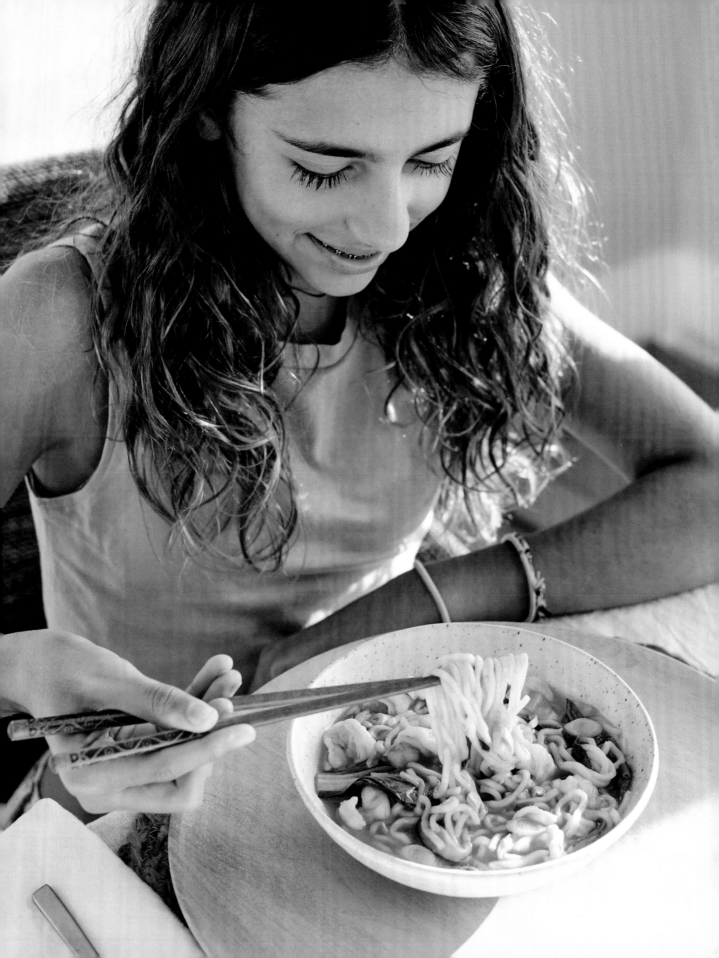

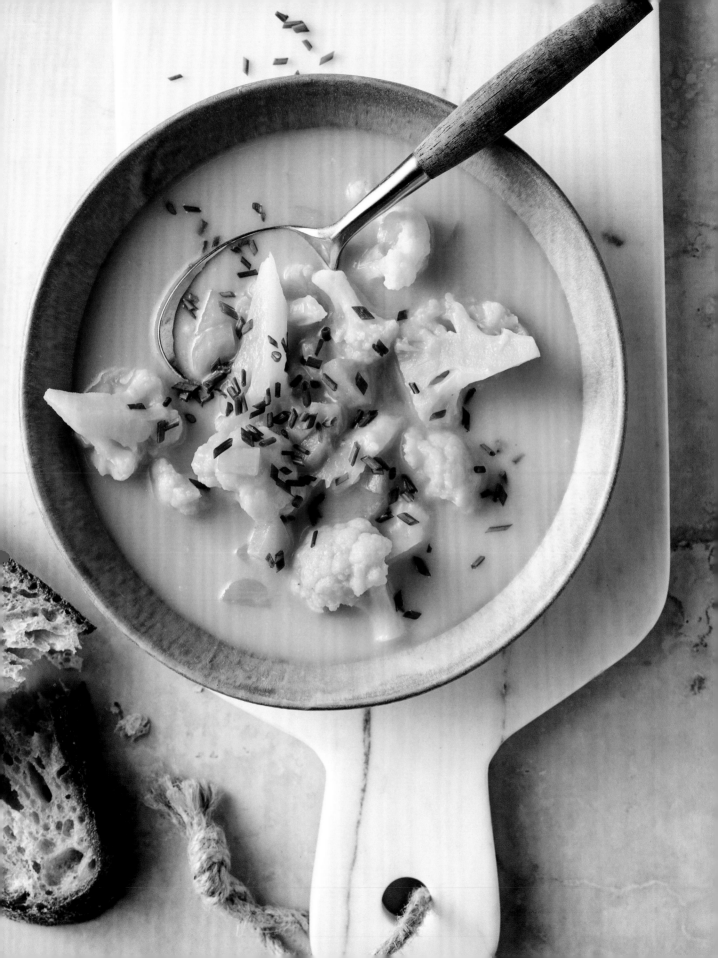

Cauliflower Cheddar Soup

SERVES 4

Q V GF

This hearty, cheesy cauliflower soup made with sharp cheddar is exactly what you want on a chilly day! It's thickened without cream by simply pureeing some of the soup, and it's ready in less than thirty minutes. Feel free to switch up the cheese (Gouda with a sprinkling of nutmeg is a great variation) and top with chopped chives if you have them. Serve with some crusty bread, a half sandwich, or a side salad to make it a meal.

1 tablespoon unsalted butter

¼ cup chopped carrot

½ cup chopped yellow onion

1 tablespoon all-purpose or gluten-free flour

4 cups reduced-sodium chicken or vegetable broth*

1 medium head cauliflower, roughly chopped (24 ounces of florets)

1 cup shredded sharp cheddar cheese

*Read the label to be sure this product is gluten-free.

In a heavy-bottomed medium pot, melt the butter over medium heat. Add the carrot and onion and cook until softened, about 5 minutes. Stir in the flour and cook until the flour is no longer raw, 1 to 2 minutes.

Add the broth and cauliflower, increase the heat to medium-high, and bring to a boil. Cover, reduce the heat to medium-low, and simmer until the vegetables are tender, 15 to 20 minutes. Remove the pot from the heat.

Transfer 2 cups of the soup (including some of the cauliflower) to a blender and puree until smooth. Pour the pureed soup back into the pot, add the cheddar, and stir until melted.

Divide the soup among bowls and season with freshly ground black pepper. Serve immediately.

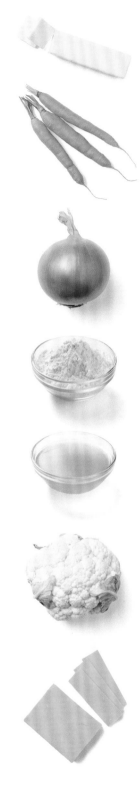

Per Serving (1½ cups) ● Calories 210 ● Fat 12 g ● Saturated Fat 8 g ● Cholesterol 37 mg
Carbohydrate 13 g ● Fiber 4 g ● Protein 14 g ● Sugars 5 g ● Sodium 780 mg

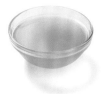

Stracciatella Tortellini Soup

SERVES 4

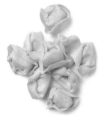

This comforting soup is like a warm hug in a bowl! It's perfect to soothe someone who's feeling under the weather. With just five ingredients, it's a great back-pocket recipe to keep in your repertoire. I love it with tortellini, but mini ravioli, cooked orzo, ditalini, or stars can be used in their place.

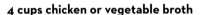

4 cups chicken or vegetable broth

**1 (9-ounce) package refrigerated cheese tortellini
 (I like Buitoni Three Cheese)**

2 large eggs

**¼ cup freshly grated Pecorino Romano cheese, plus more
 (optional) for serving**

2 cups baby spinach

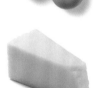

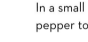

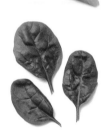

In a large pot, combine the broth with 1½ cups water and bring to a boil over medium-high heat. Add the tortellini to the pot and cook until tender, 6 to 7 minutes, or according to the package directions.

In a small bowl, whisk the eggs with the grated Pecorino and freshly ground black pepper to taste.

Reduce the heat to medium and slowly stream the eggs into the pot, stirring the broth constantly with a fork. The eggs will set and form ribbons. Stir in the baby spinach and cook until wilted, 1 to 2 minutes more.

Serve immediately with more cheese for topping, if desired.

Per Serving (1⅓ cups) ● Calories 276 ● Fat 10 g ● Saturated Fat 3.5 g ● Cholesterol 124 mg
Carbohydrate 30 g ● Fiber 3 g ● Protein 17 g ● Sugars 3 g ● Sodium 948 mg

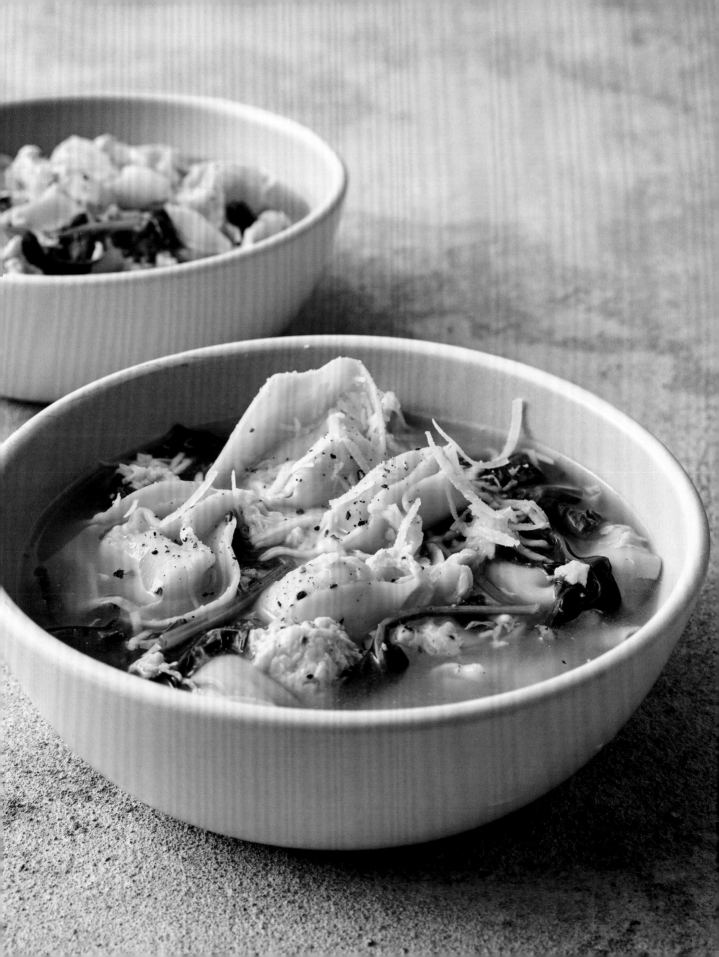

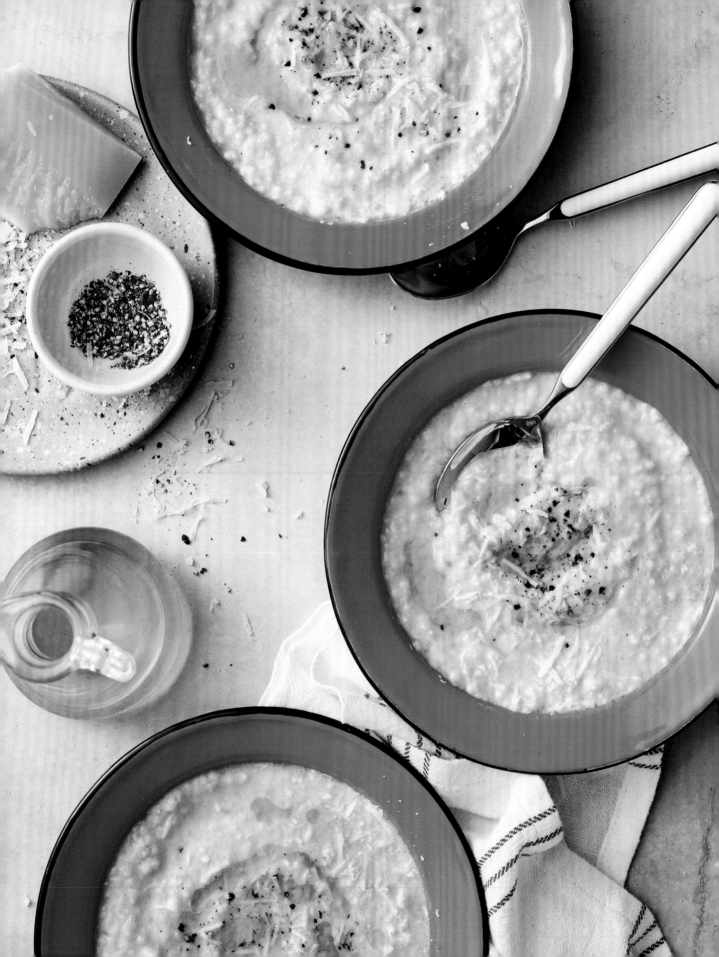

Creamy Pastina Soup

SERVES 4

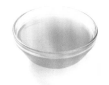

Is there anything more comforting than a warm bowl of pastina pasta? Pastina with lots of butter and cheese was one of my favorite pasta dishes as a kid. This soup sneaks in some veggies with riced cauliflower, but it's fully camouflaged, so if you have picky eaters, they'll never know!

6 cups reduced-sodium chicken or vegetable broth

1 Parmesan or Pecorino Romano rind

1 cup pastina or acini di pepe pasta

1½ cups frozen cauliflower rice

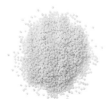

1 tablespoon unsalted butter

3 large eggs

¼ cup freshly grated Parmesan or Pecorino Romano cheese, plus more (optional) for serving

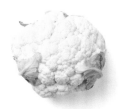

In a large pot, combine the broth and cheese rind and bring to a boil over high heat. Add the pasta, cauliflower rice, and butter and cook according to the pasta package directions until the pasta is tender.

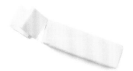

In a small bowl, beat the eggs. Beat in ¼ cup of the hot broth to warm the eggs, then whisk in the grated cheese. Add the egg/cheese mixture to the soup and whisk until creamy. Remove the pot from the heat.

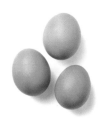

Serve the soup topped with a drizzle of extra-virgin olive oil, freshly ground black pepper to taste, plus extra grated cheese, if desired.

Per Serving (1²/₃ cups) ● Calories 347 ● Fat 10 g ● Saturated Fat 4 g ● Cholesterol 153 mg
Carbohydrate 45 g ● Fiber 3 g ● Protein 19 g ● Sugars 5 g ● Sodium 1,031 mg

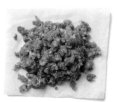

Italian Wedding Soup

SERVES 6

Wedding soup is a delicious bowl of tiny meatballs and escarole simmered in a rich broth with small pasta, such as acini di pepe or orzo. It's an Italian American classic and so tasty and comforting on cold nights. For an extra punch of flavor, mince 2 cloves of garlic and add to the meatball mixture.

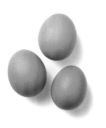

1 pound ground beef (90% lean) or a mixture of beef and turkey

2/3 cup seasoned bread crumbs, regular or gluten-free

1/2 cup freshly grated Parmigiano-Reggiano cheese, plus more (optional) for serving

1 large egg

8 cups low-sodium chicken broth*

6 cups (10 ounces) chopped escarole (from about 1/2 medium head) or other leafy greens

3/4 cup (4 1/2 ounces) small pasta (such as acini di pepe or orzo) or gluten-free orzo

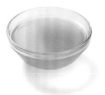

*Read the label to be sure this product is gluten-free.

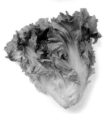

In a large bowl, combine the beef, bread crumbs, Parmigiano, egg, 1/2 teaspoon kosher salt, and freshly ground black pepper to taste and use a fork to mix everything thoroughly. Roll the mixture into 48 small meatballs, about 1 inch in diameter and 1/2 ounce each. Set aside on a sheet pan.

In a large pot, combine the broth and 1/2 cup water and bring to a boil over high heat. Reduce the heat to low for a gentle simmer, then carefully drop in the meatballs and add the escarole. Stir gently to combine. Cover the pot and cook until the meatballs are fully cooked through and the escarole is tender, about 15 minutes.

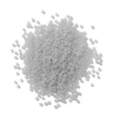

Stir in the pasta and increase the heat to medium. Cook the pasta to al dente according to the package directions. Taste and season with more salt, if needed. Serve hot, with additional grated Parmigiano on the side, if desired.

Per Serving (1 3/4 cups) ● Calories 342 ● Fat 13 g ● Saturated Fat 4.5 g ● Cholesterol 91 mg
Carbohydrate 30 g ● Fiber 3.5 g ● Protein 26 g ● Sugars 3 g ● Sodium 817 mg

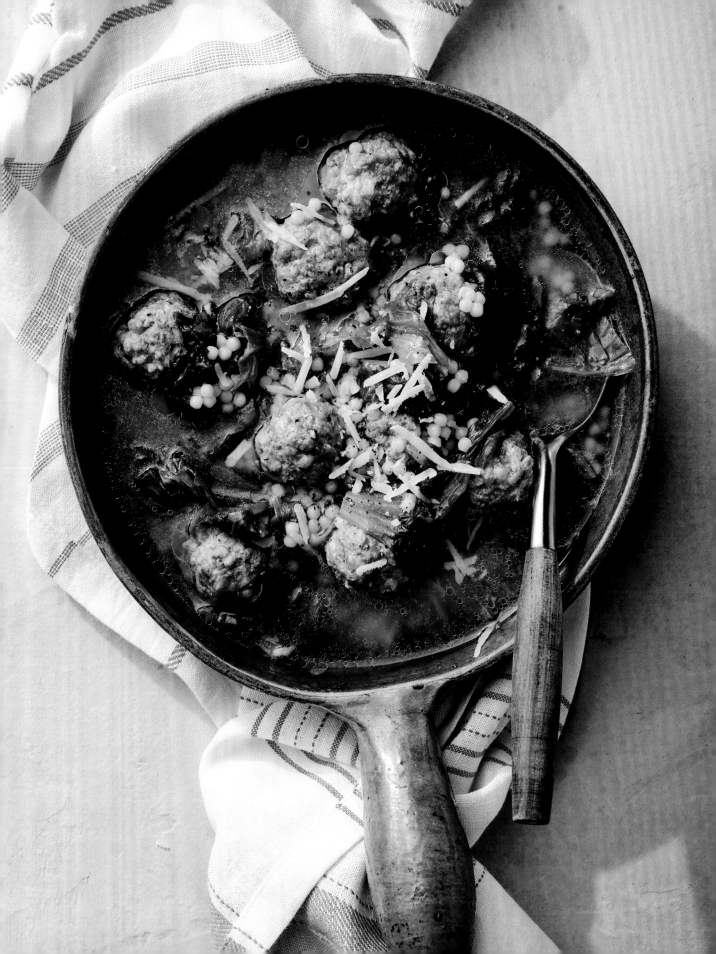

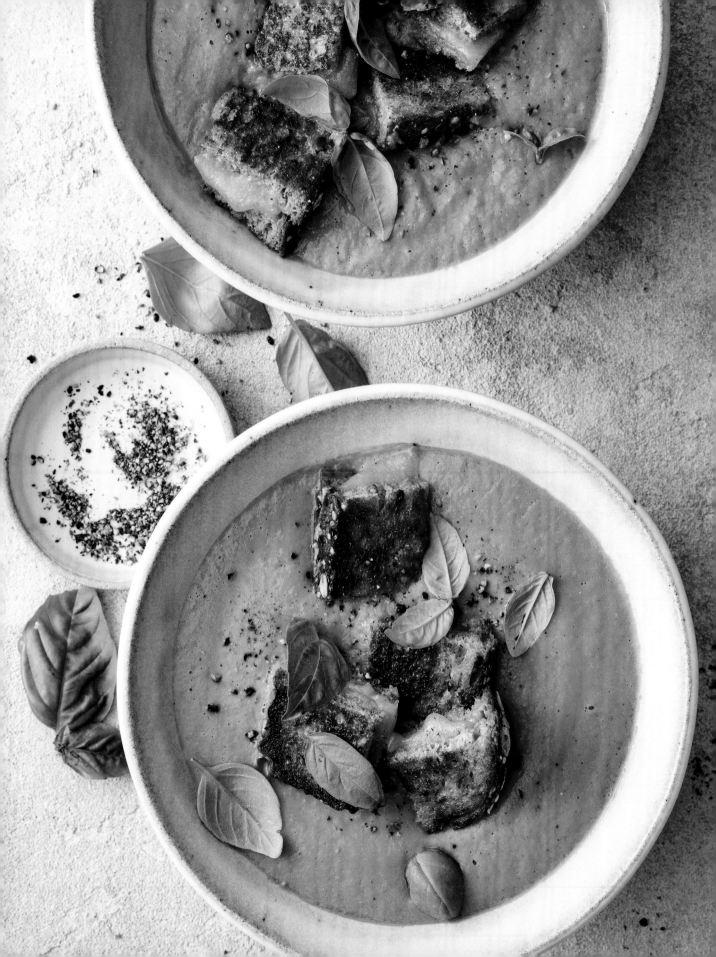

Sheet Pan Tomato Soup
with Grilled Cheese Croutons

SERVES 4

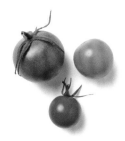

This simple tomato soup is extra rich and creamy, but without any cream! Roasting the vegetables creates a silky soup that pairs perfectly with grilled cheese croutons, which may be the best part. We all know tomato soup and grilled cheese are a classic duo, but when you turn the sandwich into cheesy, crispy bites to top your soup? Game over.

1½ pounds cherry tomatoes

1 yellow onion, quartered

1 head garlic

4 (1-ounce) slices whole-grain or gluten-free bread

4 slices cheddar cheese or vegan cheddar (such as Violife)

1½ cups vegetable broth*

Chopped fresh herbs, such as basil or chives, for garnish

*Read the label to be sure this product is gluten-free.

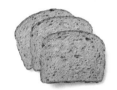

Preheat the oven to 400°F.

Spread the cherry tomatoes and onion on a sheet pan. Sprinkle with ¾ teaspoon kosher salt and freshly ground black pepper to taste, then drizzle with 1 tablespoon extra-virgin olive oil and toss everything together.

Remove the papery outer layers of the head of garlic and cut the top ¼ inch or so off the head, to expose the individual cloves. Spray with olive oil, wrap the head of garlic in foil, and place it on the baking sheet with the tomatoes.

Roast until the tomatoes have softened and burst and the garlic is golden, about 35 minutes.

(recipe continues)

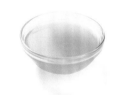

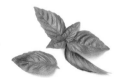

Per Serving (1 cup soup + ¼ of the croutons) ● Calories 274 ● Fat 15 g ● Saturated Fat 6 g
Cholesterol 28 mg ● Carbohydrate 27 g ● Fiber 6 g ● Protein 12 g ● Sugars 8 g ● Sodium 707 mg

Meanwhile, heat a griddle over medium-low heat. Spray olive oil over one side of each bread slice. Turn the slices over, top 2 of the bread slices with 2 slices cheddar each, and place the remaining 2 slices of bread on top, oiled sides up. Add the sandwiches to the griddle and cook until the bread is golden and the cheese has melted, 3 to 4 minutes per side. Transfer the sandwiches to a plate or cutting board and cut into 1-inch cubes.

When the vegetables are ready, carefully remove the garlic from the foil. Transfer the tomatoes and onion to a blender. Squeeze the garlic cloves out of the head of garlic and add them to the blender. Pour in the vegetable broth and blend until smooth. (The soup can be refrigerated for up to 4 days or frozen for up to 6 months.)

Divide the soup among four bowls, garnish with herbs, and serve immediately with the grilled cheese croutons on top.

Thai-Inspired Chicken, Lemongrass, Mushroom Soup

SERVES 5

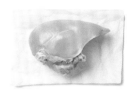

Tom yum is a light and refreshing Thai soup traditionally made with makrut lime leaves, galangal, and a chile paste called *nam prik pao*, giving it its distinctive hot and sour flavor. This rendition takes its inspiration from those dynamic flavors and makes smart use of food scraps—lime rind, cilantro stems, and mushroom stems—to enrich the broth while the chicken gently cooks. Don't skip the lemongrass, as it imparts a citrusy, herby dimension to the soup; you can usually find it with the other packaged herbs in the produce section.

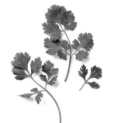

1½ pounds bone-in chicken breasts or thighs, skin removed

½ bunch cilantro

8 ounces fresh shiitake mushrooms

2 limes

3 (4- to 6-inch) stalks lemongrass, cut into 2-inch pieces

1½ tablespoons Sriracha sauce, plus more for serving

2 teaspoons fish sauce

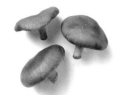

Pat the chicken dry and season all over with ½ teaspoon kosher salt and set aside.

Remove the cilantro leaves from the stems, reserving both separately (you'll have about 1 cup leaves). Trim the mushroom caps from the stems and reserve both separately as well. Juice one of the limes into a small bowl and reserve the spent rind. Cut the second lime into wedges and set aside until serving.

In a Dutch oven or large heavy-bottomed pot, heat 2 tablespoons olive oil over medium-high heat until it starts to shimmer, about 2 minutes. Add the chicken breasts to the pot and let cook undisturbed until browned, 3 to 5 minutes. Carefully flip the chicken and reduce the heat to medium-low.

(recipe continues)

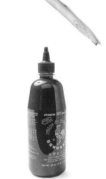

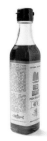

Per Serving (1½ cups) ● Calories 245 ● Fat 9 g ● Saturated Fat 1.5 g ● Cholesterol 99 mg
Carbohydrate 8 g ● Fiber 1.5 g ● Protein 32 g ● Sugars 2 g ● Sodium 602 mg

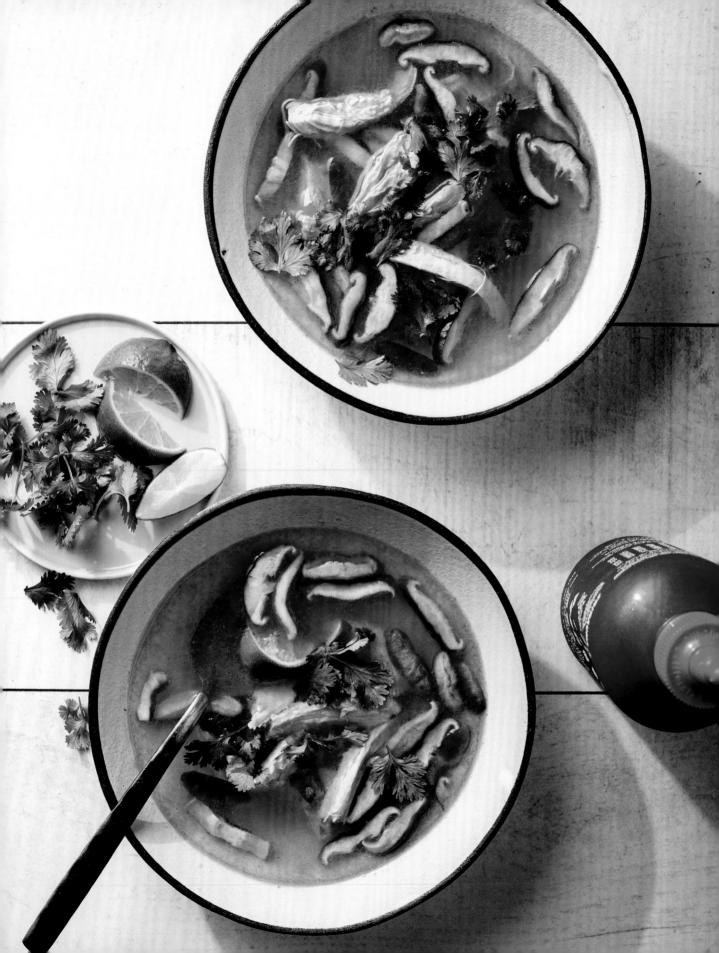

Use the side of your knife to smash the pieces of lemongrass. Add them to the pot along with 6 cups water, the cilantro stems, mushroom stems, reserved lime rind, Sriracha, and fish sauce. Increase the heat to high and bring the soup to a boil. Reduce the heat to low, cover, and simmer until the chicken reaches an internal temperature of 165°F or its juices run clear, 30 to 40 minutes (depending on the size of the chicken breasts).

Use a slotted spoon to carefully transfer the chicken to a plate. Scoop out and discard the solids from the pot. Add the shiitake mushroom caps and let the soup gently simmer over low heat while you prep the chicken.

When the chicken is cool enough to handle, use two forks to pull the meat off the bone and shred into bite-size pieces. Stir the chicken into the pot with the lime juice and ½ teaspoon kosher salt. Garnish with the cilantro leaves and serve right away, with the reserved lime wedges and Sriracha on the side.

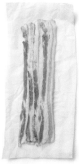

Brussels Sprouts Salad with Grated Egg

SERVES 2

This crave-worthy salad has wonderfully contrasting creamy and crunchy textures. The raw Brussels sprouts are first shaved with a knife and tossed with crisp bacon and a simple Dijon vinaigrette. But it gets even better! A hard-boiled egg is grated over the top to fall like snow over the salad. The light and fluffy grated egg is the perfect contrast to the crunchy raw veggies.

SKINNY SCOOP: You can buy Brussels sprouts preshredded, or slice them very thinly with a knife or in a food processor.

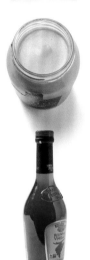

4 slices center-cut bacon

1 tablespoon Dijon mustard

1 tablespoon red wine vinegar

3½ cups shredded Brussels sprouts (about 7 ounces; see Skinny Scoop)

2 small scallions, chopped

2 large eggs, hard-boiled

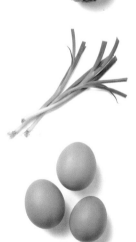

In a medium skillet, cook the bacon over medium-low heat until crisp, 3 to 5 minutes. Transfer to paper towels to drain, then crumble and set aside.

Meanwhile, in a large bowl, whisk together 2 tablespoons olive oil, the mustard, vinegar, and a pinch each of kosher salt and freshly ground black pepper. Add the Brussels sprouts and season with ¼ teaspoon salt and black pepper to taste.

Add half of the bacon and half of the scallions to the bowl of Brussels sprouts and toss well. Divide the salad between two wide bowls. Using a coarse Microplane, grate one hard-boiled egg over each bowl. Top with the remaining scallion and bacon, and a pinch of salt and black pepper, and serve.

Per Serving (1 salad) ● Calories 312 ● Fat 24 g ● Saturated Fat 5 g ● Cholesterol 191 mg
Carbohydrate 10 g ● Fiber 4 g ● Protein 15 g ● Sugars 2 g ● Sodium 743 mg

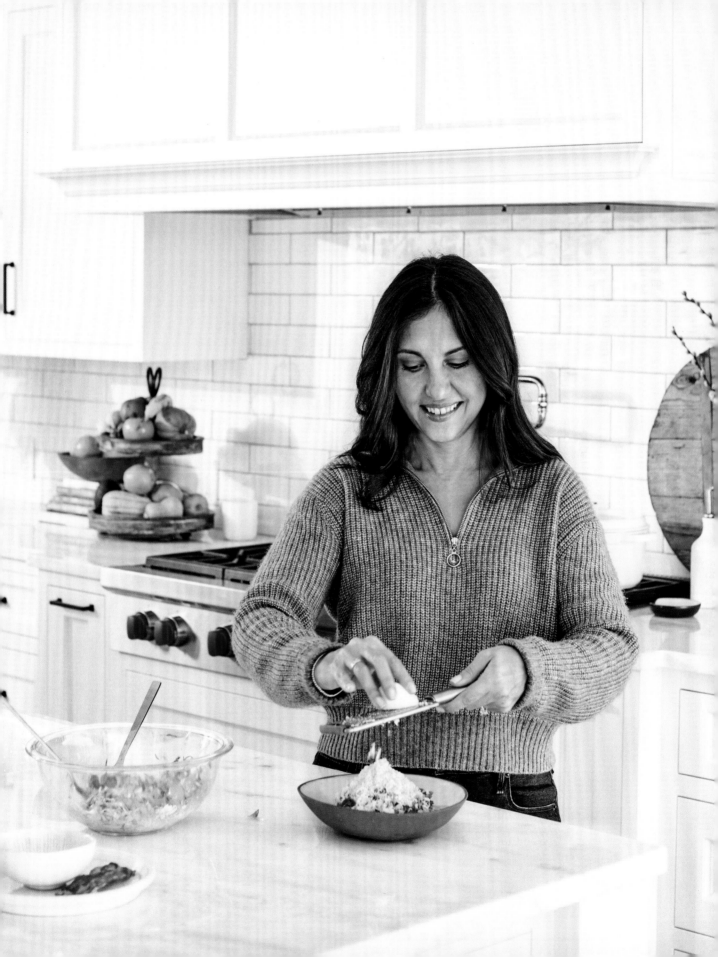

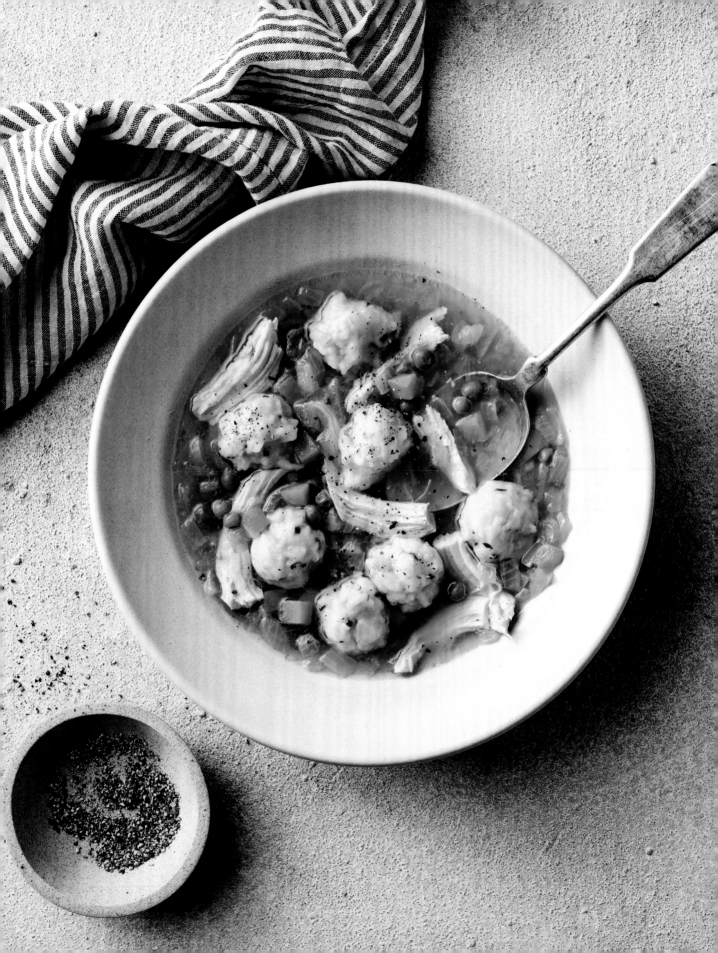

Chicken Soup
with Yogurt-Chive Dumplings

SERVES 6

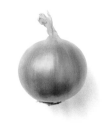

When I worked in New York City, one of my favorite soups when I went out for lunch was a chicken and dumpling one from a local mom-and-pop shop. This soup gives me those same cozy feelings, and the dumplings couldn't be easier to make. For a variation, you can swap the frozen peas and carrots for frozen mixed vegetables or use diced fresh carrots and celery instead.

SKINNY SCOOP: If you can't find self-rising flour, make your own by combining 2 cups all-purpose flour and 1½ teaspoons baking powder instead. Then measure the amount needed.

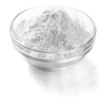

1 medium yellow onion, chopped

2/3 cup plus 2 tablespoons self-rising flour (see Skinny Scoop)

6 cups low-sodium chicken broth

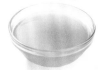

2 bone-in chicken breasts, skin removed (about 14 ounces each)

2/3 cup plain nonfat yogurt (not Greek)

2 tablespoons chopped fresh chives

1 (12-ounce) bag frozen peas and carrots (no need to thaw)

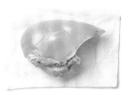

Heat a large pot over medium-high heat and add 1 teaspoon extra-virgin olive oil. Add the onion and ½ teaspoon kosher salt and cook, stirring occasionally, until the onion is soft and translucent and just starting to turn golden, about 10 minutes. Add 1 tablespoon of the flour and cook, stirring, until no longer raw, about 1 minute.

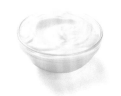

Add the chicken broth and the chicken and season with lots of freshly ground black pepper. Bring the broth to a boil, then reduce the heat to medium-low so that it bubbles gently. Cover and simmer until the chicken is cooked through, about 25 minutes.

Meanwhile, in a medium bowl, combine the remaining 2/3 cup plus 1 tablespoon flour, the yogurt, chives, and ½ teaspoon kosher salt. The dough will be very sticky, which is fine.

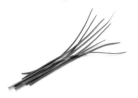

When the chicken has cooked through, remove it from the pot but leave the heat on under the simmering broth. Transfer the chicken to a cutting board and shred or cut the meat (discard the bones). Return the chicken to the pot along with the frozen peas and carrots. Using two small spoons, spoon the dumpling dough into the soup, a teaspoon at a time. Cover the pot and simmer undisturbed for 20 minutes. Gently stir the dumplings and continue to cook, uncovered, until the soup has thickened and the dumplings are tender and cooked through, 10 to 15 minutes more. Serve immediately.

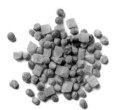

Per Serving (1⅓ cups) ● Calories 301 ● Fat 6 g ● Saturated Fat 1 g ● Cholesterol 102 mg
Carbohydrate 26 g ● Fiber 2.5 g ● Protein 36 g ● Sugars 6 g ● Sodium 622 mg

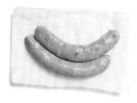

Cabbage Soup
with Sausage and White Beans

SERVES 8

On dreary days or in the dead of winter, I love a hearty cabbage soup, and this one couldn't be easier! Spicy chicken or turkey sausage (or even chorizo) team up with easy canned beans for a flavorful, stick-to-your-ribs soup. If you don't like spice, use sweet Italian sausage instead of spicy.

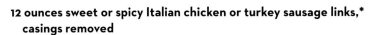

12 ounces sweet or spicy Italian chicken or turkey sausage links,*
   casings removed

1 large onion, finely diced

4 garlic cloves, minced

2 tablespoons red wine vinegar

2 (15-ounce) cans white beans,* such as navy or cannellini, rinsed and drained

2 (14.5-ounce) cans petite diced tomatoes

6 cups (12 ounces) coarsely chopped cabbage (from ½ small head)

*Read the label to be sure this product is gluten-free.

Heat a Dutch oven or large heavy-bottomed pot over medium-high heat. Add the sausage in small pieces and sear until the bottom is well browned, 2 to 3 minutes. Break it up with your spoon until it's cooked through and browned all over, 2 to 3 minutes more. Use a slotted spoon to transfer the sausage to a bowl, leaving the fat behind, if any.

Reduce the heat to medium and add ½ tablespoon olive oil and the onion. Cook, stirring, until it starts to brown, 8 to 10 minutes. Add the garlic and cook until fragrant, about 1 minute more.

Add 1 tablespoon of the vinegar and scrape the bits off the bottom of the pot to deglaze it. Stir in the white beans, 1¼ teaspoons kosher salt, reserved sausage, and tomatoes. Add the cabbage and 7 cups water. Increase the heat to high and bring to a boil, then reduce to medium-low and cook at a very gentle simmer until the cabbage is tender, 40 to 45 minutes.

Remove from the heat and stir in the remaining 1 tablespoon vinegar. Serve immediately.

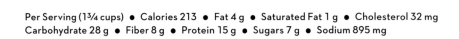

Per Serving (1¾ cups) ● Calories 213 ● Fat 4 g ● Saturated Fat 1 g ● Cholesterol 32 mg
Carbohydrate 28 g ● Fiber 8 g ● Protein 15 g ● Sugars 7 g ● Sodium 895 mg

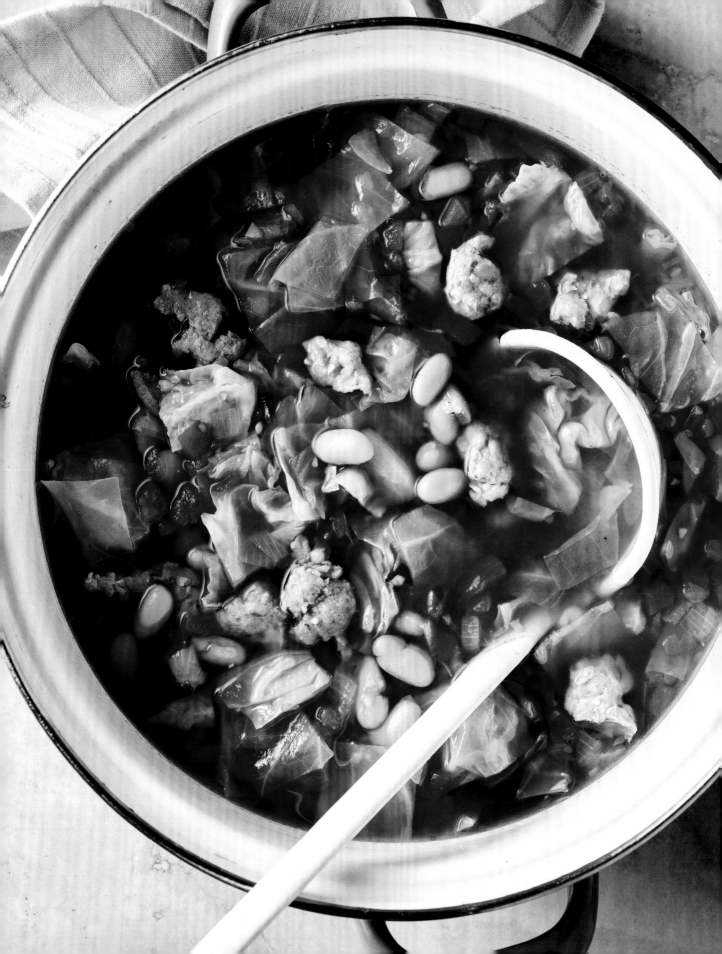

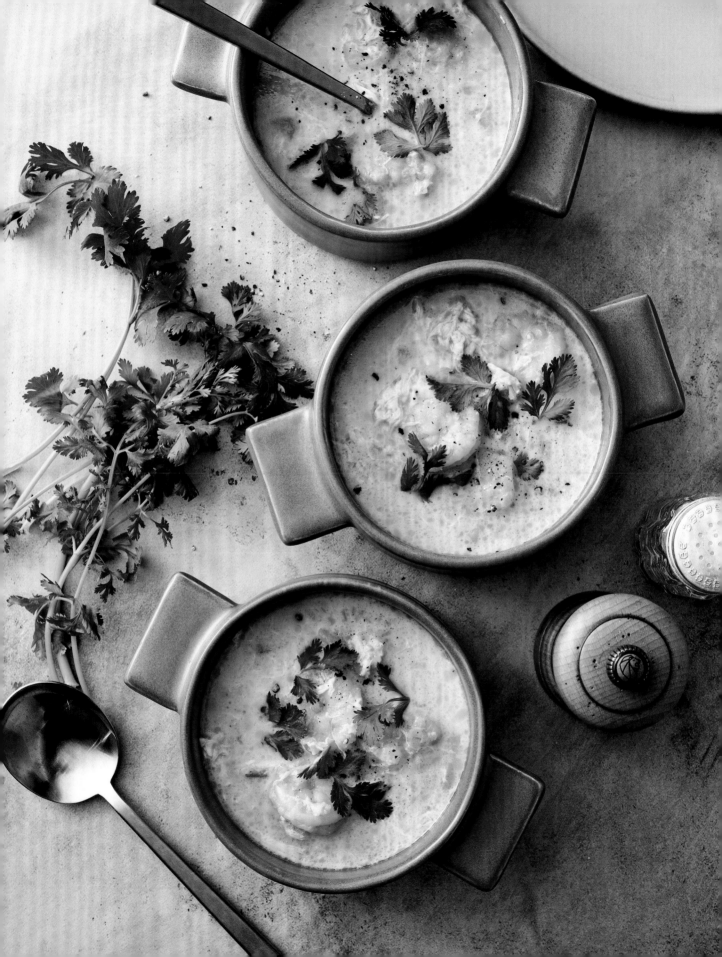

Mom's Instant Pot Creamy Shrimp and Rice Soup

SERVES 8

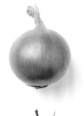

My mom has been making her version of this shrimp soup every Christmas for as long as I can remember! Although it's made with only a few ingredients, it's a special-occasion dish because it takes her more than 2 hours to prepare it. But good news: I streamlined her recipe for the Instant Pot, and now it can be ready in a fraction of the time. Garnish with fresh parsley, if you have it, for extra freshness.

1 small yellow onion, finely chopped

1 plum tomato, peeled, seeded, and finely chopped

1 medium waxy potato (such as white or red varieties), peeled and cut into ½-inch cubes (about 1 cup)

¼ cup uncooked long-grain white rice

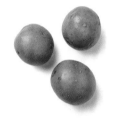

1 pound medium shrimp, peeled and deveined (halved if large)

1 (12-ounce) can evaporated milk

6 large eggs

Press the sauté button on an electric pressure cooker and heat 2 tablespoons olive oil. Add the onion and tomato and sauté, stirring often, until the onion is translucent, about 5 minutes. Press cancel.

Add 7½ cups water, 2 teaspoons kosher salt, the potato, rice, and shrimp and stir to combine. Seal and cook on high pressure for 30 minutes. Natural release, then open when the pressure subsides. Press sauté and stir in the evaporated milk. Once boiling, cook until the flavors meld, stirring often so the bottom doesn't burn, about 5 minutes.

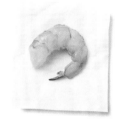

Meanwhile, crack the eggs into a large measuring cup or a bowl with a spout. Break the yolks with a fork and lightly mix (you'll want to see the separate whites and yellows). While stirring, slowly pour the egg mixture into the boiling soup to create ribbons. Simmer, stirring often so it doesn't burn, until the soup is thickened and the rice has completely dissolved, about 10 minutes. Serve immediately.

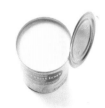

NO PRESSURE COOKER? NO PROBLEM! To make this on the stove, in a large soup pot, heat the oil over medium heat and sauté the onion and tomato. Add 8 cups water, the potato, rice, and salt and bring to a boil over high heat. Reduce the heat to low and cook until the potatoes and rice are soft, about 40 minutes. Add the shrimp and cook until the soup thickens, 40 minutes longer. Then proceed with adding the milk and eggs as written.

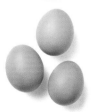

Per Serving (1½ cups) ● Calories 250 ● Fat 11 g ● Saturated Fat 4 g ● Cholesterol 236 mg Carbohydrate 16 g ● Fiber 1 g ● Protein 20 g ● Sugars 7 g ● Sodium 451 mg

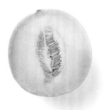

Summary Mozzarella Prosciutto Salad

SERVES 4

This chilled salad is so fresh and light, it's perfect to eat alfresco on summer nights, or to pack for a picnic on the beach or at a park. If you're entertaining, this makes a great appetizer that you can serve along with your favorite cheese board. Melon and prosciutto are a classic combo, but I really love the addition of the sweeter and juicer tropical papaya. Marinating all the fruit in lime juice and fresh mint is the best way to enjoy them, in my opinion! Serve with some grilled bread on the side if you want to make this salad more substantial.

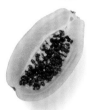

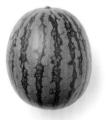

½ medium honeydew melon, seeded

½ medium papaya, seeded

½ small seedless watermelon

2 tablespoons fresh lime juice plus the grated zest of 1 lime

1 teaspoon chopped fresh mint, plus more for garnish

8 ounces baby mozzarella balls

4 ounces sliced prosciutto, torn into bite-size pieces

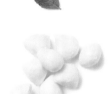

Using a 1¼-inch melon baller, scoop 24 balls of honeydew, 24 balls of papaya, and 24 balls of watermelon and transfer to a large bowl. If you don't have a melon baller, cut the fruit into 1-inch cubes. You will need about 2 cups of each. Add the lime juice, lime zest, and mint and toss to combine. Keep chilled until ready to eat.

Arrange the marinated fruit on a platter with the mozzarella and prosciutto. Garnish with fresh mint and serve.

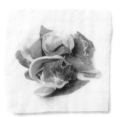

Per Serving (1½ cups fruit salad + 2 ounces mozzarella + 1 ounce prosciutto) ● Calories 298
Fat 19 g ● Saturated Fat 11 g ● Cholesterol 70 mg ● Carbohydrate 13 g ● Fiber 1.5 g
Protein 21 g ● Sugars 9 g ● Sodium 1,013 mg

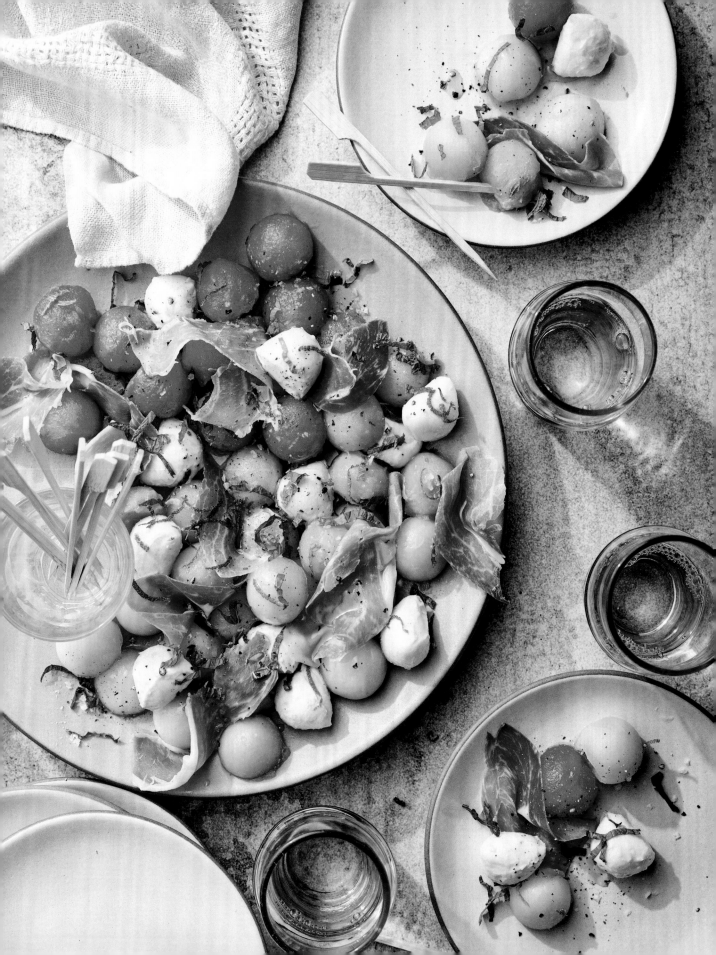

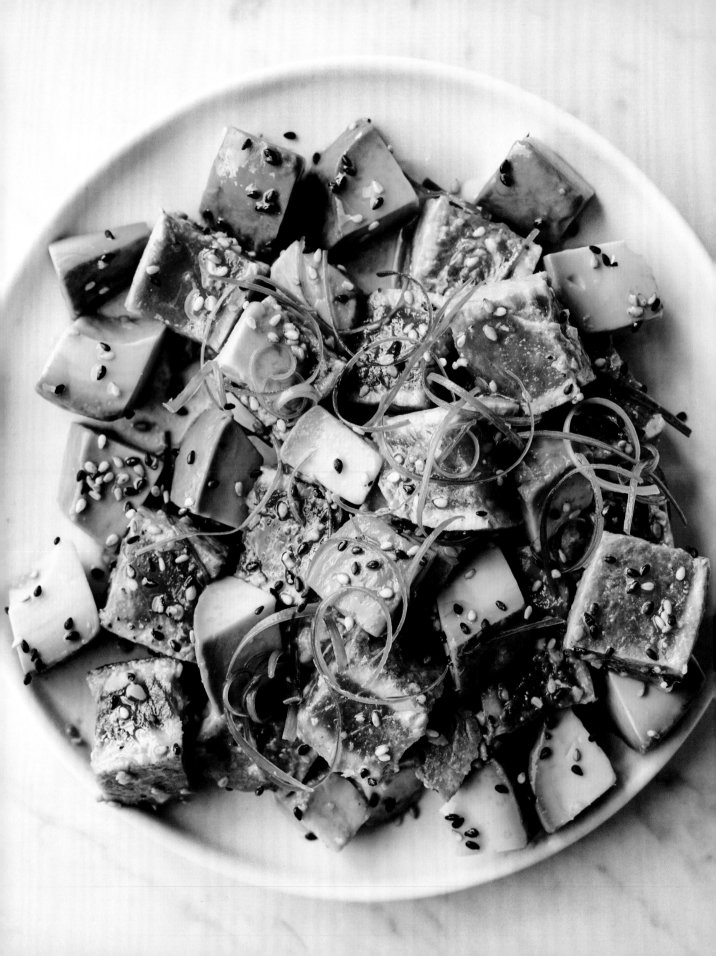

Seared Tuna and Avocado Salad

SERVES 2

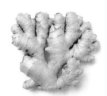

Whenever my lovely neighbors go tuna fishing, they almost always share their catch with me! I often use the tuna to make this fresh salad: It takes less than 10 minutes to prepare, and it's downright delicious. It's an ideal light meal as is, but you can also serve it over a bed of rice if you're craving more grains. Ask your fishmonger for sushi-grade tuna, and plan to make this salad the same day you buy your fish for the freshest flavor. Scallions are great as a garnish, and if you like spice like I do, feel free to add some Sriracha for heat.

½ tablespoon grated fresh ginger

Juice of ½ lime

2 tablespoons reduced-sodium soy sauce or gluten-free tamari

1 teaspoon toasted sesame oil

2 sushi-grade tuna fillets (6 ounces each)

5 ounces diced avocado (from about 1 medium)

1 teaspoon black and white sesame seeds

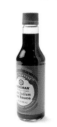

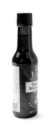

In a medium bowl, combine the ginger, lime juice, soy sauce, and sesame oil.

Place a large skillet over medium-high heat and spray with olive oil. Season both sides of the tuna with a pinch each of kosher salt and freshly ground black pepper. Add the tuna fillets to the skillet and sear for about 1 minute on each side until a slight crust forms but they're still rare in the middle. Transfer the tuna to a cutting board and cut into 1-inch cubes.

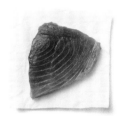

Add the tuna and the avocado to the bowl of dressing and toss to coat. Top with the sesame seeds and serve.

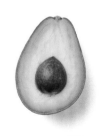

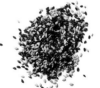

Per Serving (1½ cups) ● Calories 338 ● Fat 15 g ● Saturated Fat 2.5 g ● Cholesterol 77 mg
Carbohydrate 9 g ● Fiber 5 g ● Protein 42 g ● Sugars 1 g ● Sodium 637 mg

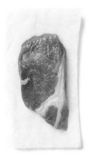

Grilled Italian Steak Salad with Arugula

SERVES 4

In the summer, after a long day at the beach or park, I love to make this steak salad and enjoy it alfresco with a glass of wine. This classic Italian tagliata salad is made with just a handful of ingredients, which means they should be the highest quality for the dish to truly shine. I usually use grass-fed sirloin beef, good-quality extra-virgin olive oil for drizzling, and freshly shaved Parmigiano-Reggiano cheese.

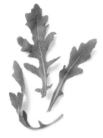

1¹/₂ pounds trimmed sirloin steaks, 1 to 1¹/₄ inches thick

7 cups baby arugula

Juice of ¹/₂ lemon, plus 1 lemon cut into wedges for serving

2 tablespoons capers, drained

¹/₂ cup shaved Parmigiano-Reggiano cheese (1 ounce)

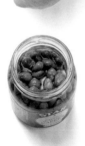

Preheat a grill or grill pan over high heat.

Spray the steak with olive oil and sprinkle both sides with 1 teaspoon kosher salt and freshly ground black pepper to taste. Place the steaks on the grill or grill pan and cook until slightly charred on one side, 3 to 4 minutes. Flip the steaks over and continue to grill 3 to 4 minutes longer, until browned and the internal temperature reads 135°F for medium-rare, 140°F for medium, or 150°F for well done (time will vary depending on thickness).

Transfer the steaks to a cutting board or platter, tent loosely with foil, and let rest for 5 minutes.

While the steaks rest, in a large bowl, toss the arugula with the lemon juice and 2 tablespoons extra-virgin olive oil. Sprinkle in ¹/₄ teaspoon kosher salt and freshly ground black pepper to taste and toss again. Divide among four plates.

Slice the steak across the grain. Top each plate of arugula with one-quarter of the sliced steak, ¹/₂ tablespoon capers, and 2 tablespoons shaved Parmigiano. Serve with lemon wedges and drizzle with more olive oil, if desired.

Per Serving (1 salad) • Calories 326 • Fat 16 g • Saturated Fat 4.5 g • Cholesterol 108 mg Carbohydrate 4 g • Fiber 1 g • Protein 41 g • Sugars 1 g • Sodium 684 mg

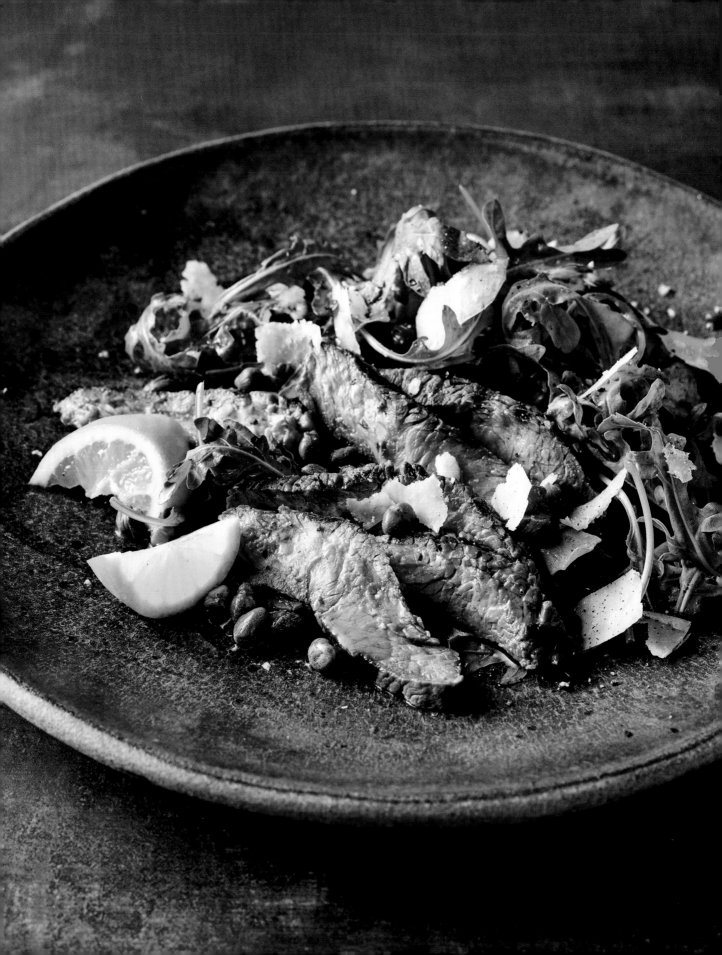

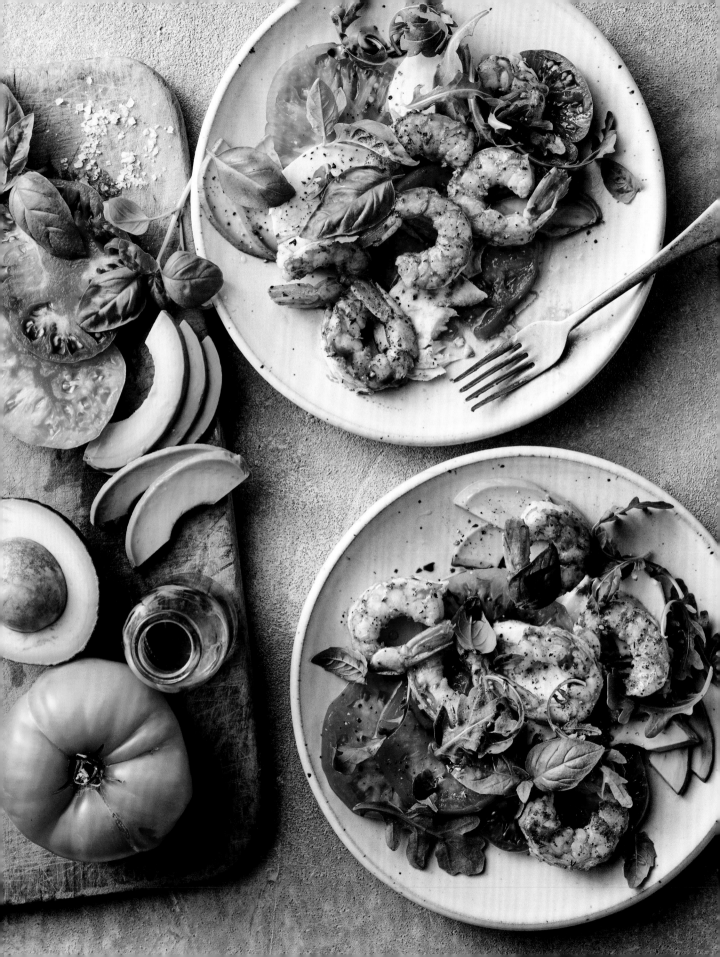

Avocado Caprese Salad with Blackened Shrimp

SERVES 4

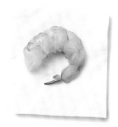

Not surprisingly, when I travel I'm all about the food, and I found my inspiration for this dish during a girls' trip to Anna Maria Island on the Gulf Coast of Florida, where they have the best seafood. I had this for dinner at a local restaurant, and I loved the idea of adding blackened shrimp (for protein) and avocado (for healthy fats) to a caprese salad to make it a main dish for lunch or a light dinner. To make this a true caprese, you can add fresh basil!

24 extra-jumbo (16/20 count) tail-on peeled and deveined shrimp (1¼ pounds total)

2 teaspoons blackened seasoning or Cajun seasoning*

4 cups baby arugula or baby lettuce

2 medium heirloom or beefsteak tomatoes, cut into 12 slices

8 ounces fresh mozzarella cheese, cut into 8 slices

5 ounces thinly sliced avocado (from about 1 medium)

2 tablespoons balsamic glaze

*Read the label to be sure this product is gluten-free.

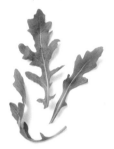

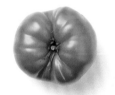

In a medium bowl, season the shrimp with the blackened seasoning. Heat a large nonstick skillet over medium-high heat and spray with oil. Add the shrimp and cook, flipping halfway, until pink and cooked through in the center, 2 to 3 minutes. Set aside.

Assemble the salad by placing 1 cup arugula on each plate, then divide and layer the slices of tomato, mozzarella, and avocado. Drizzle the salads with a total of 1 tablespoon extra-virgin olive oil and season with ¼ teaspoon kosher salt and freshly ground black pepper, to taste. Drizzle with the balsamic glaze and top with the shrimp. Serve immediately.

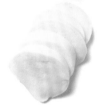

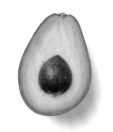

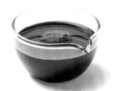

Per Serving (1 salad) ● Calories 432 ● Fat 21 g ● Saturated Fat 8.5 g ● Cholesterol 240 mg
Carbohydrate 13 g ● Fiber 3.5 g ● Protein 46 g ● Sugars 8 g ● Sodium 413 mg

Veggie
Mains

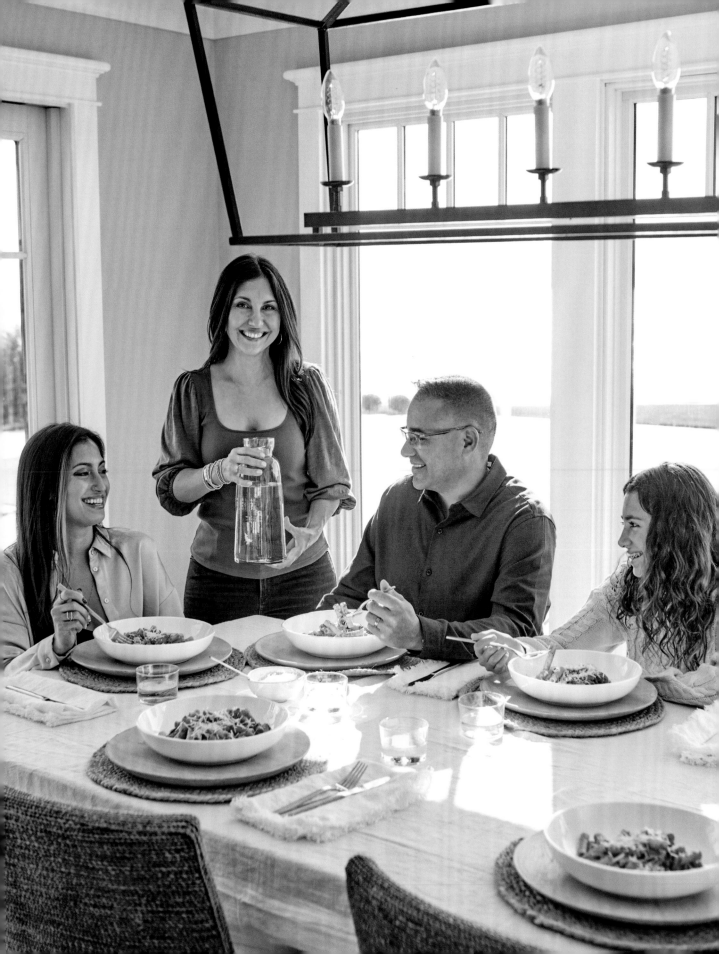

Instant Pot "Baked" Ziti with Spinach

SERVES 4

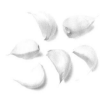

There are so many things to love about this one-pot dinner. It's quick, using one pot means fewer dishes to wash, and since the pasta cooks with the sauce, you honestly can't tell that the pasta is whole wheat. But for me the biggest win is just that Tommy loves it so much—and he's not always easy to please! If you want to add meat to make it even heartier, use a meat sauce instead of marinara, or add some leftover chopped-up turkey meatballs (see The Juiciest Italian Turkey Fried Meatballs Ever, page 146).

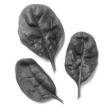

3 garlic cloves, smashed with the side of a knife

2 cups chopped baby spinach

**10 ounces (about 3 cups) whole wheat pasta (I like DeLallo),
 such as ziti or cavatappi**

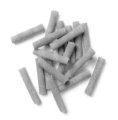

2 cups good-quality marinara sauce

½ cup part-skim ricotta cheese

¼ cup freshly grated Pecorino Romano cheese

1 cup shredded part-skim mozzarella cheese

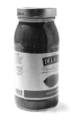

Press the sauté button on an electric pressure cooker. When hot, add 1 teaspoon olive oil and the garlic. Cook, stirring, until golden, about 1 minute. Press cancel.

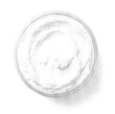

Stir in 2 cups water and ¾ teaspoon kosher salt, scraping the bottom of the pot to deglaze it and making sure the garlic is not stuck to the bottom.

Stir in the spinach and pasta. Pour in the marinara sauce, making sure it evenly covers all the pasta. (Do not stir or you will get a burn message.)

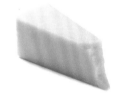

Seal and cook on high pressure for 7 minutes. Quick release, then open when the pressure subsides and give everything a big stir. Top with dollops of ricotta and sprinkle with the Pecorino and mozzarella. Cover with the lid until the cheese melts, 3 to 4 minutes. Serve immediately.

NO PRESSURE COOKER? NO PROBLEM! In a large heavy pot, heat 1 teaspoon olive oil over medium heat. Add the garlic and cook until golden, about 1 minute. Add the water and salt and bring to a boil. Stir in the spinach, pasta, and marinara sauce. Reduce the heat to low. Cover and cook until the pasta is tender, 20 to 25 minutes, stirring every 5 minutes so the bottom doesn't burn. Top with the cheeses, cover, and cook until melted, 4 to 6 minutes.

Per Serving (1½ cups) ● Calories 463 ● Fat 13 g ● Saturated Fat 6 g ● Cholesterol 33 mg
Carbohydrate 61 g ● Fiber 5.5 g ● Protein 22 g ● Sugars 8 g ● Sodium 850 mg

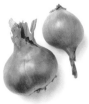
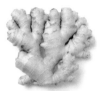
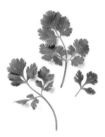

Coconut Red Curry Lentils

SERVES 6

Lentils are my top go-to ingredient for extra fiber because they don't take a long time to cook, and they're so nutritious and delicious! This creamy coconut red curry is comforting and flavorful. I like to serve it with rice or garlic naan, and it's also great for meal prep, as it reheats well throughout the week. If you want to add some vegetables, toss in a few handfuls of baby spinach or frozen peas at the end and let them cook for 5 minutes.

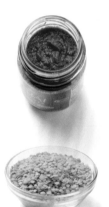

2 large shallots, chopped

1 tablespoon minced fresh ginger

¼ cup chopped fresh cilantro, plus more for garnish

2 tablespoons Thai red curry paste

1½ cups uncooked red lentils, rinsed

3 cups vegetable broth*

½ cup canned full-fat coconut milk, plus more (optional) for drizzling

*Read the label to be sure this product is gluten-free.

In a large pot, heat 1 teaspoon olive oil over medium heat. Add the shallots and cook, stirring occasionally, until translucent, 3 to 5 minutes. Add the ginger and cilantro and cook until soft and fragrant, 1 to 2 minutes more. Stir in the curry paste.

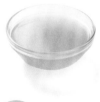

Add the lentils, vegetable broth, coconut milk, and 1 cup water and stir to combine. Increase the heat to high and bring to a boil. Reduce the heat to medium-low and simmer, stirring occasionally, until the lentils thicken and are tender, 20 to 24 minutes. If the mixture is too thick, add a little water to thin it out.

Serve warm topped with additional cilantro and a drizzle of coconut milk, if desired.

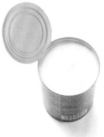

Per Serving (¾ cup) ● Calories 236 ● Fat 5 g ● Saturated Fat 3.5 g ● Cholesterol 0 mg
Carbohydrate 35 g ● Fiber 6 g ● Protein 13 g ● Sugars 3 g ● Sodium 352 mg

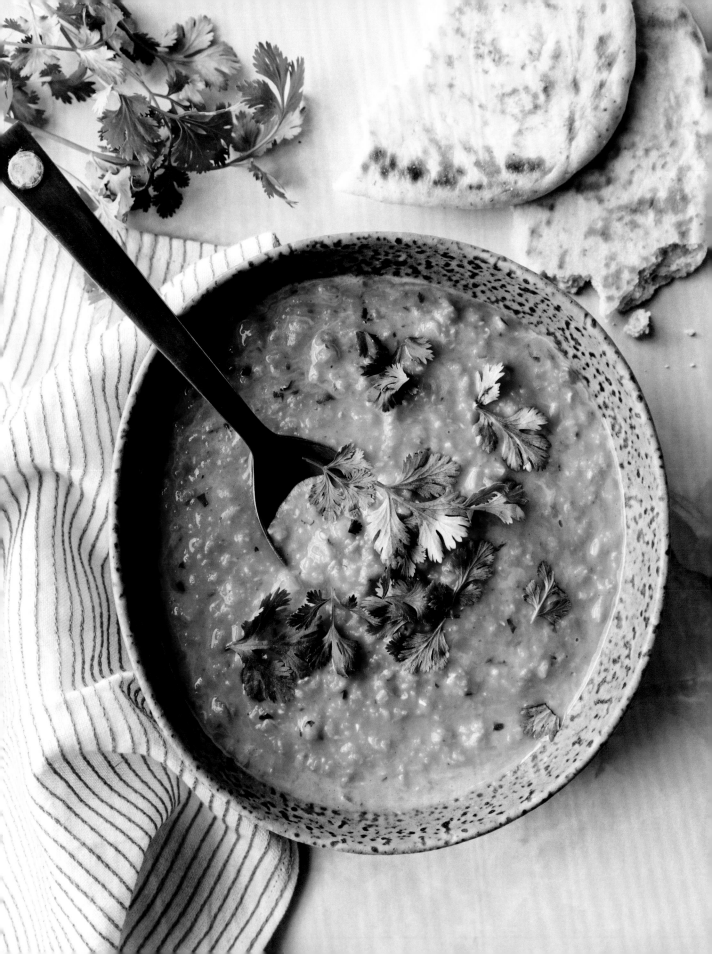

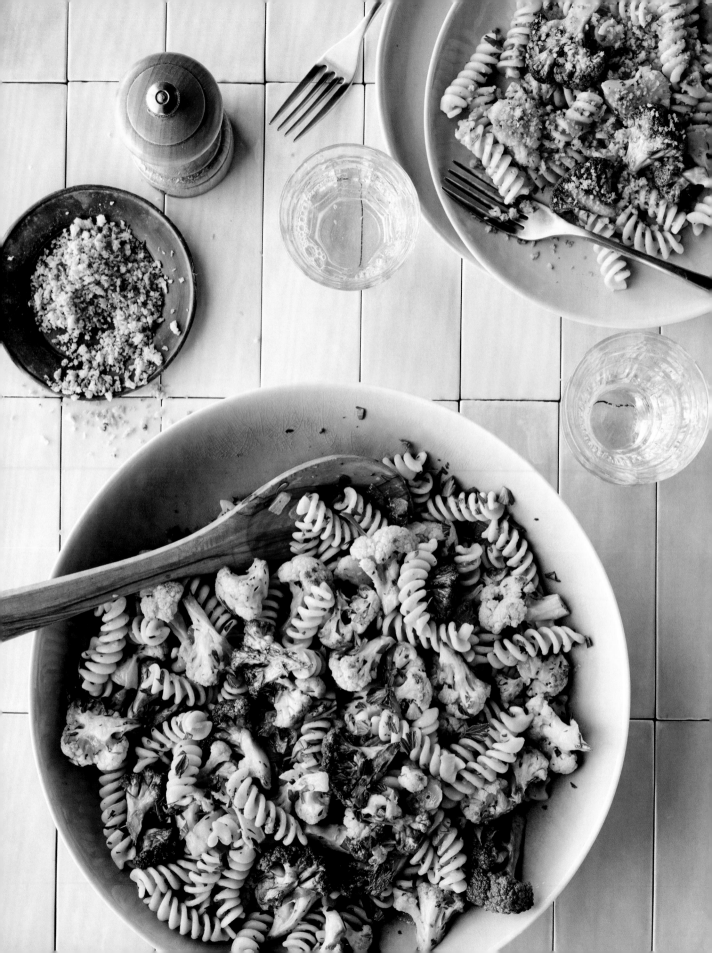

Pasta with Roasted Cauliflower and Garlicky Toasted Bread Crumbs

SERVES 4

I love cauliflower prepared in lots of different ways, but there's something special about roasting it that brings out its natural nuttiness. The anchovy fillets dissolve easily into the oil, and it's a simple way to add savory flavor to pasta dishes without tasting fishy at all. I like using colorful cauliflower, if I can find it, for an extra punch of color. The best part, though, is the toasted bread crumb topping, which gives the pasta the perfect crunchy bite. To take the bread crumbs up a notch, add some red pepper flakes and ¼ cup chopped fresh parsley.

1 garlic clove, minced

3 tablespoons seasoned bread crumbs, regular or gluten-free

5 anchovy fillets

1 medium head cauliflower (about 1 pound), cut into ½-inch pieces

1 small onion, roughly chopped

8 ounces fusilli or any short pasta shape, regular or gluten-free

¼ cup freshly grated Pecorino Romano cheese, plus more (optional) for serving

Preheat the oven to 450°F.

Bring a large pot of water with 2 tablespoons kosher salt to a boil over high heat.

Spray an ovenproof medium skillet (preferably cast-iron) with olive oil and set over medium low heat. Add the garlic and bread crumbs and toast, stirring often to prevent burning, until golden, 1½ to 2 minutes. Transfer the bread crumbs to a bowl and set aside.

(recipe continues)

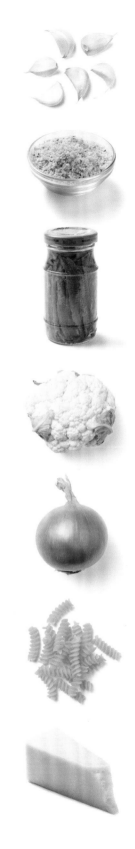

Per Serving (1½ cups) ● Calories 392 ● Fat 12 g ● Saturated Fat 2.5 g ● Cholesterol 10 mg
Carbohydrate 59 g ● Fiber 6 g ● Protein 15 g ● Sugars 9 g ● Sodium 434 mg

Wipe out the skillet and return it to medium-low heat. Add 2 tablespoons extra-virgin olive oil and add the anchovies. Cook, stirring, until they begin to dissolve, about 1 minute. Add the cauliflower, increase the heat to medium-high, and stir to coat. Cook, undisturbed, until the bottom of the cauliflower starts to brown, 3 to 4 minutes. Stir and continue to cook until light brown all over, 1 to 2 minutes more. Add the onion and cook until lightly golden, about 1 minute, then give the cauliflower one last stir and transfer the pan to the oven. Roast until the cauliflower is tender and browned all over, 6 to 8 minutes. Return the skillet to the stove.

Meanwhile, add the pasta to the boiling water and cook to al dente according to the package directions. Reserving 1 cup of the cooking water, drain the pasta.

Place the skillet with the cauliflower mixture over high heat. Add the drained pasta, Pecorino, and ⅓ to ½ cup of the reserved pasta water and cook, stirring, until the pasta is well coated, adding more pasta water if needed, 30 to 60 seconds. Drizzle with 1 teaspoon olive oil and stir once more.

Divide the pasta evenly among four plates. Top each with the toasted bread crumbs and serve with additional Pecorino, if desired.

Lentils and Rice with Caramelized Onions

SERVES 4

Inspired by the traditional Middle Eastern dish *mujaddara*, this delicious combination of rice, lentils, and caramelized onions takes pantry staples to a whole new level! Bonus: Combining rice with lentils (or beans) provides a complete protein—giving your body all the essential amino acids it needs in one delicious meal. If you'd like, add a cinnamon stick to the rice along with the cumin for some warmth.

1 cup uncooked green lentils, rinsed and drained

3 medium yellow onions, halved and cut into ⅛-inch-thick slices

1 cup uncooked basmati rice, rinsed

1½ teaspoons ground cumin

2 cups vegetable or chicken broth*

¼ cup chopped fresh cilantro or parsley, plus more for garnish

6 tablespoons 2% plain Greek yogurt

*Read the label to be sure this product is gluten-free.

In a small saucepan, combine the lentils and 2 cups water. Bring to a boil over high heat. Reduce the heat to low, cover, and simmer until the lentils are parboiled (slightly softened but with a bite), about 15 minutes. Drain and set aside.

Meanwhile, heat a large deep skillet over medium-high heat. Add 1 tablespoon extra-virgin olive oil, the onions, and ¼ teaspoon kosher salt and cook, tossing often to allow for even cooking, until they start to brown, about 12 minutes. Reduce the heat to medium-low and continue to cook, stirring often, until the onions are soft and caramelized, 15 to 17 minutes more. Remove two-thirds of the onions from the pan and set aside for topping.

To the remaining onions in the pan, add the lentils, rice, 2 teaspoons kosher salt, cumin, and ⅛ teaspoon freshly ground black pepper. Add the broth and mix thoroughly, scraping the bottom of the pan with a wooden spoon. Bring to a boil over high heat, then reduce the heat to low, cover, and cook for 20 minutes. Remove from the heat and let it sit, covered, for 5 more minutes to let the steam finish cooking the rice.

Add the cilantro and gently mix into the rice and lentils, fluffing with a fork. Top with the reserved caramelized onions and garnish with more cilantro or parsley. Dollop the yogurt on top.

Per Serving (1¾ cups) ● Calories 473 ● Fat 5 g ● Saturated Fat 1 g ● Cholesterol 2.5 mg Carbohydrate 89 g ● Fiber 9 g ● Protein 20 g ● Sugars 15 g ● Sodium 914 mg

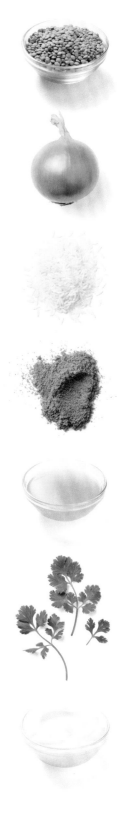

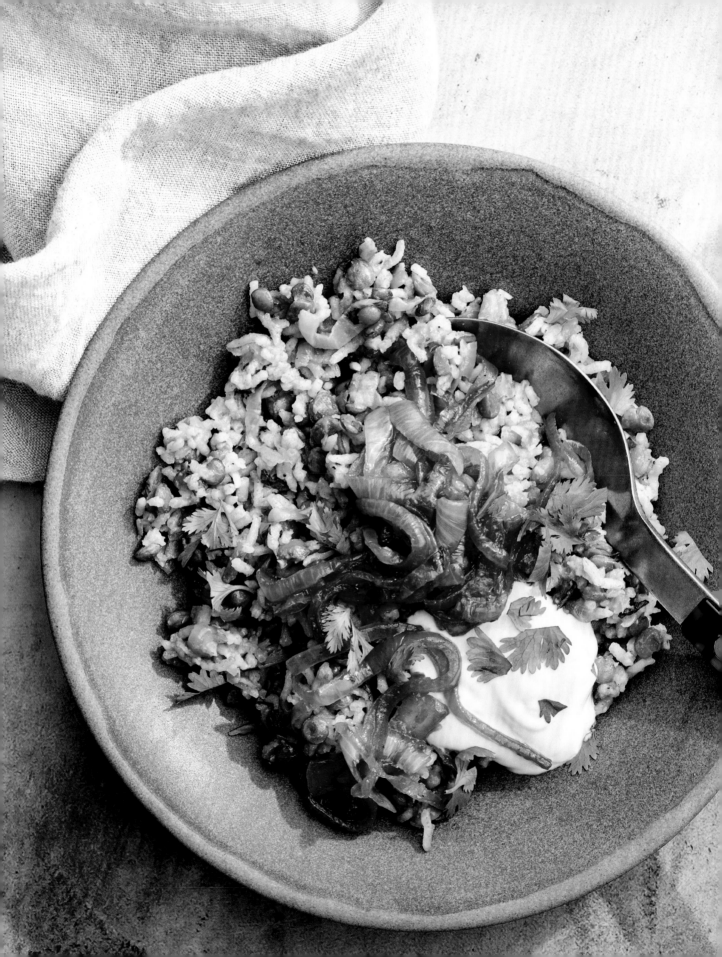

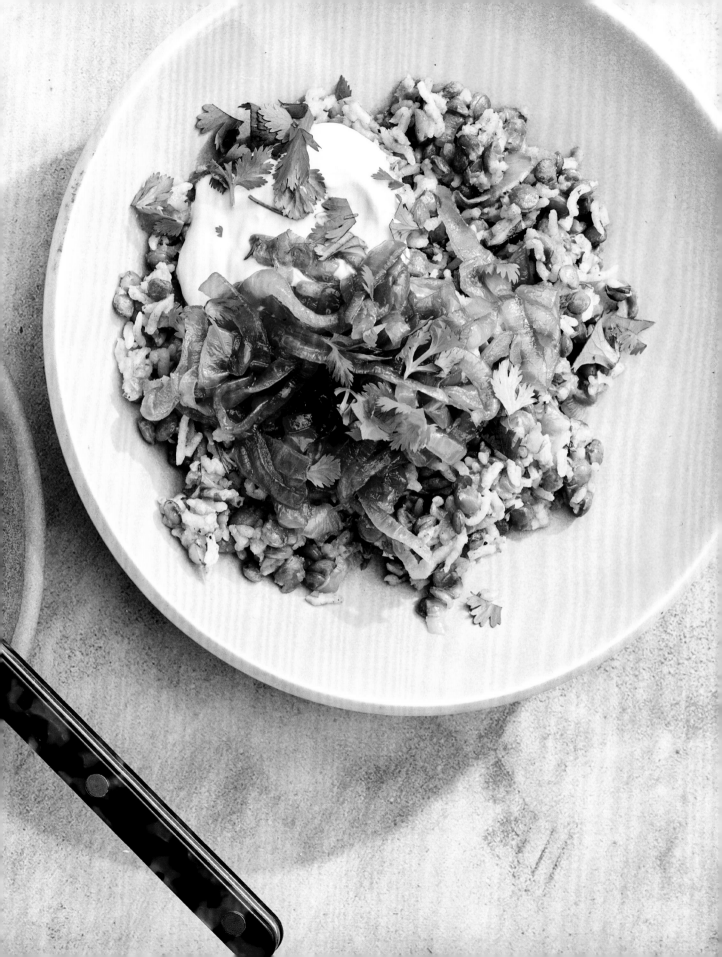

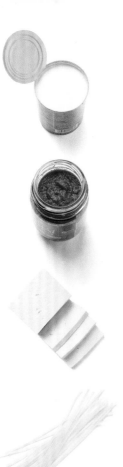

Peanut Butter Curry Noodles

SERVES 4

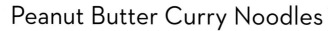

Q V GF DF

Rice noodles are simmered in a quick, creamy sauce made with a few pantry staples—canned coconut milk, peanut butter, and red curry paste. I love topping the dish with Sriracha, chopped scallions, or cilantro, but you decide if you want to stick to 7 ingredients here! If you're not a fan of tofu, you can use chicken or shrimp.

1 cup canned light coconut milk

¼ cup plus 1 tablespoon Thai red curry paste

1 (14-ounce) package firm tofu, pressed and cut into ½-inch cubes

6 ounces dried rice noodles

3 tablespoons smooth peanut butter

6 ounces baby spinach

1 lime, halved

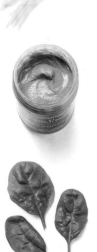

In a medium bowl, whisk together 2 tablespoons of the coconut milk, 1 tablespoon of the red curry paste, and ¼ teaspoon kosher salt until smooth. Add the tofu and marinate for 10 minutes.

Meanwhile, bring a medium pot of water to a boil over high heat and cook the noodles according to the package directions. The noodles should be soft (but still chewy and not mushy) after boiling. Drain the noodles, rinse them with cold water, and set aside.

Heat a large deep skillet over medium heat and spray with oil. Add the tofu in a single layer and cook until browned on the bottom, about 1½ minutes. Flip and repeat until browned on the other side. Transfer the tofu to a plate and set aside.

To the skillet, add ½ cup water, the peanut butter, and the remaining ¾ cup plus 2 tablespoons coconut milk and ¼ cup red curry paste. Bring to a boil over medium-high heat, whisking to combine, then reduce the heat to low so that the mixture simmers gently. Whisk until the peanut butter is totally dissolved.

Stir in the spinach, cover, and cook until the spinach is wilted, about 2½ minutes. Remove the skillet from the heat. Add the noodles and tofu to the skillet and stir to coat. Squeeze in the juice of ½ lime and season with ¼ teaspoon kosher salt.

Cut the remaining lime half into wedges. Serve with the lime wedges on the side.

Per Serving (1½ cups) ● Calories 393 ● Fat 15 g ● Saturated Fat 5 g ● Cholesterol 0 mg
Carbohydrate 42 g ● Fiber 3.5 g ● Protein 16 g ● Sugars 3 g ● Sodium 677 mg

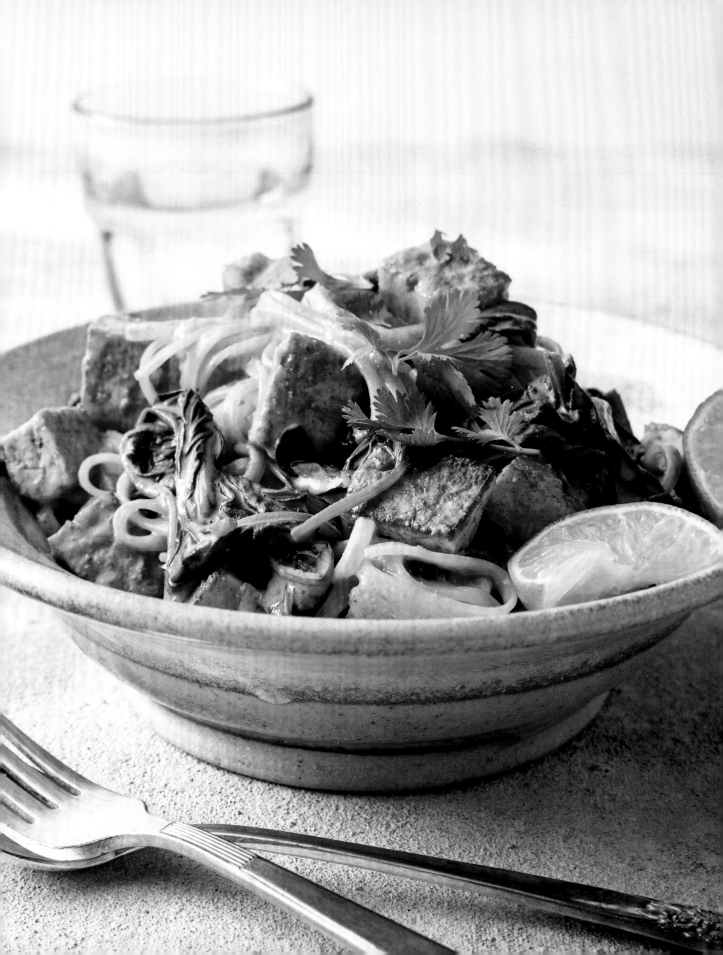

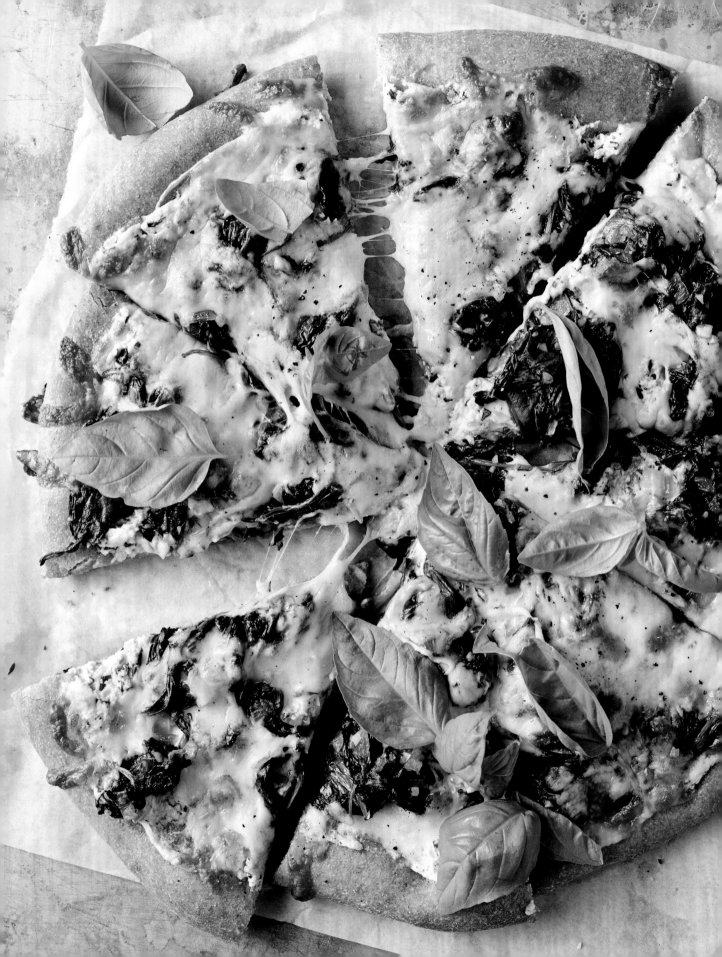

White Pizza with Spinach

SERVES 4

White pizzas typically don't include tomato sauce, and in this delicious version I use a creamy, basil-infused ricotta as the base and top it with garlicky spinach and shallots. The toppings contain more moisture than your typical pizza toppings, so it's important to parbake the crust to ensure that it won't get soggy. Never fear, though. The sheet pan technique I use to form and bake the crust makes it easy, mess-free, and quick—no flour or rolling pin needed!

12 ounces store-bought whole wheat pizza dough

3 large garlic cloves, minced

1/2 cup diced shallots (from 2 small)

5 ounces baby spinach

1/2 cup part-skim ricotta cheese, drained

2 tablespoons chopped fresh basil, plus more for garnish

1/2 cup shredded part-skim mozzarella cheese

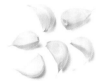

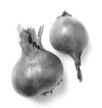

Allow the dough to come to room temperature, about 20 minutes.

Meanwhile, preheat the oven to 425°F. Spray a large sheet pan or round nonstick pizza pan with olive oil.

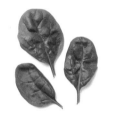

Stretch the pizza dough with your hands, then place it on the prepared sheet pan. Press and stretch it with your fingers on the sheet pan into a thin even 10-inch round. Poke it all over with a fork, then transfer to the oven to parbake until it's dry and partially cooked but not browned, 6 to 8 minutes.

Meanwhile, heat a large deep skillet over medium heat. Add 2 tablespoons extra-virgin olive oil, the garlic, and the shallots and cook until golden, about 1 minute. Add the spinach, 1/2 teaspoon kosher salt, and black pepper to taste. Cook until the spinach is wilted and the garlic and shallots begin to brown, about 4 minutes. Drain, if watery.

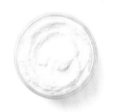

In a small bowl, combine the ricotta, basil, 1/4 teaspoon kosher salt, and black pepper to taste.

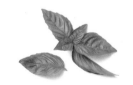

Once the crust is parbaked, spread the ricotta mixture evenly over the surface, leaving a 1-inch border all around. Top with the spinach mixture, then sprinkle with the mozzarella. Return to the oven and bake until the edges are golden and the cheese is melted, 8 to 10 minutes. Garnish with additional basil, slice into 8 pieces, and serve.

Per Serving (2 slices) ● Calories 350 ● Fat 14 g ● Saturated Fat 4 g ● Cholesterol 19 mg
Carbohydrate 42 g ● Fiber 7.5 g ● Protein 14 g ● Sugars 3 g ● Sodium 619 mg

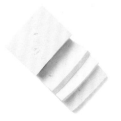

Sheet Pan BBQ Tofu and Broccoli

SERVES 2

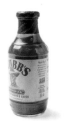

Here's a fun and easy way to prepare tofu: Slather it with BBQ sauce and cook it on a sheet pan alongside some broccoli—it doesn't get simpler than that! Since tofu is a blank slate for any flavor, the BBQ sauce gives it lots of taste without having to marinate it. A quick slaw on the side is the perfect complement.

SKINNY SCOOP: Not a fan of tofu? Use 1-inch cubes of chicken breast instead. For even easier meal prep, you can buy a bag of precut coleslaw instead of cutting the individual vegetables.

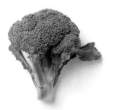

1 (14-ounce) package extra-firm tofu (see Skinny Scoop)

1/3 cup of your favorite BBQ sauce

1 large head broccoli, cut into florets (9 ounces florets)

2/3 cup shredded red cabbage

2/3 cup shredded green cabbage

1/3 cup shredded carrots

1 tablespoon apple cider vinegar

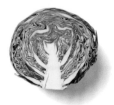

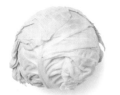

Preheat the oven to 425°F. Spray a large sheet pan with oil (if desired, for easier cleanup, line it first with foil).

Place the tofu on a clean kitchen towel or paper towels. Cover with another towel and gently press the tofu to remove as much excess moisture as possible. Transfer to a cutting board and cut into 1/2-inch cubes.

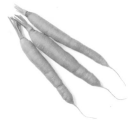

Transfer the tofu to the prepared sheet pan in an even layer. Brush half of the BBQ sauce on all sides of the tofu until completely coated, flipping the tofu as needed.

Place the broccoli in a large bowl and toss with 2 tablespoons extra-virgin olive oil and 1/2 teaspoon kosher salt. Scatter on the sheet pan around the tofu.

Roast, flipping the tofu and broccoli halfway, until the broccoli is tender, about 20 minutes. Remove from the oven and brush the remaining BBQ sauce over the tofu.

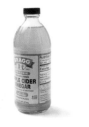

Meanwhile, in a large bowl, toss together both cabbages, the carrots, vinegar, 2 teaspoons extra-virgin olive oil, and 1/8 teaspoon kosher salt.

Serve the slaw alongside the tofu and broccoli.

Per Serving (2 cups tofu and broccoli + 2/3 cup slaw) ● Calories 507 ● Fat 29 g ● Saturated Fat 4 g
Cholesterol 0 mg ● Carbohydrate 40 g ● Fiber 8 g ● Protein 25 g ● Sugars 23 g ● Sodium 777 mg

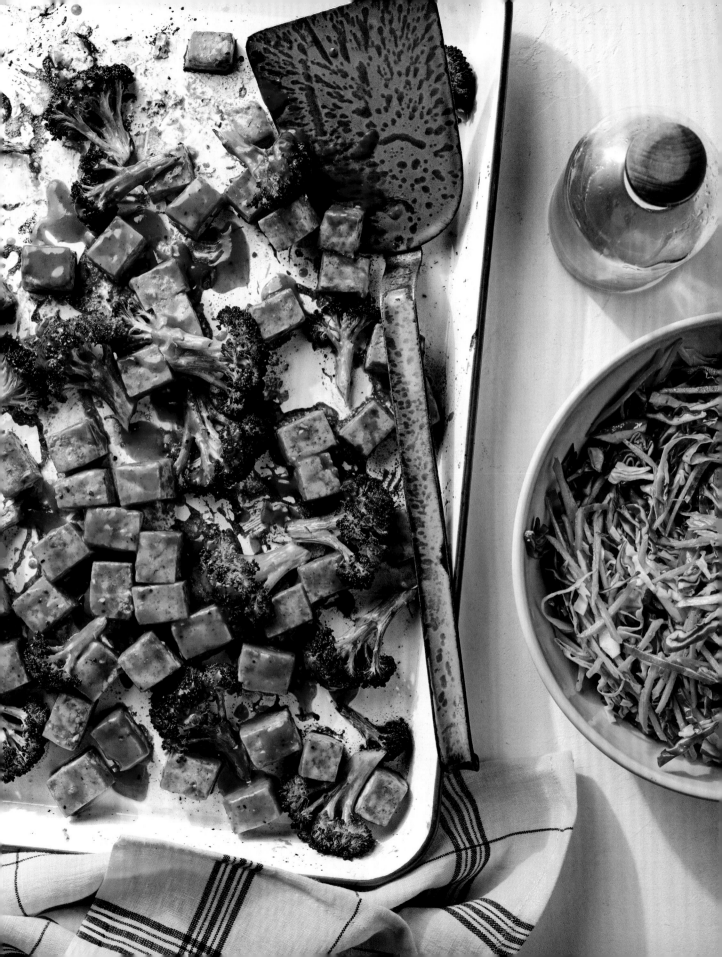

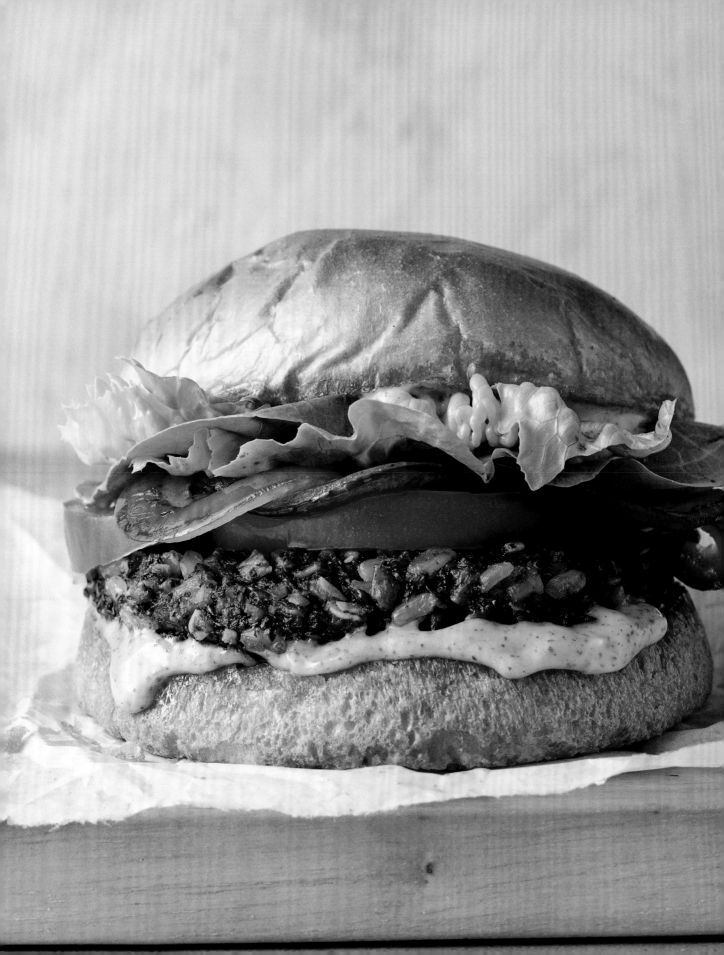

Weeknight Veggie Burgers

SERVES 4

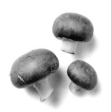

I wanted to create a veggie-loaded patty that didn't have the mealy texture of beans or chickpeas. The results are these tasty burgers loaded with sautéed mushrooms, onions, and shelled edamame for protein (usually found in the produce section or frozen). Serve them however you like your burgers: in toasted buns, topped with cheese, special sauce, ketchup, mustard, avocado, sautéed onions, lettuce, and/or tomatoes—you name it!

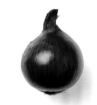

SKINNY SCOOP: If you want to make this vegetarian, look for vegan Worcestershire sauce, as many regular brands contain anchovies.

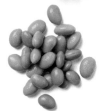

8 ounces sliced cremini mushrooms

1 medium red onion, roughly chopped

¾ cup shelled edamame, thawed if frozen

1 tablespoon cornstarch

1 tablespoon Worcestershire sauce* (see Skinny Scoop)

½ cup cooked brown rice (I love Trader Joe's frozen brown rice)

⅓ cup quick-cooking oats*

*Read the label to be sure this product is gluten-free.

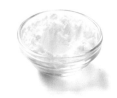

Preheat the oven to 425°F. Line a sheet pan with parchment paper.

Heat a large nonstick skillet over medium-low heat and add 2 tablespoons extra-virgin olive oil. Add the mushrooms, red onion, ¾ teaspoon kosher salt, and freshly ground black pepper to taste. Cook, stirring occasionally, until tender, about 5 minutes. Let the mixture cool for a few minutes, then transfer to a food processor and pulse a few times until finely chopped. Add the edamame, cornstarch, and Worcestershire sauce and pulse a few more times, until the edamame are finely chopped.

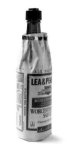

Transfer the mixture to a large bowl, add the brown rice and oats, and mix to combine. With wet hands to prevent sticking, divide the mixture into 4 equal portions and shape into flat patties about 4 inches in diameter and ½ inch thick. (At this point, you can bake them right away or freeze for another night.)

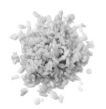

Transfer the patties to the prepared sheet pan and bake, flipping halfway through, until the burgers are golden and heated through, about 30 minutes. (To cook from frozen, add 3 more minutes on each side.) Serve immediately with your favorite fixings, if desired.

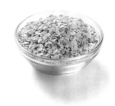

Per Serving (1 patty) ● Calories 178 ● Fat 8 g ● Saturated Fat 1 g ● Cholesterol 0 mg
Carbohydrate 21 g ● Fiber 5 g ● Protein 7 g ● Sugars 4 g ● Sodium 260 mg

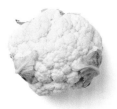

Whole Roasted Cauliflower Parmesan

SERVES 4

Here's a fun way to eat cauliflower: Roast it whole in the oven and then top it with tomato sauce and cheese! A handful of flavorful ingredients make a satisfying stovetop sauce that comes together quickly while the cauliflower roasts. Serve it as an entrée with garlic bread or a big green salad, or as a side dish with your choice of protein.

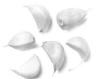

1 medium head cauliflower (about 1¼ pounds)

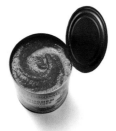

3 garlic cloves, smashed with the side of a knife

2 cups canned crushed tomatoes (I like Tuttorosso)

½ teaspoon crushed red pepper flakes

⅓ cup freshly grated Pecorino Romano or Parmesan cheese

⅓ cup shredded mozzarella cheese

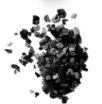

Preheat the oven to 400°F.

Trim the leaves and stem from the cauliflower, leaving the head intact. Spray evenly with olive oil and season all over with ½ teaspoon kosher salt.

Set the cauliflower in a cast-iron skillet or other ovenproof pan. Cover tightly with a few sheets of foil and roast for 20 minutes.

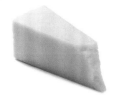

Meanwhile, in a large skillet, heat 1 teaspoon extra-virgin olive oil over medium heat. Add the smashed garlic and cook until golden on both sides, about 1 minute.

Add the crushed tomatoes and pepper flakes and season generously with freshly ground black pepper. Bring the sauce to a simmer, cover, then reduce the heat to medium-low and let it gently cook until the tomatoes no longer taste raw and the sauce has thickened a bit, about 10 minutes. Discard the garlic, then stir in half of the grated Pecorino cheese. Taste for salt (depending on the brand of tomatoes, you may need to adjust).

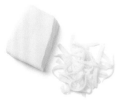

Remove the foil from the cauliflower and increase the oven temperature to 425°F. Continue to roast until you can easily pierce the center of the cauliflower with a knife, but the florets are still intact, about 20 minutes more.

Remove the skillet from the oven, pour the sauce over and around the cauliflower, and top with the mozzarella and remaining grated cheese. Return to the oven until the cheese has melted, 5 to 6 minutes more. Cut the cauliflower into 4 wedges and serve immediately.

Per Serving (¼ cauliflower head) ● Calories 142 ● Fat 6 g ● Saturated Fat 2.5 g ● Cholesterol 14 mg Carbohydrate 18 g ● Fiber 5.5 g ● Protein 9 g ● Sugars 8 g ● Sodium 650 mg

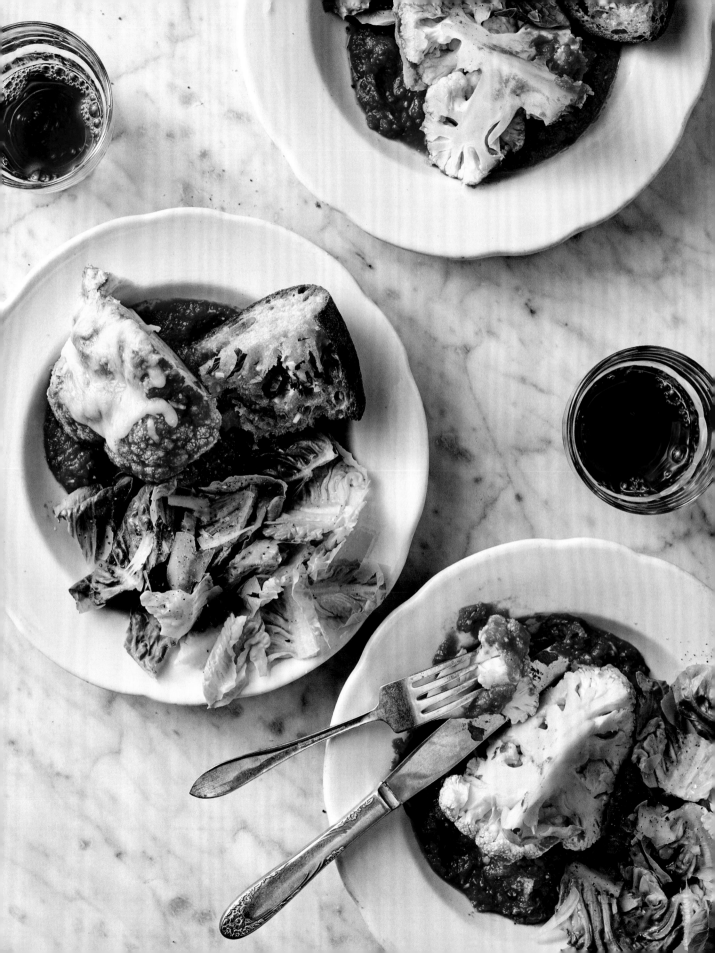

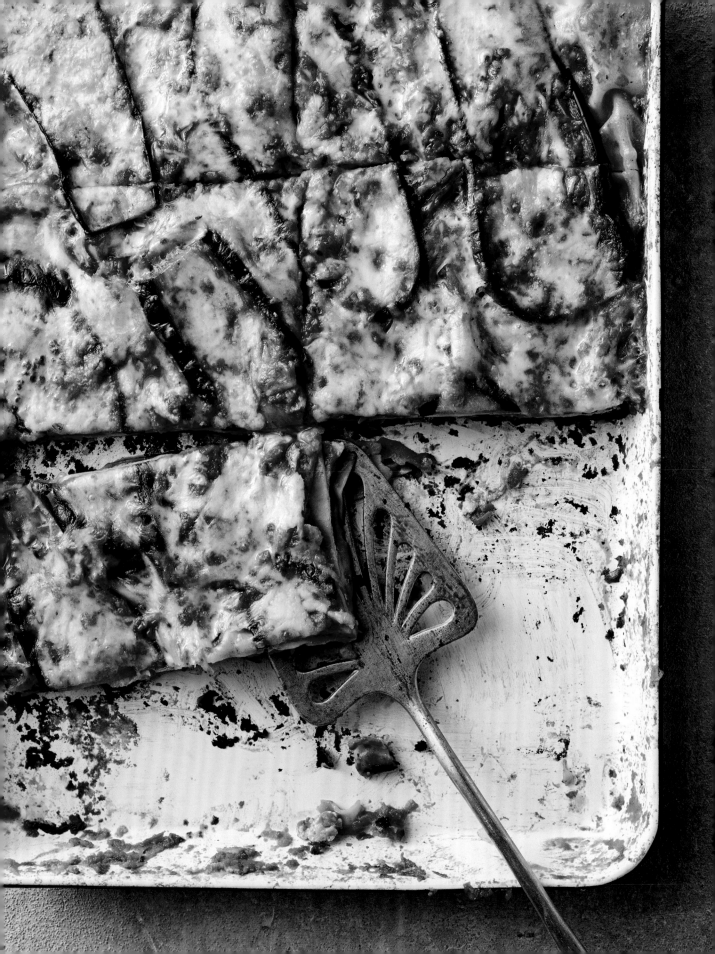

Sheet Pan Eggplant Lasagna

SERVES 8

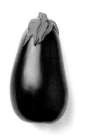

Instead of the typical sky-high pile of noodles, sauce, and cheese, this unexpected and easy lasagna layers no-boil lasagna noodles and sliced eggplant in a sheet pan, creating a thin, lightened-up version of a family favorite.

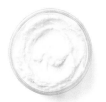

1½ pounds eggplant (2 medium or 1 large), sliced lengthwise
    into slabs ¼ inch thick

1 (15-ounce) container part-skim ricotta cheese

2 ounces Parmesan cheese, grated (½ cup)

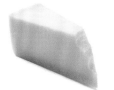

2½ cups shredded part-skim mozzarella cheese (10 ounces)

1 large egg

4 cups good-quality jarred marinara sauce

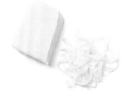

16 no-boil lasagna noodles (about 10 ounces, from 1 or 2 boxes)

Preheat the oven to 425°F. Line two large 13 x 18-inch sheet pans with parchment paper.

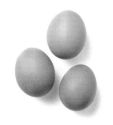

Divide the eggplant slices between the sheet pans. Spray both sides very lightly with oil and season with ¼ teaspoon kosher salt and freshly ground black pepper to taste. Cover the sheet pans tightly with foil and bake until the eggplant is tender, 10 to 12 minutes. Transfer all the eggplant to one pan and use the other for the lasagna.

Meanwhile, in a medium bowl, mix together the ricotta, Parmesan, 1 cup of the mozzarella, and the egg until thoroughly combined. Season with ¼ teaspoon kosher salt and ½ teaspoon freshly ground black pepper.

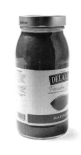

Spray the empty sheet pan lightly with oil. Spread 1 cup marinara over the bottom of the pan. Arrange half the lasagna noodles (about 8 sheets) so that they cover the whole pan (some overlap is fine), then top with half of the eggplant slices. Dollop the ricotta mixture evenly over the top, then pour over 1½ cups of the marinara sauce. Repeat with the remaining lasagna noodles, then the remaining eggplant, and finally top with the remaining 1½ cups marinara. Wrap tightly with foil.

Bake until the noodles are tender, about 30 minutes. Uncover, sprinkle with the remaining 1½ cups mozzarella, and bake until the cheese is melted and lightly browned, 5 to 7 minutes. Let the lasagna sit for 10 minutes before slicing. Cut into 8 pieces and serve immediately.

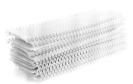

Per Serving (1 piece) ● Calories 468 ● Fat 19 g ● Saturated Fat 8.5 g ● Cholesterol 68 mg
Carbohydrate 50 g ● Fiber 5 g ● Protein 24 g ● Sugars 8 g ● Sodium 967 mg

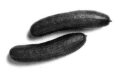

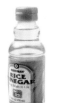

10-Minute Crispy Rice with Fried Eggs

SERVES 1

One of my favorite things to eat when I don't feel like cooking is a rice bowl topped with a runny egg. This version is loosely inspired by Korean *dolsot bibimbap*. It's traditionally served in a sizzling stone bowl that crisps up the rice, which is such a glorious thing! This very simplified version of the dish is budget-friendly and takes less than ten minutes. I top this one with chopped scallion and marinated cucumber, but it's the perfect canvas for any veggies you have on hand: wilted spinach, sautéed mushrooms, and shredded carrots are all great. If you'd like, serve it drizzled with soy sauce and sprinkled with sesame seeds.

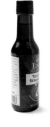

1 small Persian (mini) cucumber, quartered lengthwise and sliced crosswise into ½-inch pieces

½ teaspoon rice vinegar

½ tablespoon plus ¼ teaspoon toasted sesame oil

1 cup cooked brown rice (leftover/day-old rice or thawed from frozen)

2 large eggs

1 scallion, thinly sliced

½ tablespoon gochujang (regular or gluten-free) or Sriracha, or more to taste

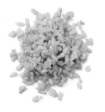

In a small bowl, season the cucumber with ⅛ teaspoon salt, the rice vinegar, and ¼ teaspoon of the sesame oil.

Add the remaining ½ tablespoon sesame oil to a medium nonstick skillet over medium heat and swirl to coat the bottom. Add the rice and spread out in an even layer. Cover and cook until the bottom of the rice is crisp and heated through, about 3 minutes. Stir the rice, then transfer to a bowl or plate.

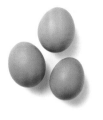

Reduce the heat to low and spray the pan with oil. Crack the eggs into the skillet, cover, and cook until the yolk is just clouded over for a runny egg, about 2 minutes. Transfer to the bowl of rice.

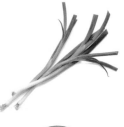

Top with the marinated cucumber, sliced scallion, and gochujang and serve.

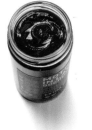

Per Serving (1 bowl) ● Calories 441 ● Fat 19 g ● Saturated Fat 4 g ● Cholesterol 372 mg
Carbohydrate 50 g ● Fiber 3.5 g ● Protein 18 g ● Sugars 5 g ● Sodium 462 mg

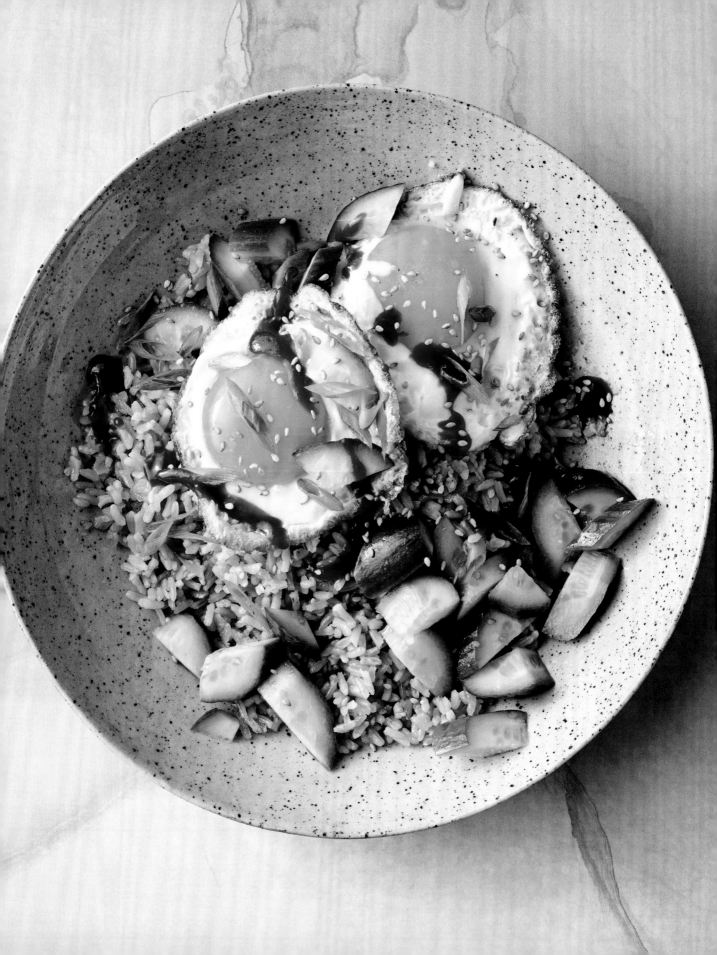

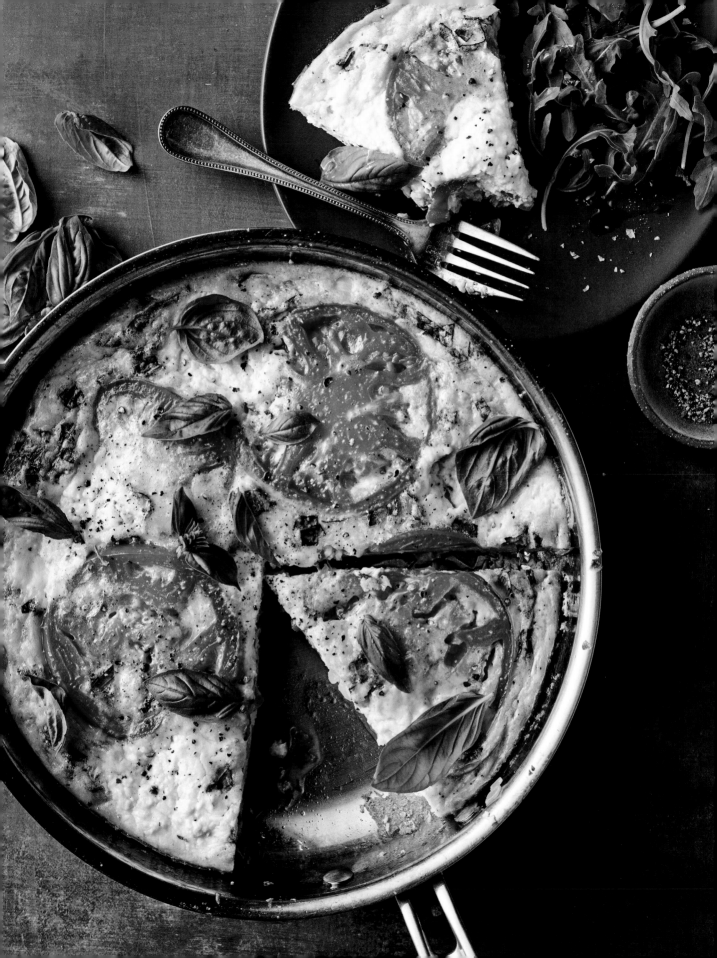

Tomato Ricotta Frittata

SERVES 4

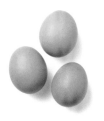

On nights when the only thing you have in your house to cook is eggs, frittatas are definitely the perfect meal to make! You can add just about anything to your frittata. Tommy's dad always adds ricotta to his (usually with sausage), which I love, but I wanted to make this meatless, so I went with tomatoes and basil instead and it's just as tasty.

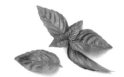

10 large eggs

8 fresh basil leaves, chopped

½ cup freshly grated Parmigiano-Reggiano cheese

½ cup whole-milk ricotta cheese, drained

1 medium yellow onion, diced

1 large vine tomato, sliced into ¼-inch-thick rounds

4 cups baby arugula

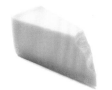

Preheat the oven to 375°F.

In a medium bowl, beat the eggs with ½ teaspoon kosher salt and freshly ground black pepper to taste. Stir in the basil and ¼ cup of the Parmigiano until well combined. In a separate small bowl, combine the ricotta and remaining ¼ cup grated cheese.

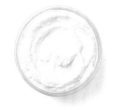

Spray a 10-inch ovenproof nonstick skillet all over with olive oil, then add 1 tablespoon extra-virgin olive oil and heat over medium heat. Add the onion and cook, stirring occasionally, until softened, 5 to 6 minutes. Spread evenly in the skillet.

Pour the eggs into the skillet. Reduce the heat to medium-low and let cook, without stirring, until the eggs begin to set around the edges of the pan, about 3 minutes. Remove from the heat.

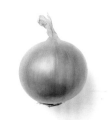

Arrange the tomato slices on top of the frittata and season them with a pinch of kosher salt. Drop tablespoons of the ricotta mixture between the tomato slices.

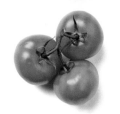

Transfer to the oven and bake until set all the way through and the top is golden, about 18 minutes. Let cool for a few minutes, then remove from the skillet and transfer to a plate or cutting board.

In a large bowl, toss the arugula with 1 teaspoon olive oil and season with ⅛ teaspoon kosher salt and freshly ground black pepper to taste. Serve with the frittata.

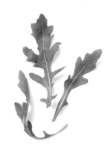

Per Serving (¼ frittata + 1 cup arugula salad) ● Calories 365 ● Fat 24 g ● Saturated Fat 9 g
Cholesterol 492 mg ● Carbohydrate 12 g ● Fiber 1.5 g ● Protein 24 g ● Sugars 6 g ● Sodium 636 mg

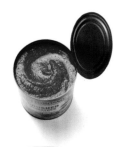

Saucy Eggs with Tomatoes

SERVES 4

When I want eggs for dinner, this is the dish I crave! I swear these eggs taste like you're having the best tasting raviolis for dinner, without all the carbs. Similar to Eggs in Purgatory, but without the heat, the eggs are poached in a Marcella Hazan–inspired tomato sauce made simply with tomatoes, butter, and onion. It's so easy and so good! Of course, bread is a must to sop up all the sauce and runny yolks.

SKINNY SCOOP: To make a shortcut version of this, use a jar of good-quality marinara instead of making the sauce from scratch. If you like heat, add ¼ to ½ teaspoon crushed red pepper flakes to the sauce along with the black pepper and finish with torn basil leaves for extra freshness.

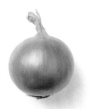

1 (28-ounce) can crushed tomatoes (I like Tuttorosso)

⅓ cup reduced-sodium chicken or vegetable broth*

2 tablespoons unsalted butter

1 small onion, peeled and quartered

8 large eggs

4 tablespoons freshly grated Pecorino Romano cheese

4 slices whole wheat or gluten-free Italian or French bread (1 ounce each)

*Read the label to be sure this product is gluten-free.

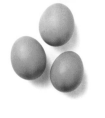

In a deep 12-inch skillet, combine the tomatoes, broth, butter, onion, ¼ teaspoon kosher salt, and freshly ground black pepper to taste (see Skinny Scoop). Bring to a boil over medium heat. Reduce the heat to medium-low, cover, and simmer until the onion quarters are soft, 20 to 25 minutes, stirring halfway.

Remove and discard the onion. Gently drop in the eggs, leaving 1 inch between them and keeping the yolks intact. Sprinkle with 2 tablespoons of the Pecorino.

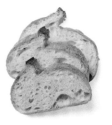

Reduce the heat to low and cover. Simmer until the egg whites are cooked but the yolks are still runny, 5 to 6 minutes, keeping a close eye so they don't overcook.

Remove from the heat and top with the remaining 2 tablespoons Pecorino, black pepper to taste, and a drizzle of extra-virgin olive oil, if desired. Serve with the bread.

Per Serving (2 eggs + ¾ cup sauce + 1 slice bread) ● Calories 369 ● Fat 18 g ● Saturated Fat 8 g
Cholesterol 392 mg ● Carbohydrate 29 g ● Fiber 5.5 g ● Protein 21 g ● Sugars 8 g
Sodium 905 mg

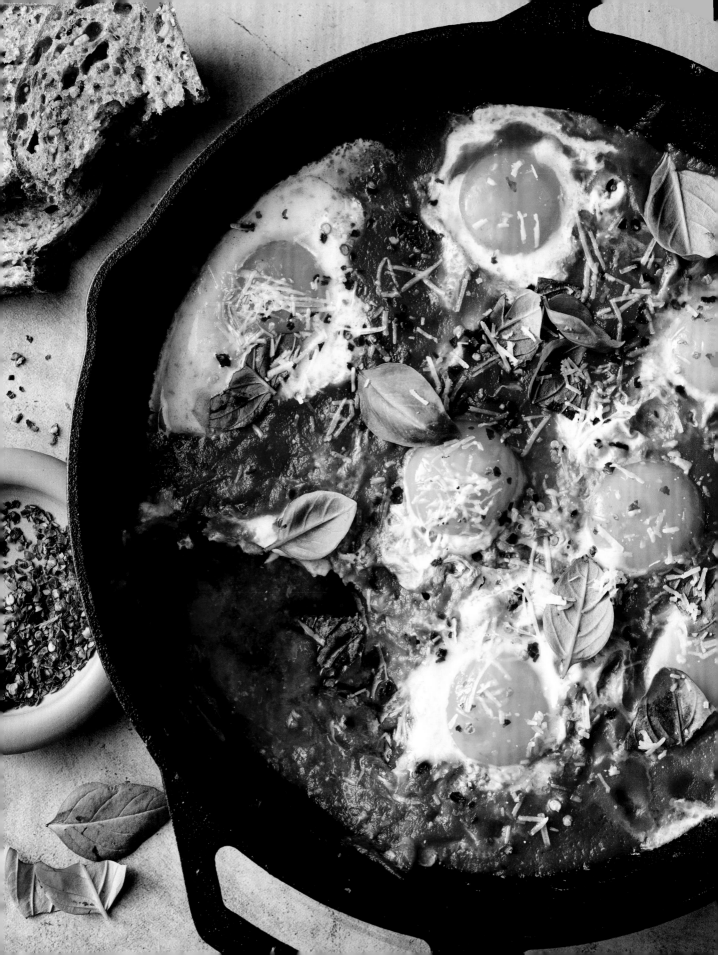

Poultry
Picks

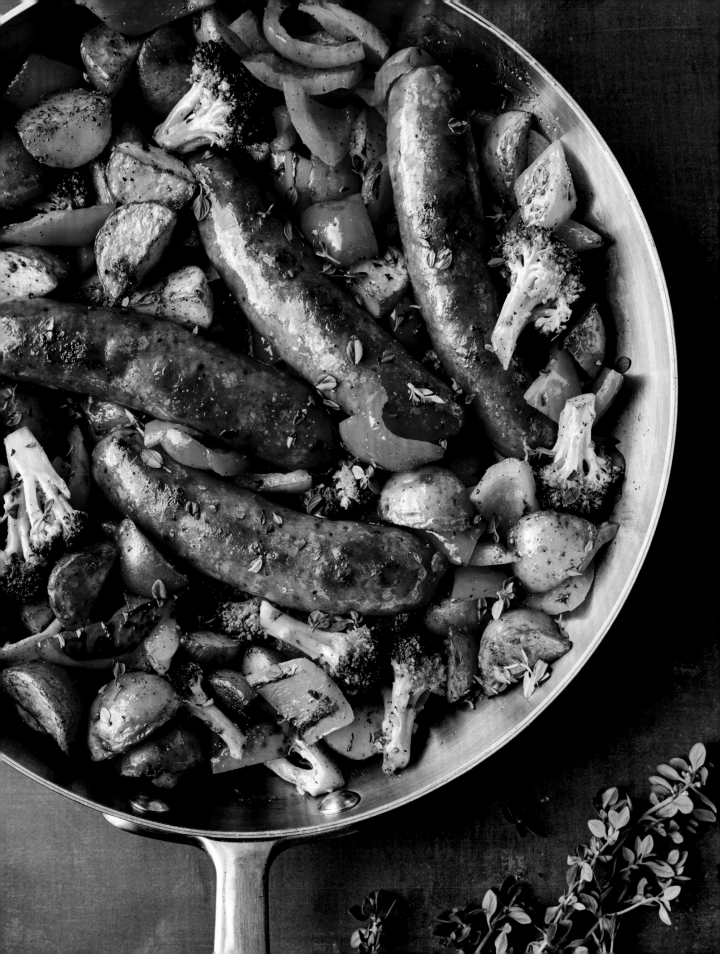

Skillet Andouille Sausage with Potatoes and Vegetables

SERVES 4

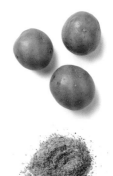

This easy one-pot skillet dinner with andouille sausage, potatoes, and vegetables is a weeknight dinner win! If you can't find turkey or chicken andouille sausage, turkey kielbasa or any smoked sausage can be used in its place.

1 pound baby red potatoes, quartered

1 teaspoon Cajun or Creole seasoning*

12 ounces fully cooked smoked turkey or chicken andouille sausage*

2 medium multicolor bell peppers (red and orange), cut into 1-inch pieces

2 cups broccoli florets (5 ounces)

2 garlic cloves, chopped

1 teaspoon fresh thyme leaves, roughly chopped

*Read the label to be sure this product is gluten-free.

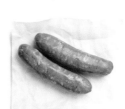

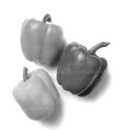

Heat a large nonstick skillet over medium-low heat and add 2 teaspoons extra-virgin olive oil. Add the potatoes and sprinkle with ½ teaspoon of the Cajun seasoning, ½ teaspoon kosher salt, and freshly ground black pepper to taste. Cover and cook until the potatoes have browned on one side, 5 to 7 minutes. Flip the potatoes, cover again, and continue to cook, stirring occasionally, until the potatoes are tender, 15 to 20 minutes. Transfer the potatoes to a plate and set aside.

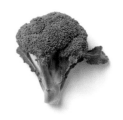

To the same skillet, over medium-low heat, add 1 teaspoon extra-virgin olive oil, the sausage, bell peppers, broccoli, garlic, and the remaining ½ teaspoon Cajun seasoning. Cover and cook until the sausages are browned and the vegetables are tender, 5 to 7 minutes.

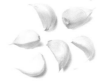

Return the potatoes to the pot and stir in the thyme. Cook for 1 minute more to allow the flavors to meld. Serve immediately.

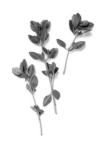

Per Serving (1¾ cups) ● Calories 302 ● Fat 15 g ● Saturated Fat 4.5 g ● Cholesterol 50 mg Carbohydrate 26 g ● Fiber 4 g ● Protein 19 g ● Sugars 6 g ● Sodium 945 mg

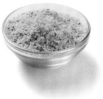

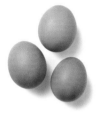

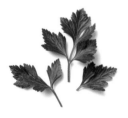

The Juiciest Italian Turkey Fried Meatballs (Ever)

SERVES 4

My Italian American father-in-law grew up in Brooklyn and loves his pasta and meatballs. These turkey meatballs are a healthier version of his fried meatballs, and they're just as delicious! Perfectly crispy on the outside, and so juicy on the inside. You can enjoy them by themselves like we do (at their house they never make it to the table!), or you can add them to any red sauce you might be making and serve with pasta.

¼ cup seasoned bread crumbs, regular or gluten-free

3 tablespoons chicken broth*

1 large egg

¼ cup chopped fresh parsley

¼ cup freshly grated Pecorino Romano cheese

2 garlic cloves, minced

1 pound ground turkey (93% lean)

*Read the label to be sure this product is gluten-free.

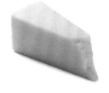

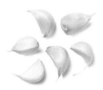

In a large bowl, combine the bread crumbs, broth, egg, parsley, Pecorino, garlic, and 1 teaspoon kosher salt and mix well to combine.

Add the turkey and use a fork to fully combine everything until well blended, being careful not to overwork the meat. Before shaping the meatballs, I like to lightly coat the palms of my hands with olive oil to prevent sticking. Form the mixture into 16 meatballs and flatten them slightly so that they are about 1 inch thick.

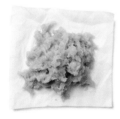

Heat a large deep skillet over medium-low heat and add 1 teaspoon extra-virgin olive oil to coat the bottom. Working in batches if needed and being careful not to overcrowd, add the meatballs in a single layer and partially cover the pan (do not fully cover because you don't want them to steam). Cook, undisturbed, until the meatballs are browned on the bottom, 5 to 6 minutes. Using tongs, flip the meatballs and cook until they are browned all over and cooked through in the center, 5 to 6 minutes more, reducing the heat as needed so the bottom of the meatballs do not burn. Serve warm.

Per Serving (4 meatballs) ● Calories 254 ● Fat 14 g ● Saturated Fat 4 g ● Cholesterol 136 mg
Carbohydrate 6 g ● Fiber 1 g ● Protein 27 g ● Sugars 1 g ● Sodium 644 mg

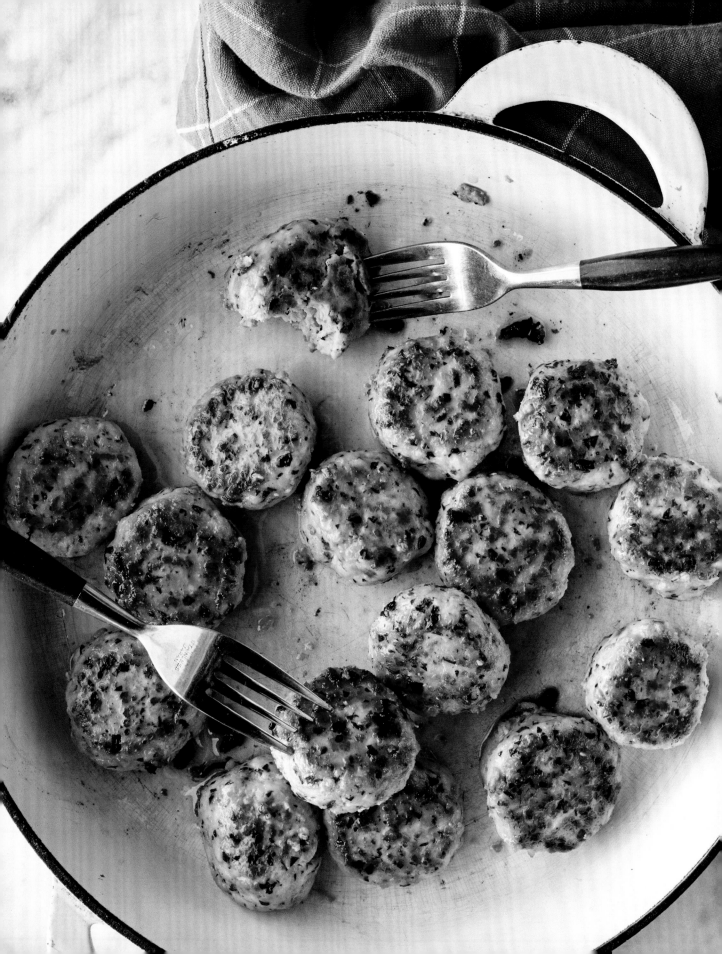

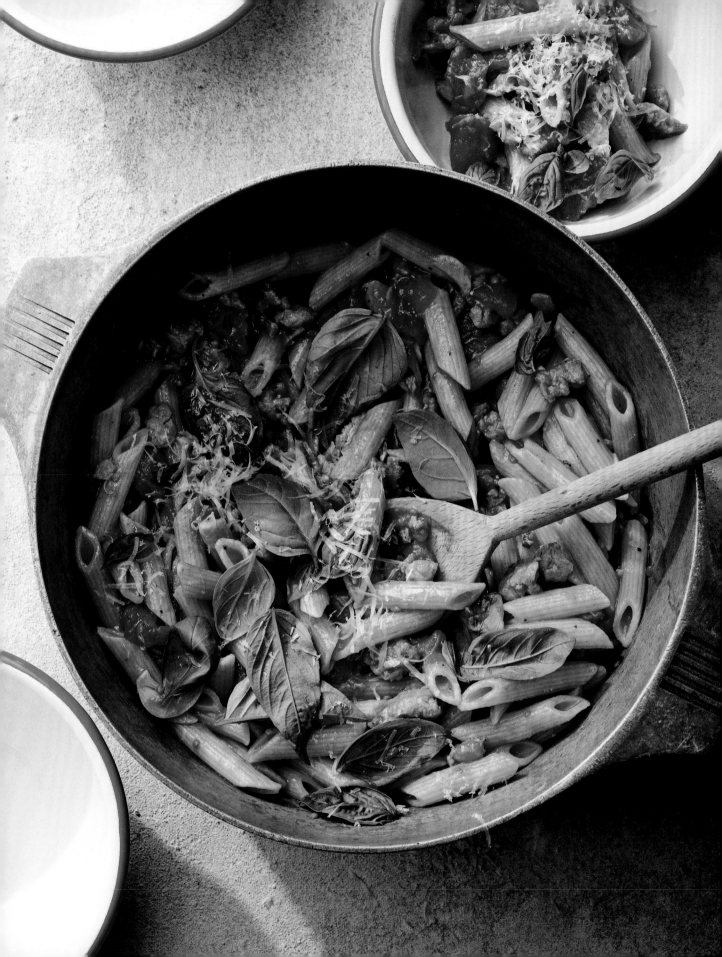

One-Pot Chicken Sausage Pasta

SERVES 4

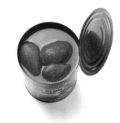

Don't you just love a one-pot pasta dinner? This simple dish is made with a flavorful Italian chicken sausage that creates a super-tasty sauce but with minimal ingredients. If you want to make it extra rich, serve topped with a dollop of ricotta. My daughter Madison gave this a big thumbs-up!

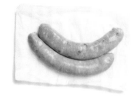

1 (28-ounce) can whole peeled tomatoes

12 ounces sweet or spicy Italian chicken sausage links,*
    casings removed

2 garlic cloves, thinly sliced

8 ounces regular or gluten-free short pasta, such as shells,
    penne rigate, or rigatoni

¼ cup freshly grated Parmesan cheese, plus more (optional) for serving

1 cup loosely packed fresh basil leaves, large leaves torn

*Read the label to be sure this product is gluten-free.

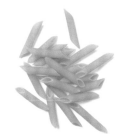

Set a fine-mesh sieve over a bowl and drain the tomatoes, reserving the liquid. Lightly press on the whole tomatoes to release any excess liquid inside the tomatoes and roughly chop them up with kitchen scissors or a knife. Pour the liquid into a measuring cup and add enough water to total 2½ cups.

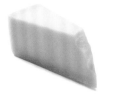

Heat a large heavy pot or Dutch oven over medium-high heat. Add 1 teaspoon extra-virgin olive oil, then crumble in the sausage. Cook, breaking the sausage up into small pieces with a wooden spoon, until the sausage is browned, 6 to 8 minutes. Add the garlic and cook until fragrant, about 2 minutes.

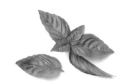

Add the tomatoes, reserved liquid, and the pasta and season with ½ teaspoon kosher salt and freshly ground black pepper to taste. Bring to a boil over high heat, then reduce the heat to medium-low so the sauce bubbles steadily. Cover the pot and cook the pasta to al dente and until the liquid is absorbed, 20 to 25 minutes, stirring every 5 minutes so the pasta cooks evenly and to make sure nothing sticks to the bottom.

Remove from the heat and stir in the Parmesan and then the basil leaves just to wilt. Serve with more Parmesan on the side, if desired.

Per Serving (1½ cups) ● Calories 418 ● Fat 11 g ● Saturated Fat 3 g ● Cholesterol 69 mg
Carbohydrate 54 g ● Fiber 3.5 g ● Protein 25 g ● Sugars 8 g ● Sodium 1,028 mg

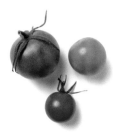

Hasselback Feta Chicken Bake

SERVES 2

GF

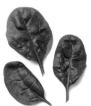

This baked chicken dish was somewhat inspired by a viral feta pasta dish from TikTok! Instead of roasting a whole block of feta with tomatoes, as in the TikTok version, I stuff chicken breasts with crumbled feta and spinach and bake it on top of tomatoes. This comes out so juicy and is delicious eaten as is, but it could also be served over orzo or pearl couscous.

10 ounces grape or cherry tomatoes, halved

3 ounces baby spinach, chopped (about 1 cup)

2 ounces feta cheese, crumbled (about 6 tablespoons)

2 garlic cloves, finely minced

2 boneless, skinless chicken breasts (about 8 ounces each)

½ teaspoon dried oregano

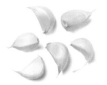

Preheat the oven to 400°F.

Place the tomatoes in a 9 × 13-inch baking dish, drizzle with 1 teaspoon extra-virgin olive oil, and season with ¼ teaspoon kosher salt and freshly ground black pepper to taste. Roast until the tomatoes just begin to soften, about 15 minutes.

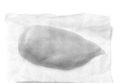

Meanwhile, spray a medium skillet with olive oil and heat over medium heat. Add the spinach and 1 teaspoon water and cook, stirring occasionally, until the spinach is slightly wilted, 2 to 3 minutes. Remove the skillet from the heat and let the spinach cool for 5 minutes. Stir in the feta and garlic.

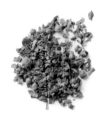

Cut slits into the tops of the chicken breasts about 75 percent of the way down, ½ inch apart, being careful not to cut all the way through (it will look like a hasselback potato). Season the chicken with ¼ teaspoon kosher salt and ground black pepper to taste.

Stuff the spinach and feta mixture into the slits. Remove the tomatoes from the oven and stir, then nestle the chicken in the center of the baking dish. Sprinkle the chicken with the oregano and more black pepper, then drizzle the top with ½ tablespoon extra-virgin olive oil.

Bake until the tomatoes burst and are saucy and the chicken is cooked through, about 25 minutes. Serve immediately.

Per Serving (1 stuffed breast + ¼ cup tomatoes) ● Calories 432 ● Fat 18 g ● Saturated Fat 6.5 g Cholesterol 191 mg ● Carbohydrate 9 g ● Fiber 2.5 g ● Protein 57 g ● Sugars 5 g Sodium 666 mg

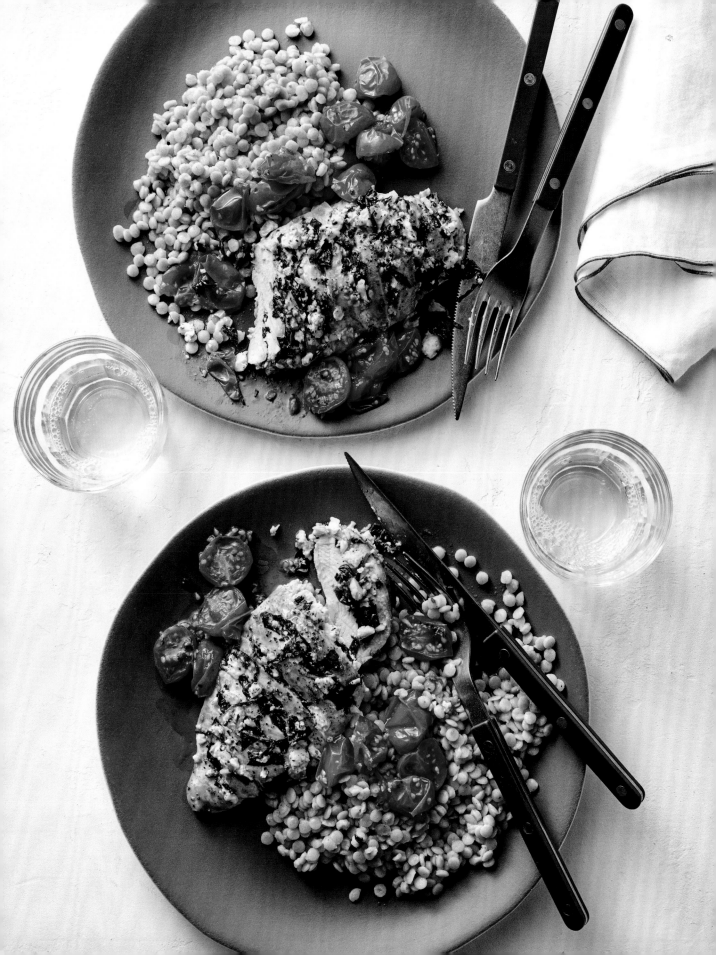

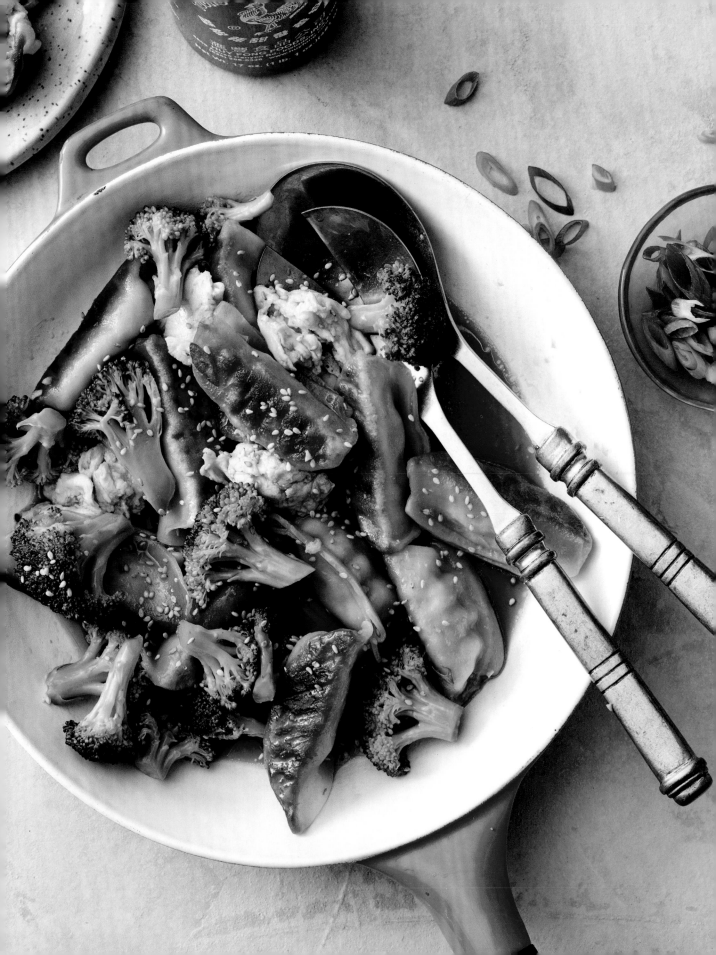

Pot Sticker Stir-Fry

SERVES 2

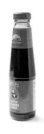

We *love* Asian dumplings in my house! We order them every time we get Chinese food, so I figured why not take a favorite appetizer and turn it into a quick meal? I added an egg for more protein and broccoli as the veggie, but you can use whatever you like—sub in bok choy, mushrooms, or even a bag of mixed stir-fry veggies. If you have scallions or toasted sesame seeds on hand, use as a garnish and serve with Sriracha if you like heat like I do!

SKINNY SCOOP: Choose your favorite frozen dumplings with whatever filling you like; I like Annie Chun's or Trader Joe's. Note that you may need more than one bag, depending on the brand.

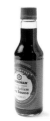

1 tablespoon oyster sauce

1 tablespoon reduced-sodium soy sauce

1 large garlic clove, minced

2 large eggs, lightly beaten

1 tablespoon toasted sesame oil

14 frozen chicken or veggie dumplings (see Skinny Scoop)

3 cups bite-size broccoli florets

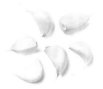

In a medium bowl, whisk together the oyster sauce, soy sauce, garlic, and 2 tablespoons water.

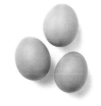

Heat a 12-inch nonstick skillet over medium heat and spray with oil. Add the eggs and a pinch of kosher salt and scramble until the eggs are just cooked, 1 to 1½ minutes. Transfer the eggs to a plate and wipe the skillet clean.

Add the sesame oil and the frozen potstickers to the skillet in a single layer and cook, turning often, until both sides are golden, 4 to 5 minutes.

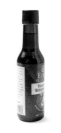

Add the broccoli and 2 tablespoons water. Cover and steam until the dumplings are heated through and the broccoli is crisp-tender, 1½ to 2 minutes.

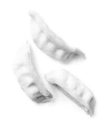

Uncover the skillet, pour in the sauce, and stir gently to coat. Add the eggs and cook until combined and heated through, about 30 seconds more. Serve right away.

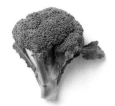

Per Serving (2¾ cups) ● Calories 389 ● Fat 17 g ● Saturated Fat 4 g ● Cholesterol 206 mg
Carbohydrate 42 g ● Fiber 7.5 g ● Protein 21 g ● Sugars 3 g ● Sodium 1,214 mg

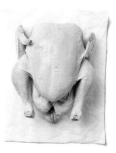

Sheet Pan Spatchcock Chicken with Brussels Sprouts

SERVES 4

This is the ultimate one-pan chicken meal, ready in 45 minutes. Spatchcocking (opening and flattening) your bird allows it to cook much more quickly. You can ask your butcher to do this for you, but it's really not hard to do yourself. Lemon slices impart citrusy brightness to this easy weeknight meal. If you're not a fan of Brussels sprouts, swap them out for broccoli florets. Serve this with a nice green salad to make it a meal.

1 (3½-pound) whole chicken

1 lemon, halved

1 teaspoon sweet paprika

1 teaspoon garlic powder

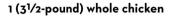

2 large sprigs of fresh rosemary, plus ¼ teaspoon minced

1½ pounds large Brussels sprouts, trimmed and halved

To spatchcock the chicken, lay the chicken on a cutting board breast side down. Use sharp kitchen shears to remove the backbone by cutting through the ribs right next to the spine, along both sides. Flip the chicken over, breast side up, then use the palm of your hand to push firmly down on the breastbone until you hear it crack to ensure that the chicken lies completely flat.

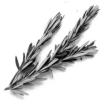

Pat the chicken dry with paper towels, then squeeze the juice from one lemon half all over the chicken. Season all over with 1½ teaspoons kosher salt, the paprika, garlic powder, and a generous pinch of freshly ground black pepper. Let the chicken come to room temperature while the oven preheats.

Preheat the oven to 450°F. Spray a sheet pan with olive oil.

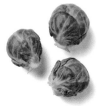

Slice the remaining lemon half into thin slices and arrange them in the center of the prepared sheet pan. Top with the rosemary sprigs and place the chicken on top, skin side up. Sprinkle with the minced rosemary.

(recipe continues)

Per Serving (¼ skinless chicken + 6 ounces Brussels sprouts) ● Calories 370 ● Fat 13 g ● Saturated Fat 3.5 g ● Cholesterol 127 mg ● Carbohydrate 17 g ● Fiber 7 g ● Protein 47 g ● Sugars 4 g Sodium 725 mg

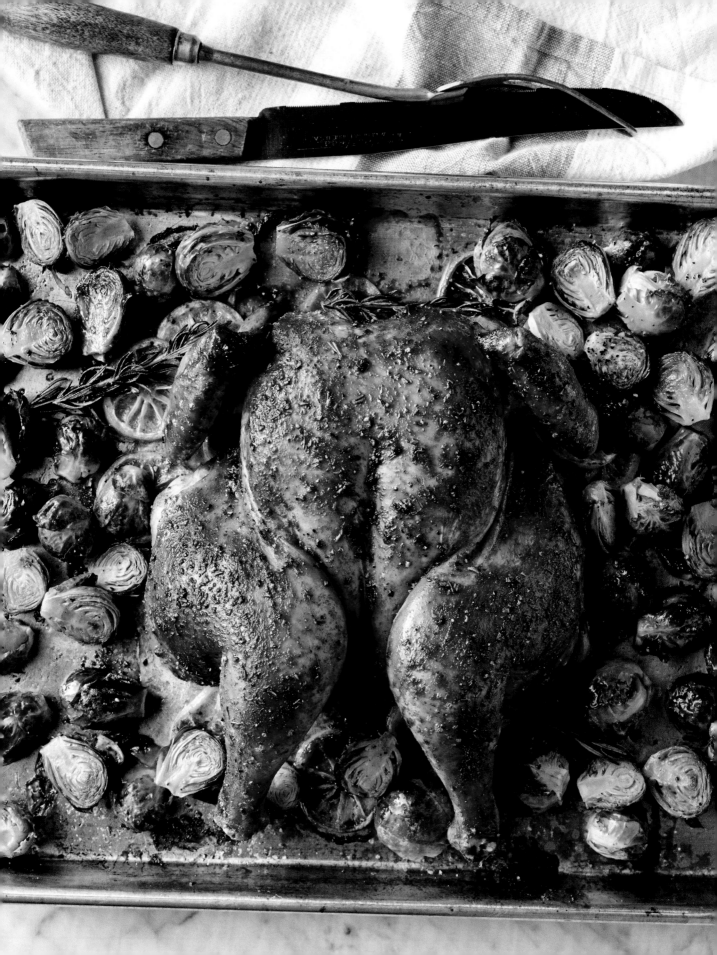

Partially roast the chicken for 25 minutes, then remove the sheet pan from the oven and add the Brussels sprouts, scattering them all around the chicken. Drizzle the Brussels sprouts with 2 teaspoons extra-virgin olive oil and season with ½ teaspoon kosher salt. Return the sheet pan to the oven and continue to roast until the chicken is golden brown, an instant-read thermometer inserted into the thickest part of the thigh registers 165°F, and the Brussels sprouts are tender and golden, 20 to 25 minutes more.

Let the chicken rest for 10 minutes before carving. Discard the skin, if desired. Serve immediately with the roasted Brussels sprouts.

Sweet Potato Turkey Burgers

SERVES 4

This turkey burger recipe couldn't be any easier. It's one of each: 1 roasted sweet potato, 1 pound of ground turkey, and 1 teaspoon each of the spices. The burgers are perfect for meal prep and are great on a bun, with a side of grains, or (my favorite) simply with chopped romaine, cherry tomatoes, and Marinated Red Onions (page 159), because I love how the zip of the onions contrast with the savory-sweet burgers.

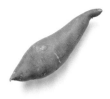
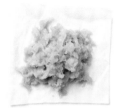
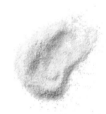
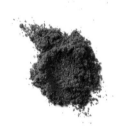
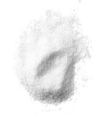

1 medium sweet potato (about 6 ounces)

1 pound ground turkey (93% lean)

1 teaspoon garlic powder

1 teaspoon chili powder*

1 teaspoon onion powder

Marinated Red Onions (optional; recipe follows)

*Read the label to be sure this product is gluten-free.

Preheat the oven to 425°F.

Poke holes all over the sweet potato with a fork. Place on a small sheet pan and bake the sweet potato until tender, 45 to 50 minutes. (Alternatively, cook the sweet potato in a preheated air fryer at 370°F for 35 to 45 minutes.)

Remove and discard the skin from the sweet potato and transfer to a large bowl. Mash with a fork until smooth. Add the turkey, garlic powder, chili powder, onion powder, and 1 teaspoon kosher salt and stir until well combined. Form the mixture into 8 flat patties (they will plump up as they cook).

Heat a large nonstick skillet or grill pan over low heat. When the skillet is hot, spray it with oil and add the burger patties. Cook until the centers are cooked through, about 5 minutes per side. (Alternatively, use an air fryer: Spray the air fryer basket with oil, add the burgers, and cook at 370°F for 5 to 6 minutes per side, until the burgers are cooked through in the center and slightly browned on the outside.)

Serve immediately with Marinated Red Onions, if desired.

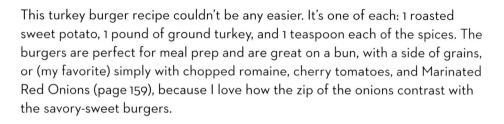

(recipe continues)

Per Serving (2 patties) ● Calories 201 ● Fat 10 g ● Saturated Fat 2.5 g ● Cholesterol 84 mg Carbohydrate 9 g ● Fiber 1 g ● Protein 22 g ● Sugars 2 g ● Sodium 331 mg

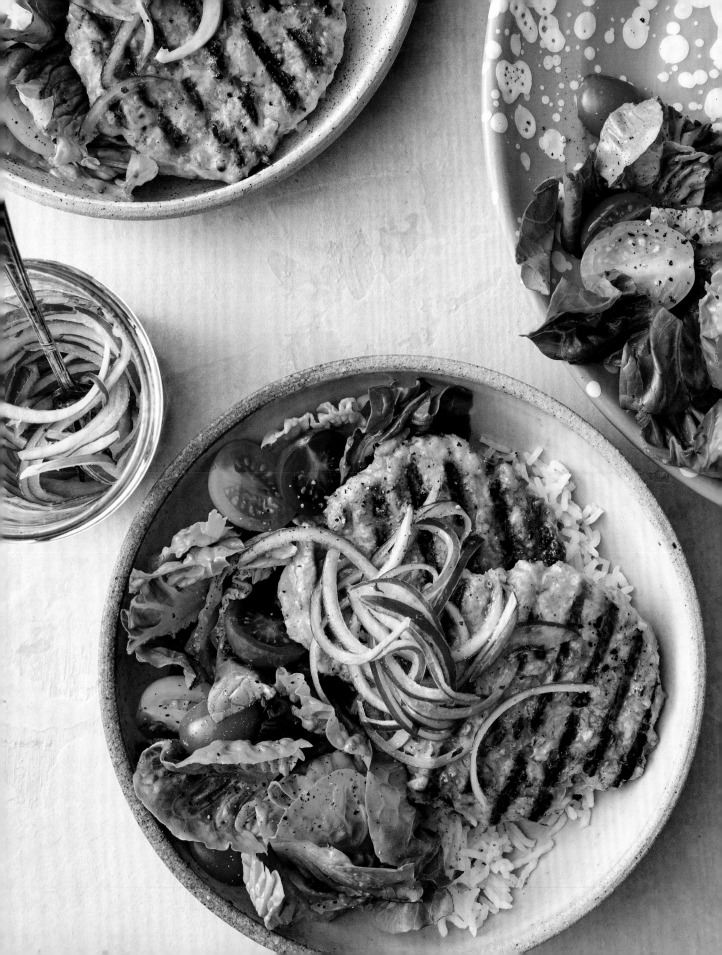

Marinated Red Onions

MAKES ABOUT 1 CUP

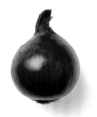

If you've been following me a long time, you've probably seen me use these onions as the base for my weekly house salads. In fact, I have a recipe called My House Salad, Made with Love in my first cookbook, where I do something similar, only with chopped onions. I learned the trick to taking the bite out of the onions from my mother-in-law years ago, and I have never stopped using it since. These onions are not only ideal for salads but also great on burgers, sandwiches, you name it!

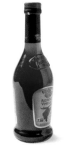

1 medium red onion, thinly sliced

3 tablespoons red wine vinegar

½ teaspoon garlic powder

½ teaspoon dried parsley flakes

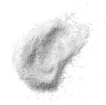

Place the onion slices in a shallow bowl and sprinkle with ½ teaspoon kosher salt. Drizzle with 3 tablespoons extra-virgin olive oil, the vinegar, garlic powder, dried parsley, and freshly ground black pepper to taste and toss to combine. Let the mixture sit on the counter for at least 1 hour to marinate, or as long as 4 days in an airtight container in the refrigerator.

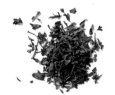

Per Serving (2 tablespoons/about ⅛ medium onion) ● Calories 12 ● Fat 0.5 g ● Saturated Fat 0 g ● Cholesterol 0 mg ● Carbohydrate 1 g ● Fiber 0.5 g ● Protein 0 g ● Sugars 0.5 g Sodium 71 mg

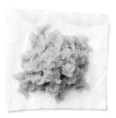

Turkey Unstuffed Pepper Bowls

SERVES 4

 Q GF DF FF

I love stuffed peppers, but I don't make them as often as I'd like because they take so much time to prepare. My simple solution is to turn them into rice bowls! It's so much faster and easier to simply chop all the ingredients I usually use in my stuffed peppers and just serve them over rice. They're also great for meal prep!

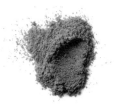

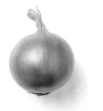

1⅓ pounds ground turkey (93% lean)

1 teaspoon ground cumin

1 small yellow onion, diced

3 small bell peppers (multicolor), cut into ½-inch pieces

3 garlic cloves, minced

1 (8-ounce) can tomato sauce

4 cups cooked white or brown rice, for serving

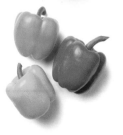

Set a large skillet over high heat and spray with olive oil. Add the turkey and season with the cumin and 1 teaspoon kosher salt. Cook, breaking the meat up, until the turkey is cooked through, about 5 minutes. Transfer to a medium bowl and set aside.

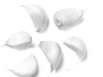

Using the same pan, heat ½ tablespoon olive oil over medium heat. Add the onion and bell peppers and season with ¼ teaspoon kosher salt and freshly ground black pepper to taste. Cook until softened, 5 to 6 minutes. Add the garlic and cook until fragrant, about 1 minute. Add the cooked ground turkey, tomato sauce, and ½ cup water. Cover and simmer, stirring occasionally, until the flavors meld and the sauce thickens, about 20 minutes.

Divide the rice among shallow bowls, top each with the turkey mixture, and serve.

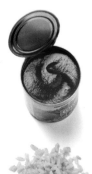

Per Serving (1 cup turkey/pepper sauce + 1 cup rice) ● Calories 504 ● Fat 16 g
Saturated Fat 3.5 g ● Cholesterol 112 mg ● Carbohydrate 57 g ● Fiber 6 g ● Protein 35 g
Sugars 9 g ● Sodium 733 mg

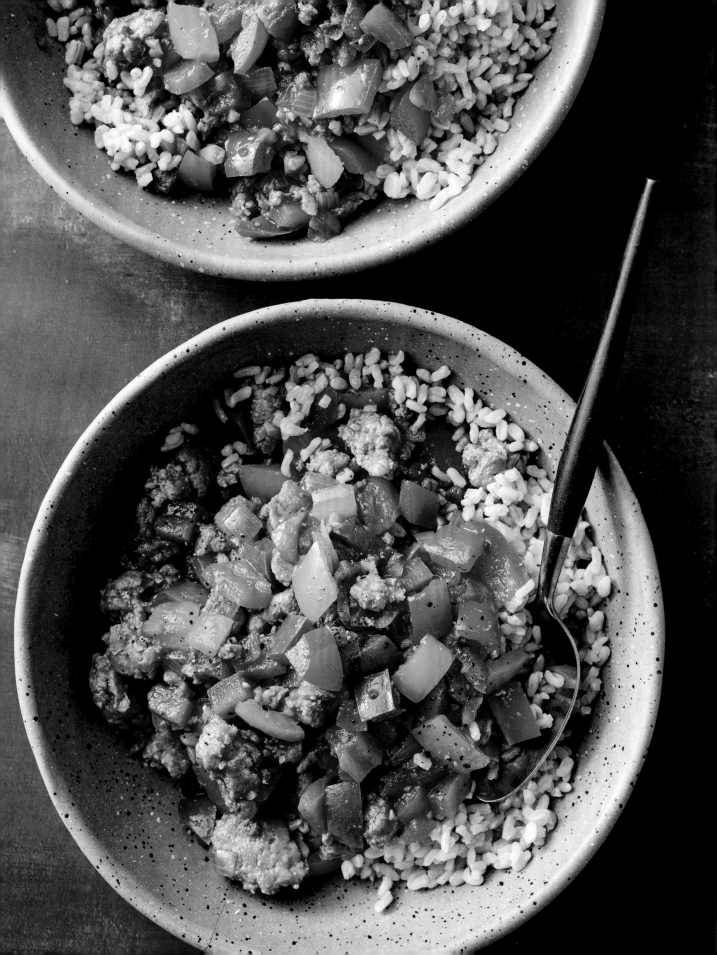

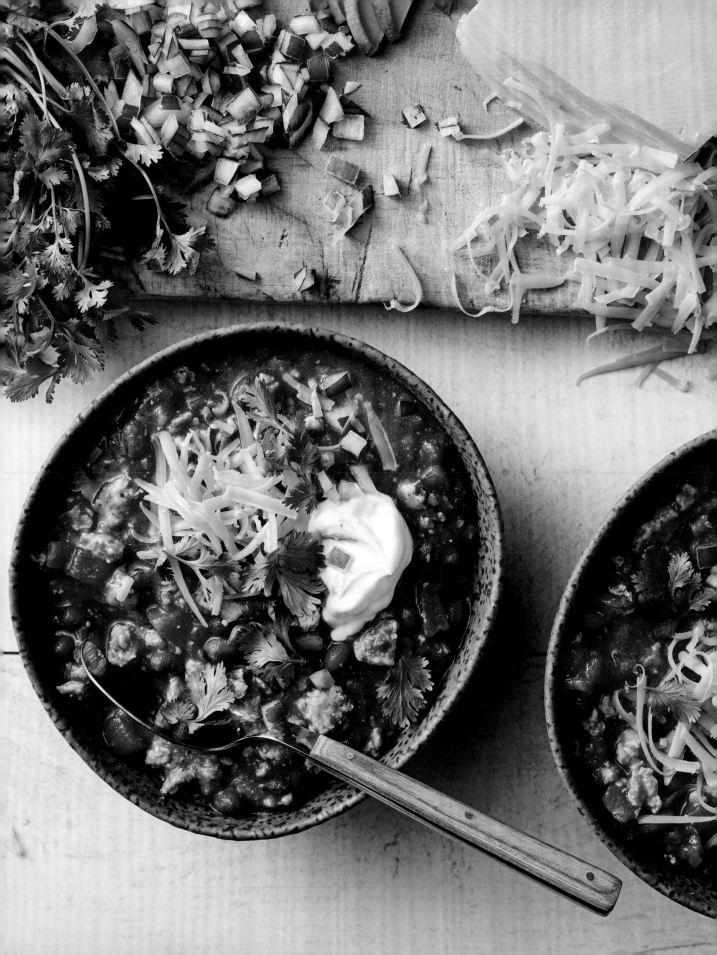

15-Minute Turkey-Bean Chili

SERVES 4

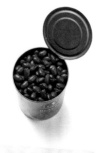

Do you know the secret ingredient to making a quick chili that tastes like it's been simmering for hours? Puree a can of beans. It thickens the chili without all the time on the stovetop, so you can whip this up in less than fifteen minutes. Bonus, it's high in protein and fiber, and leftovers make a great lunch. Ground chicken, beef, or veggie crumbles also work great here, and taco seasoning eliminates the need for a pantry full of spices. Top it with your favorite chili fixings, like avocado, chopped cilantro, and/or tortilla chips.

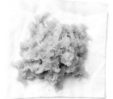

2 (15-ounce) cans low-sodium black or red beans (or use one of each), rinsed and drained

1 pound ground turkey (93% lean)

¼ cup diced red onion, plus more for garnish

1 (10-ounce) can Ro-Tel diced tomatoes and green chilies

3 tablespoons reduced-sodium taco seasoning

½ cup shredded cheddar cheese (2 ounces)

¼ cup whole-milk Greek yogurt or sour cream, for topping

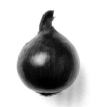

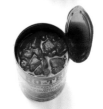

Place 1 can of beans in the blender with ¾ cup water and puree until smooth.

Set a large pot over medium heat and spray with olive oil. Add the turkey and cook, breaking it up with a wooden spoon, until cooked through, 4 to 5 minutes. Add the red onion and cook until softened, 2 to 3 minutes. Add the tomatoes, second can of beans, the pureed beans, and taco seasoning. Bring to a boil over medium heat. Reduce the heat to low, cover, and simmer until thickened, 10 to 15 minutes.

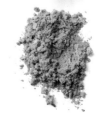

Serve topped with the cheddar, yogurt, and some chopped red onion.

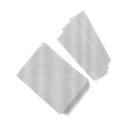

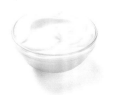

Per Serving (1¼ cups) ● Calories 469 ● Fat 16 g ● Saturated Fat 6 g ● Cholesterol 100 mg
Carbohydrate 43 g ● Fiber 16 g ● Protein 39 g ● Sugars 3 g ● Sodium 893 mg

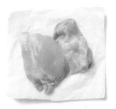

Puerto Rican Pinchos de Pollo (Grilled Chicken Skewers)

SERVES 4

When I spent summers as a kid in Puerto Rico, *pinchos* were one of my favorite street foods—because how can you not love meat on a stick!? My cousin makes these at her barbecues and she shared her recipe with me. They traditionally serve the *pinchos* with a slice of grilled Italian bread on the end of the stick, as I do here. They're great as is or with rice, tostones, and/or a salad alongside.

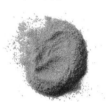

1½ pounds boneless, skinless chicken thighs, cut into 1-inch pieces

1 teaspoon adobo seasoning

1 (5-gram) packet sazón seasoning with achiote (about ½ tablespoon)

1 teaspoon garlic powder

3 tablespoons BBQ sauce

2 teaspoons yellow mustard

4 slices Italian bread (about 1 ounce each)

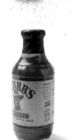

Place the chicken in a medium bowl, spray with olive oil, and season with the adobo, sazón, garlic powder, and ¼ teaspoon kosher salt. Mix thoroughly to coat. Cover and marinate in the refrigerator for at least 1 hour or as long as overnight.

In a small bowl, combine the BBQ sauce, mustard, and about 2 tablespoons water to thin it out. (You want a light coating on the chicken that's not too thick.)

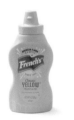

Preheat an outdoor grill to medium heat. Thread the chicken pieces along 4 metal skewers. Oil the grates and grill the chicken, turning the skewers occasionally, until golden brown and cooked through in the center, about 15 minutes. (Alternatively, to broil the chicken, preheat the broiler with the oven rack set 6 inches from the heating element. Oil a wire rack and set it inside a sheet pan. Place the chicken skewers on top of the wire rack and cook as directed.)

Brush the BBQ sauce mixture evenly over the chicken and continue to cook, turning a few times, until golden, taking care not to burn, about 2 more minutes.

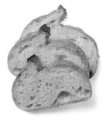

Spray the bread with olive oil and grill (or broil) until warmed and slightly toasted, 30 to 60 seconds on each side. Place each slice on the end of the pincho and serve.

Per Serving (1 skewer) ● Calories 313 ● Fat 8 g ● Saturated Fat 2 g ● Cholesterol 160 mg
Carbohydrate 21 g ● Fiber 1.5 g ● Protein 36 g ● Sugars 6 g ● Sodium 944 mg

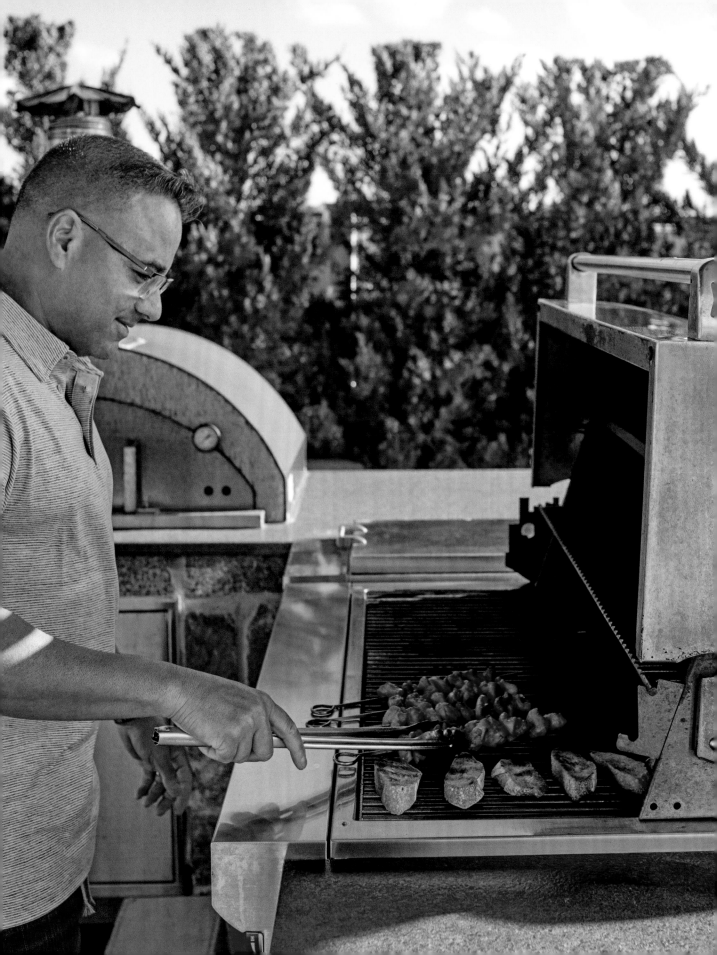

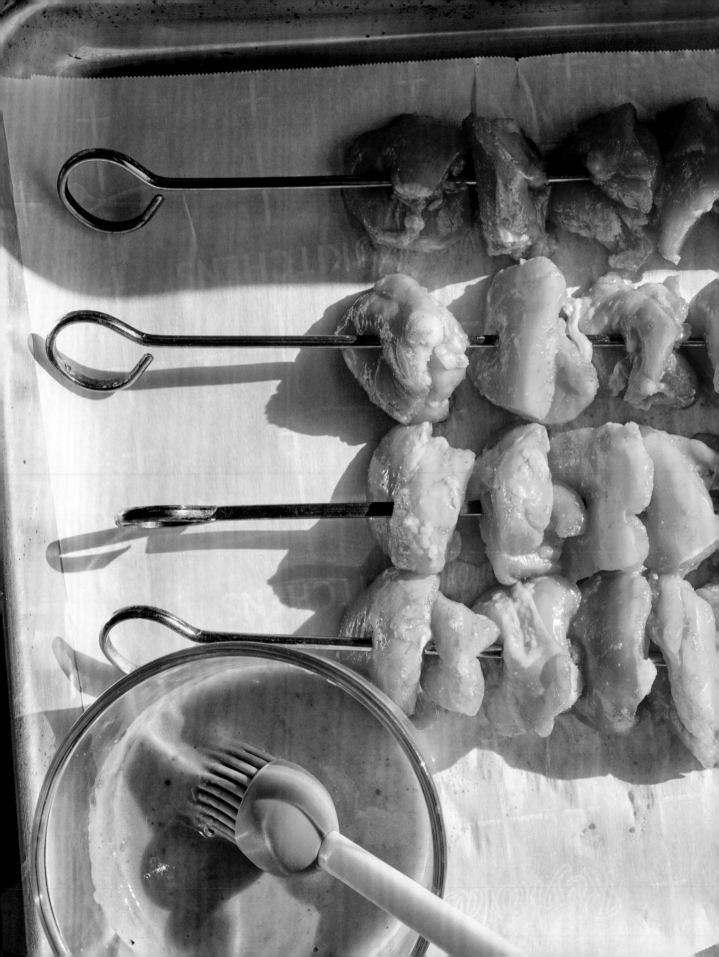

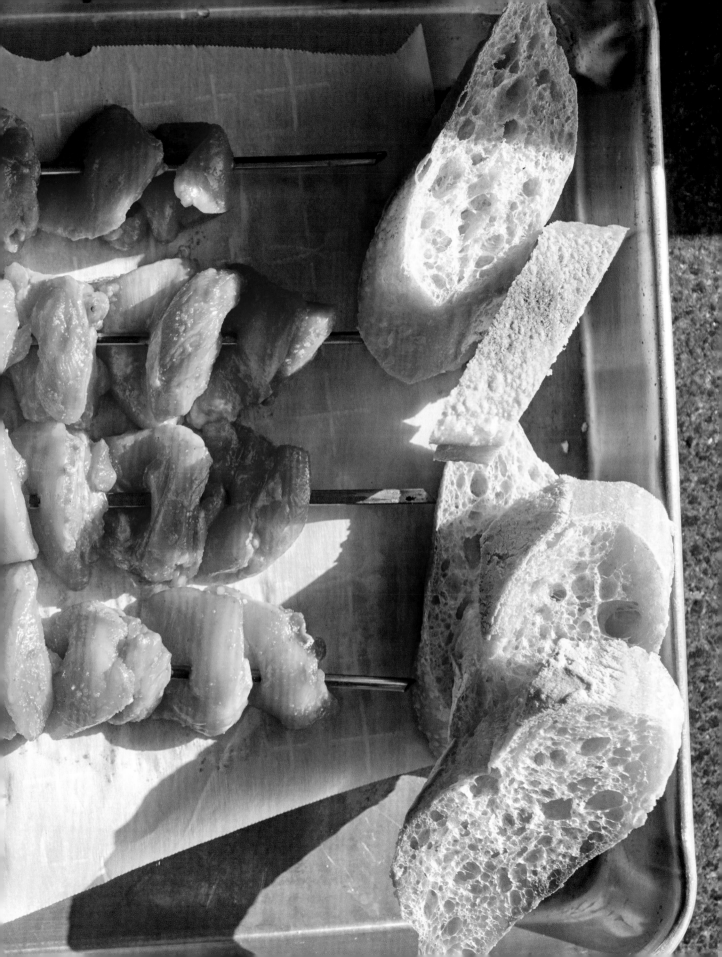

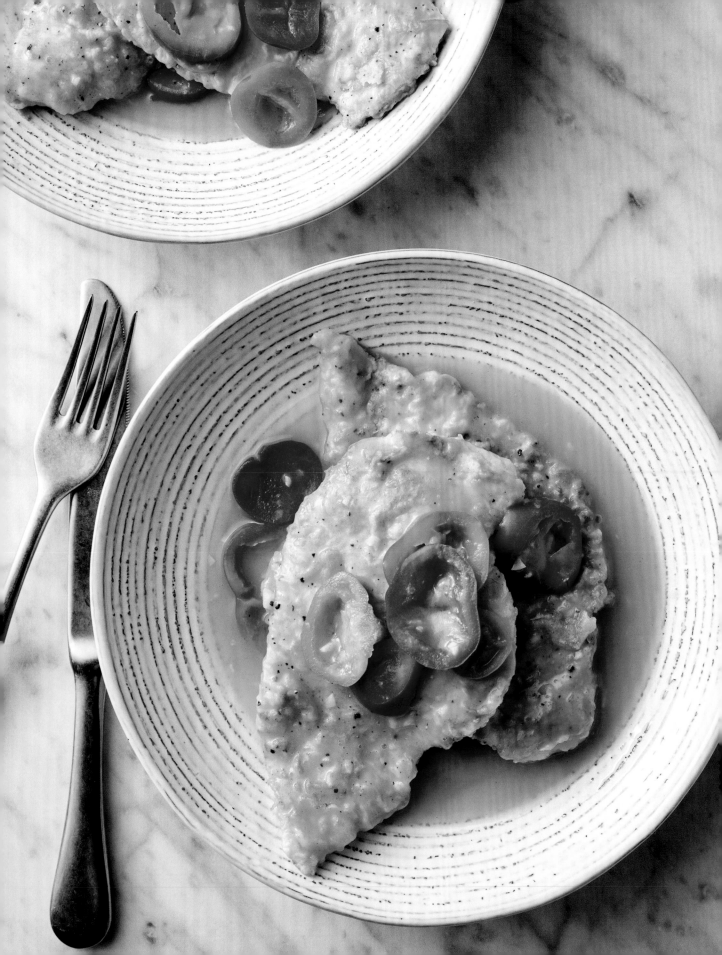

Chicken with Hot Cherry Peppers

SERVES 4

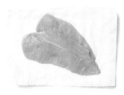

If you like spicy food, pickled hot cherry peppers are the perfect addition to pretty much anything, especially sandwiches and salads. So why not add them to chicken? The delicious results are spicy, salty, slightly acidic … and did I mention spicy? This is great served over pasta or rice, with a salad on the side.

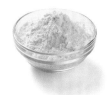

8 thin-sliced chicken breast cutlets (about 4 ounces each)

⅓ cup plus 1 tablespoon all-purpose flour

2 large eggs

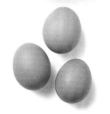

1½ cups low-sodium chicken broth

2 garlic cloves, minced

¾ cup jarred sliced multicolor hot cherry peppers, drained

¼ cup white wine

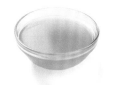

Season the chicken on both sides with 1 teaspoon kosher salt and black pepper to taste.

Place ⅓ cup of the flour in a shallow bowl. In another shallow bowl, beat the eggs with 1 tablespoon water.

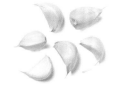

Heat a large nonstick pan over medium heat and add 1 teaspoon extra-virgin olive oil to lightly coat the bottom of the pan.

Lightly flour a chicken cutlet, shaking off the excess. Dip in the beaten egg, letting the excess drip off, then add to the hot pan. Repeat with more cutlets, fitting them in a single layer (you will need to work in batches). Cook the chicken until cooked through and lightly browned, 2 to 3 minutes per side. Transfer to a plate and repeat with 1 teaspoon more oil and the remaining chicken. Set aside.

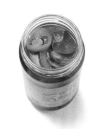

In a small bowl, whisk the broth and remaining 1 tablespoon flour until well combined.

Add 1 teaspoon oil to the empty skillet (no need to wipe it out) over medium heat. Add the garlic and cook until fragrant, about 30 seconds. Add the hot cherry peppers and white wine. Cook until the liquid is reduced by half, then add the chicken broth mixture. Bring to a boil, then reduce the heat to medium and simmer until slightly reduced and thickened, 2 to 3 minutes. Return the chicken to the pan to combine with the sauce and cook just until heated through, about 30 seconds. Serve immediately.

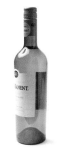

Per Serving (2 chicken cutlets with sauce) ● Calories 408 ● Fat 12 g ● Saturated Fat 2.5 g
Cholesterol 260 mg ● Carbohydrate 13 g ● Fiber 1 g ● Protein 56 g ● Sugars 1 g ● Sodium 746 mg

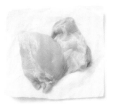

Sweet and Spicy Gochujang Chicken Bowls

SERVES 4

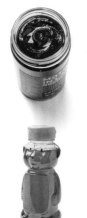

Gochujang is a delicious sweet and spicy Korean condiment made of fermented chiles. It's an amazing ingredient to keep in your refrigerator because it instantly adds complex, savory flavor to dishes. Combined with honey, it makes an irresistible glaze that doubles as a sauce for drizzling over these chicken bowls.

SKINNY SCOOP: As with all bowls, feel free to substitute your favorite cooked grain or use chopped greens instead to make a hearty salad.

8 boneless, skinless chicken thighs (about 4 ounces each), trimmed of fat

3 tablespoons gochujang, regular or gluten-free

3 tablespoons honey

3 cups cooked brown rice or jasmine rice (see Skinny Scoop)

4 Persian (mini) cucumbers, sliced

2 teaspoons toasted sesame seeds

4 scallions, green tops only, thinly sliced on an angle

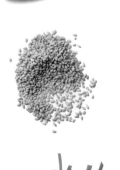

Adjust an oven rack to 6 inches from the heating element and preheat the broiler to high. Line a sheet pan with foil.

Pat the chicken dry all over and season with 1 teaspoon kosher salt. Place on the prepared sheet pan and broil until lightly browned on both sides and cooked through in the center, about 5 minutes per side.

Meanwhile, in a small bowl, combine the gochujang, honey, and 1 tablespoon extra-virgin olive oil and stir until combined. Set aside half of the glaze for serving.

When the chicken is done, use a spoon or brush to coat both sides of the thighs with the remaining glaze. Switch the broiler setting to low. Return the pan to the oven and broil the chicken until the glaze starts to form a crust and the edges start to brown, 2 to 3 minutes.

Divide the rice among four bowls. Slice the chicken and top the rice bowls. Arrange the cucumbers next to the chicken and season with a pinch of kosher salt. Drizzle the reserved glaze over the chicken. Top with the sesame seeds and scallion greens and serve.

Per Serving (2 thighs + ¾ cup rice + 1 cucumber) • Calories 544 • Fat 15 g • Saturated Fat 3 g Cholesterol 213 mg • Carbohydrate 53 g • Fiber 3 g • Protein 49 g • Sugars 18 g • Sodium 712 mg

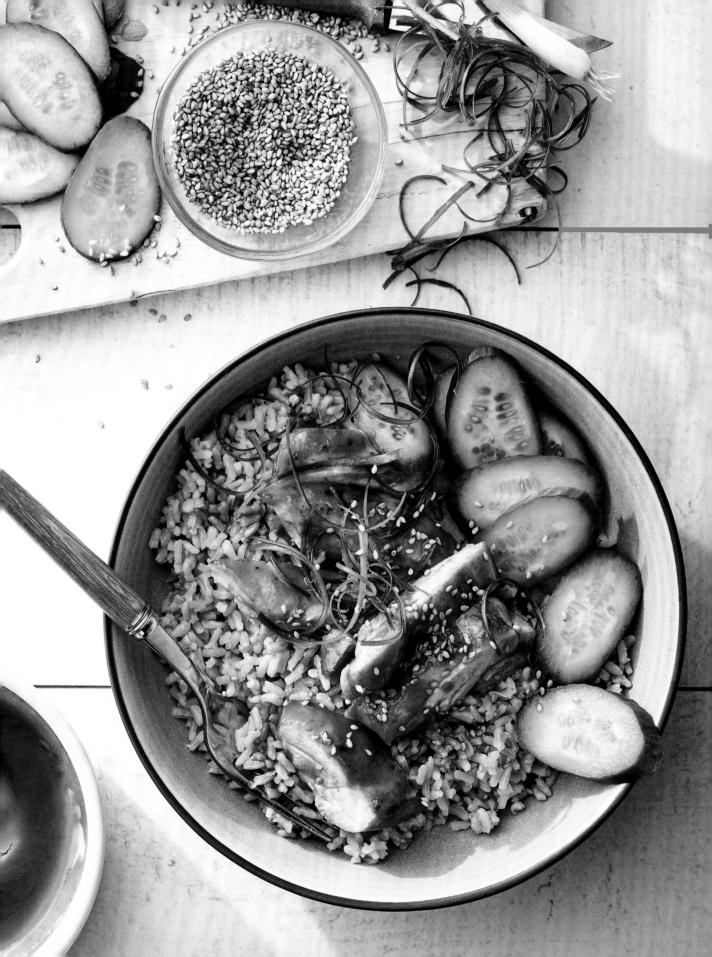

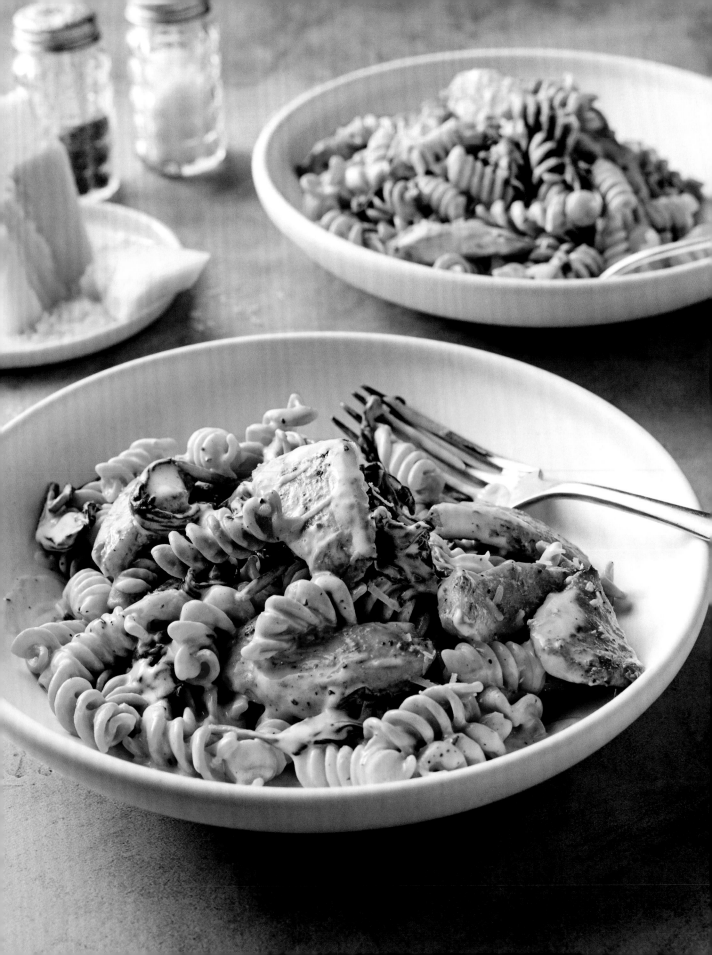

Creamy Chicken and Spinach Tri-Colore Pasta

SERVES 4

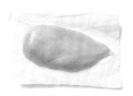

 Q GF

This creamy pasta dish is the ultimate comfort meal. I used tricolor pasta to give it some visual appeal, and lots of spinach for a nutritional boost. The sauce is lightened up with reduced-fat milk and cream cheese instead of heavy cream, but trust me, you won't miss it! You can even add some diced tomatoes if you want more veggies or top with fresh herbs like basil. Tommy gave this dish his seal of approval!

SKINNY SCOOP: I use my own homemade poultry seasoning (see page 177) that's super flavorful but without the added salt. If you use store-bought, be careful of the sodium levels. Or swap the poultry seasoning for Cajun seasoning.

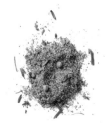

1 pound boneless, skinless chicken breasts, cut into ½-inch pieces

3 teaspoons Kickin' Chicken Poultry Seasoning (page 177) or store-bought poultry seasoning

1 cup reduced-fat (2%) milk

⅓ cup freshly grated Pecorino Romano cheese

3 tablespoons ⅓-less-fat cream cheese (I like Philadelphia)

3 cups packed baby spinach (about 5 ounces)

8 ounces tricolor rotini, bow ties, or any short pasta shape, regular or gluten-free

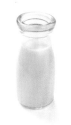

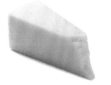

Bring a large pot of salted water to a boil over high heat.

Meanwhile, in a medium bowl, season the chicken with 2 teaspoons of the poultry seasoning.

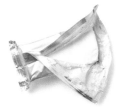

In a small blender, combine the milk, ¼ cup of the Pecorino, the cream cheese, and the remaining 1 teaspoon poultry seasoning and blend until smooth. Set aside.

(recipe continues)

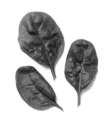

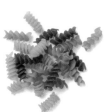

Per Serving (1½ cups) ● Calories 485 ● Fat 10 g ● Saturated Fat 4.5 g ● Cholesterol 102 mg Carbohydrate 53 g ● Fiber 3.5 g ● Protein 41 g ● Sugars 4 g ● Sodium 914 mg

Heat a deep 12-inch skillet over high heat. When the pan is very hot, spray it with oil and add the chicken in a single layer. Cook, undisturbed, until the bottom browns, 2 to 3 minutes. Flip and cook the other side until browned and cooked through, 2 to 3 minutes. Reduce the heat to medium-low and add the cream mixture and baby spinach. Stir until the spinach wilts, 2 to 3 minutes.

Meanwhile, cook the pasta to al dente according to the package directions. Reserve ½ cup of the cooking water, drain the pasta.

Add the pasta to the skillet with the chicken and stir to combine. Reduce the heat to low and cook, stirring, until the sauce coats the pasta, about 1 more minute. Add some of the reserved cooking water to loosen the sauce if it gets too thick. Remove from the heat and top with the remaining Pecorino and freshly ground black pepper to taste. Serve immediately.

Air Fryer Chicken Drumsticks

SERVES 4

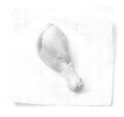

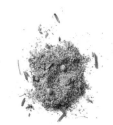

My mother-in-law whipped up these juicy drumsticks in the air fryer for dinner one night, and they were so simple and tasty, they're now in my weekly dinner rotation. I re-created her poultry seasoning for this recipe, but honestly you can use any poultry seasoning you like. I usually season the chicken a few hours before (or even as long as overnight) for a deeper flavor.

8 skin-on medium chicken drumsticks

**1 tablespoon Kickin' Chicken Poultry Seasoning (page 177)
or store-bought poultry seasoning**

In a large bowl, season the chicken all over with the seasoning. (Not a must, but if you have time, do this the night before so it's more flavorful.)

Working in batches if needed, place the chicken in an air fryer basket in a single layer. Cook at 400°F until the skin is golden and crisp and the chicken is cooked through, 20 to 22 minutes, flipping halfway.

Serve immediately.

NO AIR FRYER? NO PROBLEM! Place the chicken on a sheet pan and bake in a preheated 425°F oven for 40 minutes, flipping halfway.

(recipe continues)

Per Serving (2 drumsticks) ● Calories 432 ● Fat 25 g ● Saturated Fat 6.5 g ● Cholesterol 248 mg Carbohydrate 1 g ● Fiber 0 g ● Protein 48 g ● Sugars 0 g ● Sodium 563 mg

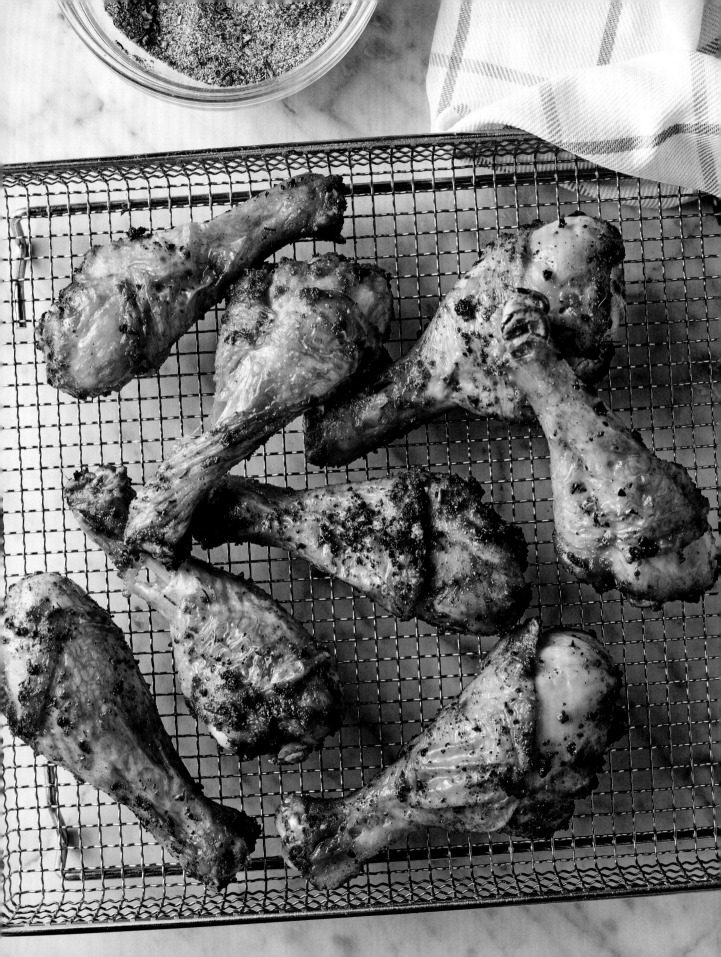

Kickin' Chicken Poultry Seasoning

MAKES ¾ CUP

I use this flavorful poultry seasoning mix anytime I want to pump up the flavor of chicken. It's great on Air Fryer Chicken Drumsticks (page 175), Creamy Chicken and Spinach Tri-Colore Pasta (page 173), and for a whole roasted chicken. You can adjust the salt to your taste, and if you like your poultry spicy, add some cayenne pepper to the mix.

2 tablespoons garlic powder

2 tablespoons onion powder

2 tablespoons sweet paprika

2 teaspoons dried oregano

1 teaspoon ground cumin

1 teaspoon ground sage

1 teaspoon dried thyme

Combine all the ingredients with ¼ cup kosher salt and ½ teaspoon freshly ground black pepper and store in an airtight container.

Per Serving (1 teaspoon) ● Calories 5 ● Fat 0 g ● Saturated Fat 0 g ● Cholesterol 0 mg Carbohydrate 1 g ● Fiber 0 g ● Protein 0 g ● Sugars 0 g ● Sodium 374 mg

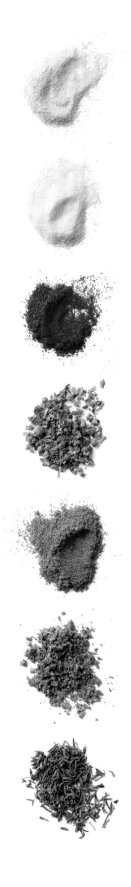

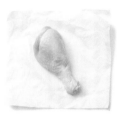

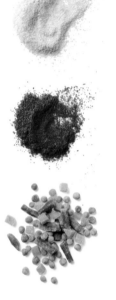

BBQ Chicken Foil Packets

SERVES 4

When you don't feel like cooking, this chicken foil packet couldn't be easier! Made with bone-in skinless chicken, your favorite BBQ sauce, and frozen veggies, they're ready in a snap. It's an easy meal-in-one, and the best part is the super-easy cleanup!

SKINNY SCOOP: The easiest way to remove the skin from the drumstick is to use one paper towel to hold the chicken and another to pull the skin right off.

4 bone-in chicken thighs and 4 drumsticks, skin removed (see Skinny Scoop)

½ teaspoon garlic powder

½ teaspoon smoked paprika

3 cups frozen mixed vegetables

½ cup BBQ sauce

Chopped fresh parsley (optional), for garnish

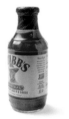

Preheat the oven to 425°F.

In a large bowl, season the chicken all over with 1 teaspoon kosher salt, the garlic powder, and smoked paprika and mix to thoroughly coat.

Cut four 18 × 12-inch pieces of heavy-duty foil and lay on a flat surface. Place ¾ cup frozen mixed veggies in the center of each piece of foil. Place 1 drumstick and 1 thigh in the middle of each foil packet. Brush both sides of the chicken with ¼ cup of the BBQ sauce.

Bring up the long sides of the foil, so the ends meet over the food, then double-fold them, leaving room for heat to circulate inside. Double-fold the two short ends to seal the packet tight, so no steam escapes.

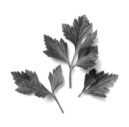

Place the foil packets on a baking sheet and bake until the chicken is cooked through and reaches an internal temperature of 160°F, 50 to 55 minutes.

Remove the baking sheet from the oven. Carefully open the foil packets and brush the chicken with the remaining ¼ cup BBQ sauce. With the foil left open, return to the oven and bake until the sauce starts to form a crust on the chicken and the edges start to brown, about 5 minutes.

Serve garnished with fresh parsley, if desired.

Per Serving (1 foil packet) ● Calories 468 ● Fat 11 g ● Saturated Fat 3 g ● Cholesterol 249 mg
Carbohydrate 31 g ● Fiber 4.5 g ● Protein 57 g ● Sugars 14 g ● Sodium 885 mg

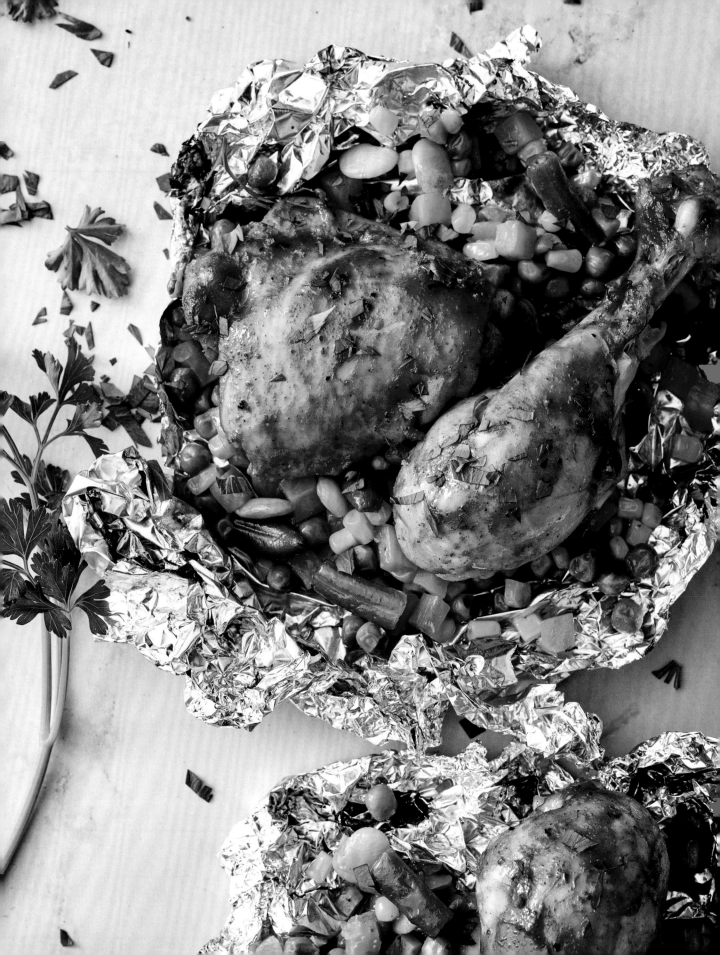

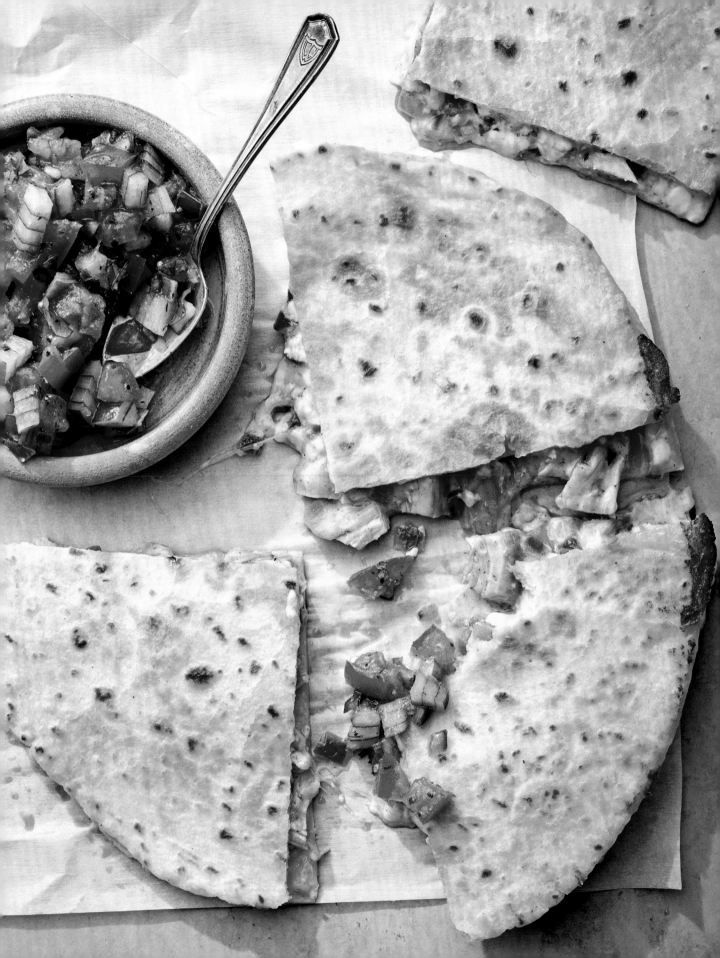

Cheesy Chicken Quesadilla

SERVES 1

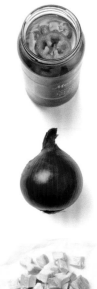

I love chicken quesadillas, but with all that cheese they're hard to make without going over my daily intake of fats. So I came up with the idea to "stretch" the shredded cheese by adding some low-fat cottage cheese to the mix, and it came out so cheesy, delicious, and super high in protein! I'll never make them any other way again. Serve them as is or with your favorite toppings like guacamole, sour cream, or pico de gallo (see the recipe from Madison's Steak Tacos with Cilantro-Lime Rice, page 201).

SKINNY SCOOP: If you don't have fajita seasoning, you can use equal parts garlic powder, onion powder, chili powder, and salt.

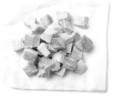

1 tablespoon pickled jalapeño slices, drained and chopped

¼ cup chopped red onion

3 ounces cooked chicken breast, chopped (⅔ cup)

¼ teaspoon fajita seasoning (see Skinny Scoop)

⅓ cup shredded reduced-fat Mexican blend cheese

3 tablespoons 2% cottage cheese

2 (7-inch) low-carb flour tortillas (I love Mission Carb Balance) or gluten-free tortillas, such as Siete

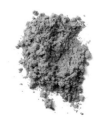

In a large skillet, heat 1 teaspoon extra-virgin olive oil over medium heat. Add the chopped jalapeño and onion and cook until softened, 2 to 3 minutes. Add the chicken, season with the fajita seasoning, and cook until heated through, about 1 minute. Transfer to a plate and wipe the pan clean.

In a small bowl, combine the shredded cheese and cottage cheese and mix well.

Spread both tortillas with the cheese mixture, leaving about 1 inch all around the edges. Top one of the tortillas with the chicken and veggies, then flip the other tortilla on top, cheese side down.

Set the skillet over medium heat and spray with olive oil. Transfer the quesadilla to the skillet and cook until it is golden and fully heated through, 2 to 3 minutes per side. Cut into wedges and serve immediately.

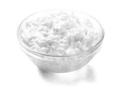

Per Serving (1 quesadilla) ● Calories 469 ● Fat 21 g ● Saturated Fat 8.5 g ● Cholesterol 127 mg Carbohydrate 45 g ● Fiber 31 g ● Protein 52 g ● Sugars 4 g ● Sodium 1,186 mg

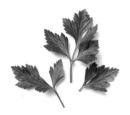

Grilled Chicken Thighs with Garlicky Chimichurri

SERVES 4

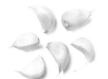

Grilled chicken can be pretty boring, but add some tasty homemade chimichurri and it's anything but! My Argentinian friend Mariella makes the best chimichurri—it's extra garlicky and amazing on anything grilled, from steaks, chicken, and sausage, to shrimp and even potatoes. Tommy can't get enough of it, so I make it on repeat all summer. Serve with white rice, roasted potatoes, or grilled vegetables to make it a meal.

SKINNY SCOOP: The chimichurri can be prepared in advance and refrigerated in an airtight container for up to 2 days.

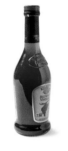

1/2 cup packed finely chopped fresh parsley leaves

6 garlic cloves, finely minced

1/4 cup red wine vinegar

1/4 teaspoon crushed red pepper flakes, or more to taste

11/2 pounds boneless, skinless thighs, trimmed of excess fat

In a small bowl, combine the parsley, garlic, vinegar, 3 tablespoons extra-virgin olive oil, the pepper flakes, 1 teaspoon kosher salt, and 1/8 teaspoon freshly ground black pepper. (See Skinny Scoop.)

In a large bowl, season the chicken with 3/4 teaspoon kosher salt and ground black pepper to taste. Pour 2 tablespoons of the chimichurri all over the chicken and let it marinate at room temperature for 10 minutes.

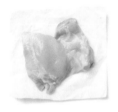

Meanwhile, preheat the grill to medium-high.

When hot, oil the grates well and grill the chicken until the juices run clear, 5 to 6 minutes per side. Transfer to a platter.

Drizzle the chicken with a little more chimichurri, then serve with the remaining chimichurri on the side.

Per Serving (41/2 ounces chicken + sauce) • Calories 308 • Fat 17 g • Saturated Fat 3.5 g
Cholesterol 160 mg • Carbohydrate 2 g • Fiber 0 g • Protein 34 g • Sugars 0 g • Sodium 658 mg

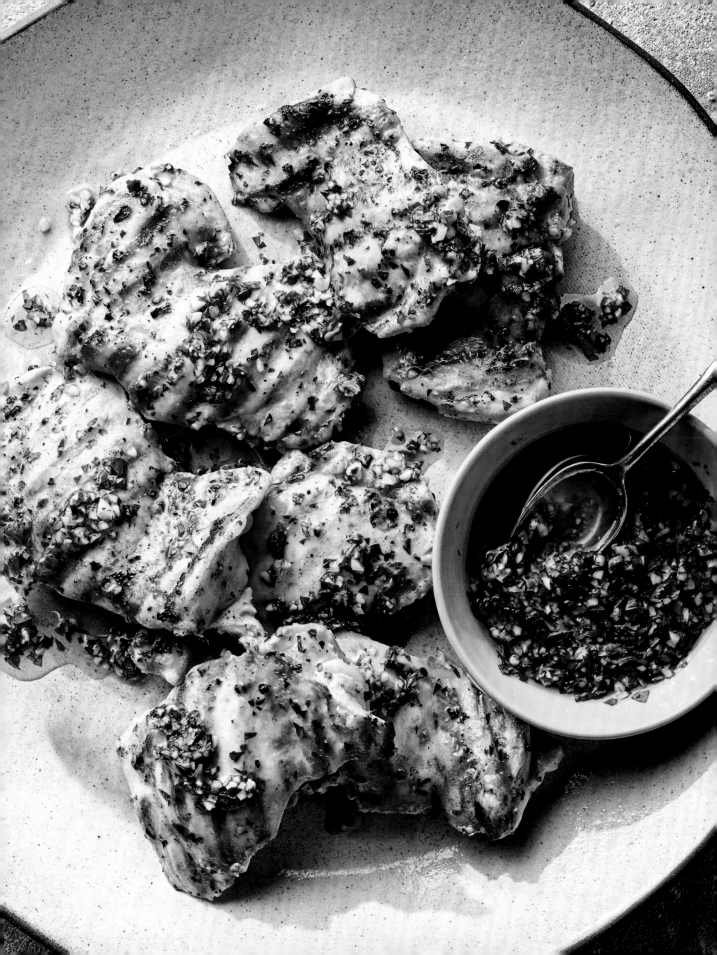

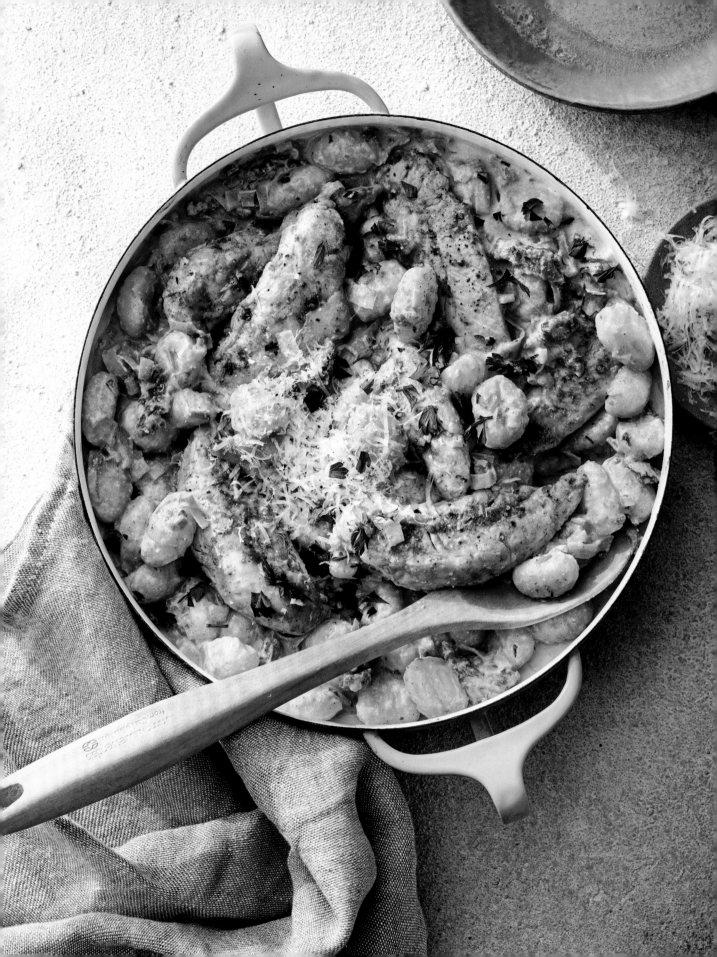

One-Pot Creamy Gnocchi with Chicken and Leeks

SERVES 4

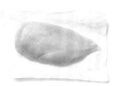

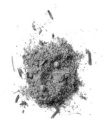

Both my kids love this gnocchi dish, and I love that it's a super-simple one-pot meal! It's so creamy and delicious, and the best part is it doesn't actually have any heavy cream. It gets creamy by cooking the gnocchi in milk along with Romano cheese, fragrant leeks, and sun-dried tomatoes. I used chicken tenderloins for protein, but boneless thighs or diced chicken breast will work, too. If you have fresh parsley for garnish, use it!

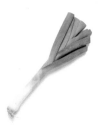

8 chicken tenders (about 2 ounces each) or diced boneless, skinless chicken breast

2½ teaspoons Kickin' Chicken Poultry Seasoning (page 177) or store-bought poultry seasoning

1 cup sliced leeks, white parts only, cut into half-moons (2 to 3 large), rinsed well

1¾ cups 2% milk

1 pound potato gnocchi

½ cup freshly grated Pecorino Romano cheese

¼ cup sun-dried tomatoes (drained), cut into ¼-inch strips

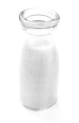

In a large bowl, season the chicken with 1½ teaspoons of the poultry seasoning.

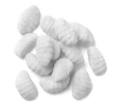

Heat a large deep nonstick skillet over medium-high heat and spray with oil. Add the chicken and cook until browned on both sides and partially cooked through, 2 minutes per side (it will finish cooking later). Transfer the chicken to a plate and set aside.

Reduce the heat to medium and add ½ tablespoon extra-virgin olive oil and the leek whites to the pan. Cook, stirring occasionally, until softened, 4 to 5 minutes.

Stir in the milk, gnocchi, Pecorino, sun-dried tomatoes, and remaining 1 teaspoon poultry seasoning. Bring to a boil over high heat. Reduce the heat to medium and cook, stirring occasionally, until the milk has reduced slightly and begins to thicken, about 3 minutes.

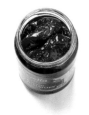

Give the mixture a big stir, then return the chicken to the skillet, slightly nestling it in. Reduce the heat to low and cook until the sauce thickens slightly and the chicken is cooked through, 3 to 4 minutes. Serve right away.

Per Serving (1 cup gnocchi + 2 chicken tenders) ● Calories 442 ● Fat 18 g ● Saturated Fat 9 g Cholesterol 122 mg ● Carbohydrate 31 g ● Fiber 2 g ● Protein 38 g ● Sugars 9 g ● Sodium 943 mg

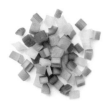

Turkey Pot Pie Noodles

SERVES 5

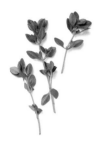

Nothing says comfort food like a cozy pot pie! Here I swapped out the crust for egg noodles, transforming classic pot pie into an easy and delicious weeknight skillet dish the kids will love. Start to finish, this takes about 20 minutes to make. It's a perfect recipe to use up leftover Thanksgiving turkey, but it's also great with a rotisserie chicken. If you want to make it dairy-free you can omit the half-and-half. Also feel free to add peas or frozen corn if you want more veggies.

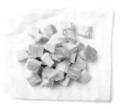

3 cups frozen or fresh mirepoix (diced onions, celery, and carrots)

1 tablespoon chopped fresh thyme and/or sage

3 cups (12 ounces) leftover cooked chopped turkey breast (or chicken)

3 cups turkey or chicken broth

2 tablespoons all-purpose flour

¼ cup half-and-half

10 ounces extra-wide egg noodles

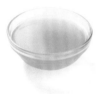

Bring a large pot of salted water to a boil over high heat.

In a large deep nonstick skillet, heat ½ tablespoon extra-virgin olive oil over medium-low heat. Add the mirepoix and thyme and/or sage and cook until the vegetables begin to soften, 3 to 4 minutes. Add the turkey, 2 cups of the broth, ¼ teaspoon kosher salt, and freshly ground black pepper to taste and bring to a gentle boil. Simmer, stirring occasionally, until the flavors meld and the vegetables are tender, about 3 minutes.

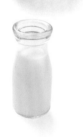

In a small bowl, combine the remaining 1 cup broth with the flour and mix to dissolve. Stir into the pot and cook until slightly thickened, about 3 minutes. Stir in the half-and-half and cook 1 minute more.

Meanwhile, cook the noodles according to the package directions.

Drain the noodles and stir into the turkey mixture. Serve immediately.

Serving Size (2 cups) ● Calories 379 ● Fat 7 g ● Saturated Fat 2 g ● Cholesterol 100 mg
Carbohydrate 51 g ● Fiber 3.5 g ● Protein 29 g ● Sugars 5 g ● Sodium 507 mg

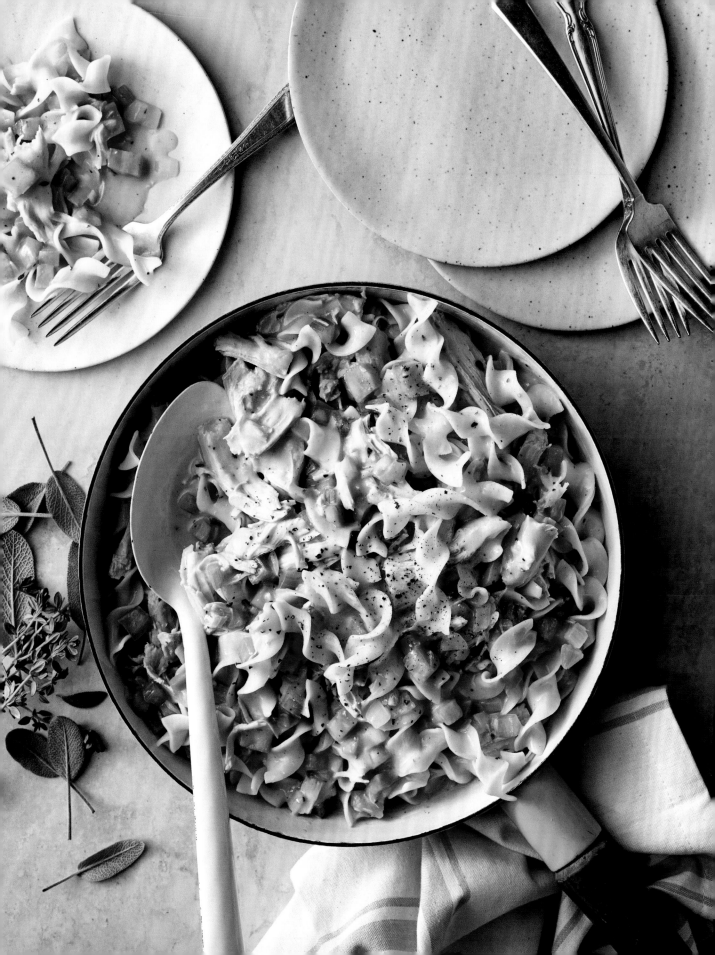

Meat
Lovers

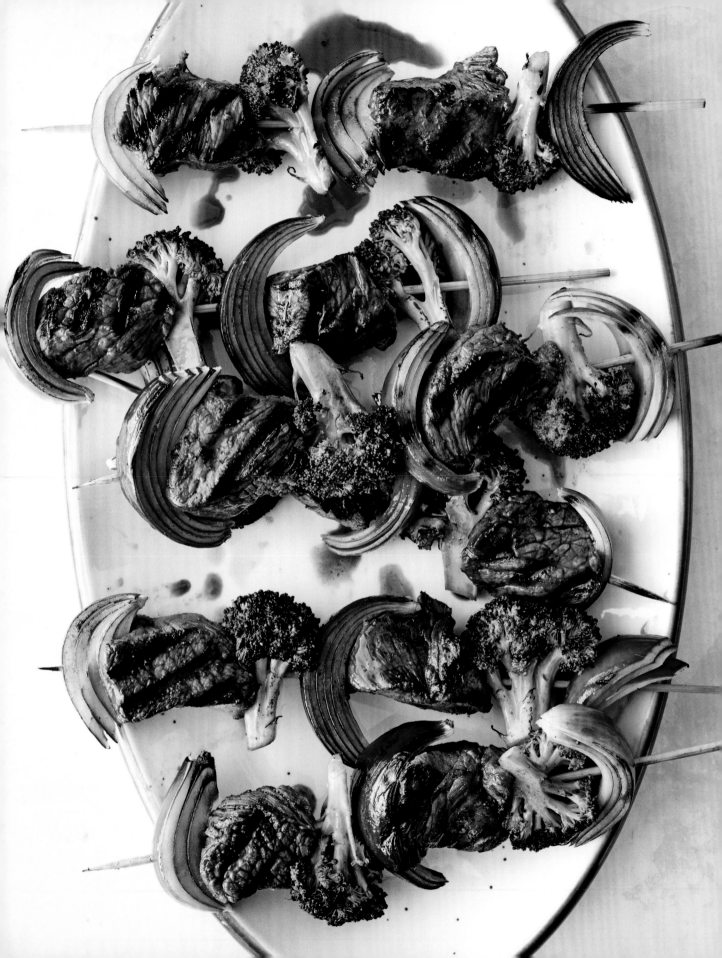

Five-Spice Beef Kebabs

SERVES 4

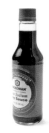

New York strip steak, which has the perfect amount of marbling, makes these Asian-inspired beef skewers flavorful and juicy. The cubed steak is threaded onto skewers with chunks of red onion and broccoli, but you can also swap in scallions, cubed eggplant, or mushrooms.

SKINNY SCOOP: If you can't find Chinese five-spice powder, feel free to use an equal amount of allspice instead.

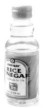

¼ cup reduced-sodium soy sauce or gluten-free tamari

2 tablespoons rice vinegar

1 tablespoon honey

1½ teaspoons Chinese five-spice powder (see Skinny Scoop)

1 pound New York strip steak, 1 inch thick, trimmed and cut into 16 cubes

2 large heads broccoli

½ medium red onion, top trimmed but root end left on

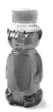

In a medium bowl, whisk together the soy sauce, vinegar, honey, five-spice powder, ½ teaspoon kosher salt, and freshly ground black pepper to taste. Add half the marinade to a separate medium bowl. Add the meat to one of the bowls and toss to coat. Set aside to marinate for 30 minutes at room temperature, stirring occasionally. (Or cover and refrigerate for up to 8 hours, tossing halfway.)

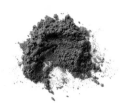

Separate the broccoli to get 16 florets (you may have some leftover broccoli). The florets should each be 1 to 2 inches, so cut any that are particularly big in half. Add the broccoli to the second bowl with the marinade and toss to coat. Let sit for up to 30 minutes.

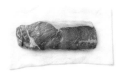

Meanwhile, soak 8 wooden skewers in water for at least 20 minutes so they don't burn on the grill (or use metal skewers). Peel the onion, then cut it lengthwise into 4 wedges.

(recipe continues)

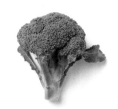

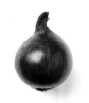

Per Serving (2 skewers) ● Calories 268 ● Fat 4 g ● Saturated Fat 1.5 g ● Cholesterol 62 mg
Carbohydrate 27 g ● Fiber 8.5 g ● Protein 36 g ● Sugars 10 g ● Sodium 853 mg

When the meat is done marinating, take 1 onion wedge and divide the layers into thirds, thread one-third onto the soaked skewer, then carefully (making sure you aren't pressing the skewer toward your hand!) thread 1 broccoli piece onto the skewer, then 1 piece of meat. Repeat with another layer of onion, broccoli, meat, then finish with the last of the onion. Repeat with all the ingredients to make 8 skewers. Place on a sheet pan and brush generously with some of the leftover marinade from the broccoli and season with a pinch each of kosher salt and freshly ground black pepper.

Preheat the grill to high heat. Grill the skewers to your desired doneness, 3 to 5 minutes per side for medium-rare. (Alternatively, to broil the skewers, adjust an oven rack to 6 inches from the heating element and preheat the broiler to high. Line a baking sheet with foil and add the skewers. Broil until the meat is cooked to your desired doneness, 4 to 5 minutes per side for medium-rare.)

Serve immediately.

Hoisin Burgers
with Quick-Pickled Cucumbers

SERVES 4

I love adding grated zucchini to my burgers. They come out so juicy and it's a great way to include more veggies in my meal! For extra zip, add 1 tablespoon of grated fresh ginger or garlic to the ground beef mixture. Serve the burgers over rice or on a toasted bun with the pickled cucumbers and a side salad.

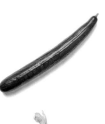

½ large English cucumber, very thinly sliced

½ medium yellow onion

1 tablespoon rice vinegar

1½ cups (6 ounces) coarsely grated zucchini (about 1 medium)

1 pound ground beef (90% lean)

¼ cup panko bread crumbs

¼ cup hoisin sauce

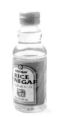

Put the cucumber in a small bowl with ½ teaspoon kosher salt and mix well. Let sit for 5 minutes.

Meanwhile, grate half of the onion to yield 1 tablespoon and set aside. Thinly slice the remaining onion. Add the sliced onion and vinegar to the cucumber. Transfer to the refrigerator to pickle while you make the burgers.

Place the grated zucchini in a clean kitchen towel and squeeze out as much of the moisture as possible. Transfer to a large bowl and add the reserved grated onion, the beef, panko, ½ teaspoon kosher salt, and freshly ground black pepper to taste and stir until combined. Divide into 4 equal portions and form into patties about 4 inches in diameter (make sure they are not too thick).

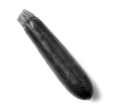

Heat a large nonstick skillet over medium-high heat and lightly spray with oil. Add the burgers and cook until browned on both sides, 4 to 5 minutes per side. Reduce the heat to low, then brush the tops of the burgers with half of the hoisin. Flip and cook about 1 minute more while brushing the other side with the remaining hoisin. Flip once more and remove the skillet from the heat to prevent the hoisin from burning. Transfer to a plate.

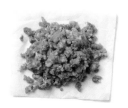

Drain the pickled cucumber and onion. Top each burger with some of the pickles and serve.

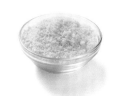

Per Serving (1 burger) ● Calories 283 ● Fat 12 g ● Saturated Fat 4.5 g ● Cholesterol 74 mg
Carbohydrate 18 g ● Fiber 1.5 g ● Protein 25 g ● Sugars 10 g ● Sodium 631 mg

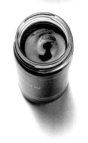

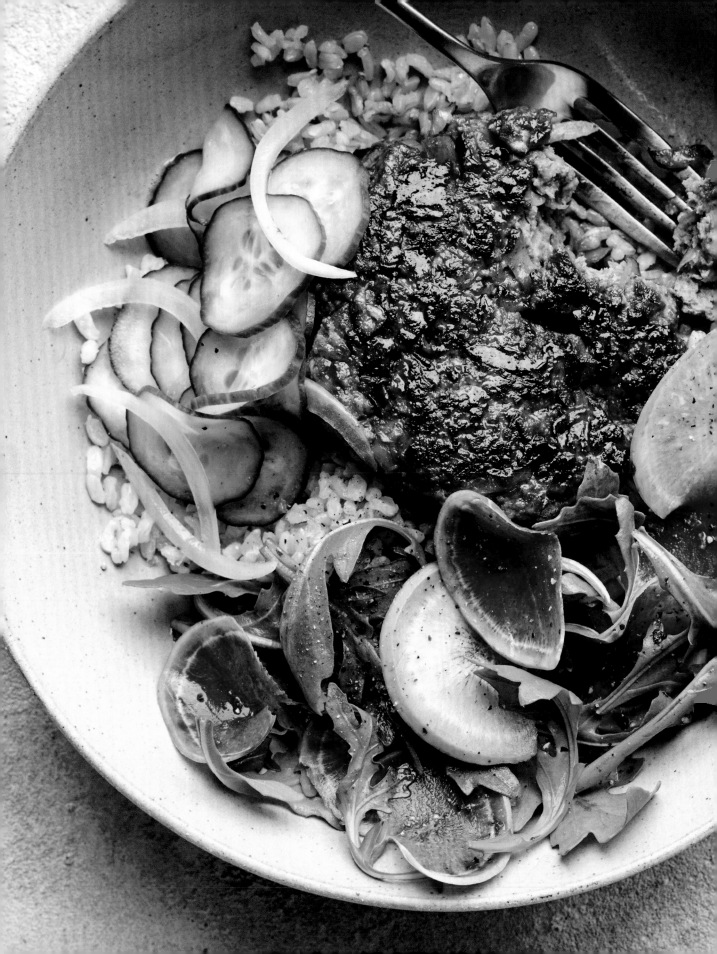

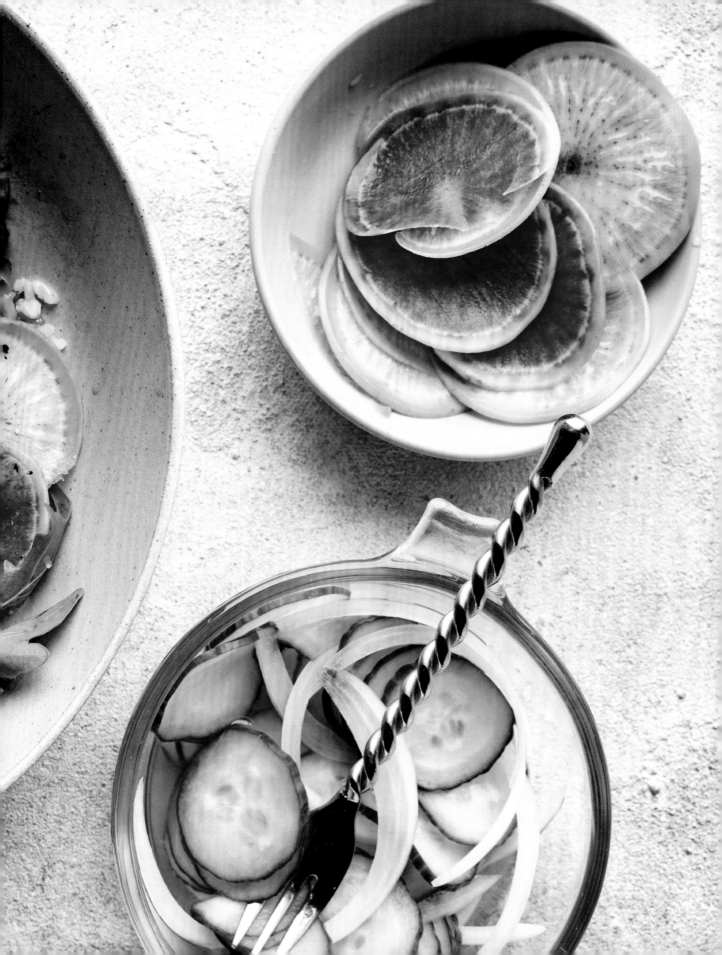

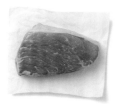

Pepper Steak and Rice

SERVES 4

Pepper steak is a dish I remember my mom made often after taking a Chinese cooking class. This family favorite of beef, peppers, and onions served over rice is ready in less than 20 minutes, and it's always a winner in my house. If you like it extra saucy, you can double the sauce ingredients. Garnish with sliced scallions if you have them on hand. Flank or skirt steak also works great instead of the top round.

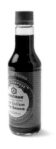

1 pound top round beef, trimmed

4 teaspoons plus 3 tablespoons reduced-sodium soy sauce or gluten-free tamari

1 tablespoon rice wine

3 teaspoons cornstarch

1 red, orange, or yellow bell pepper, thinly sliced

1 large onion, thinly sliced

3 cups cooked white or brown rice, for serving

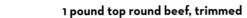

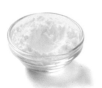

Slice the beef into thin slices with the grain. Cut each strip across the grain about 1 inch long so you have small thin slices. Place the strips in a medium bowl and add 4 teaspoons of the soy sauce, the rice wine, 1 teaspoon of the cornstarch, and ½ teaspoon freshly ground black pepper. Toss to combine.

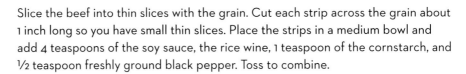

In a small bowl, whisk together 1 tablespoon water with the remaining 3 tablespoons soy sauce and 2 teaspoons cornstarch until smooth. Set aside.

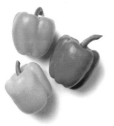

Heat a large nonstick skillet or wok over high heat. When the pan is very hot, add 2 teaspoons vegetable oil and swirl to coat the skillet. Add the beef, spreading evenly in the pan in a single layer to not overcrowd. Cook undisturbed for 20 seconds to let the beef brown, then use a spatula to stir and continue to cook, stirring, until browned all over and cooked through, about 2 minutes more. Transfer to a plate.

Add 1 teaspoon vegetable oil to the pan. When the oil is shimmering, add the bell pepper and onion and cook, stirring occasionally, until tender, 4 to 5 minutes. Return the beef to the pan and add the sauce. Stir-fry until the sauce is slightly thickened and the beef and vegetables are well coated, about 30 seconds.

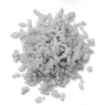

To serve, spoon ¾ cup of rice into each bowl and divide the pepper steak among the bowls.

Per Serving (1 cup pepper steak + ¾ cup rice) ● Calories 363 ● Fat 8 g ● Saturated Fat 1.5 g Cholesterol 70 mg ● Carbohydrate 41 g ● Fiber 3.5 g ● Protein 32 g ● Sugars 3 g ● Sodium 641 mg

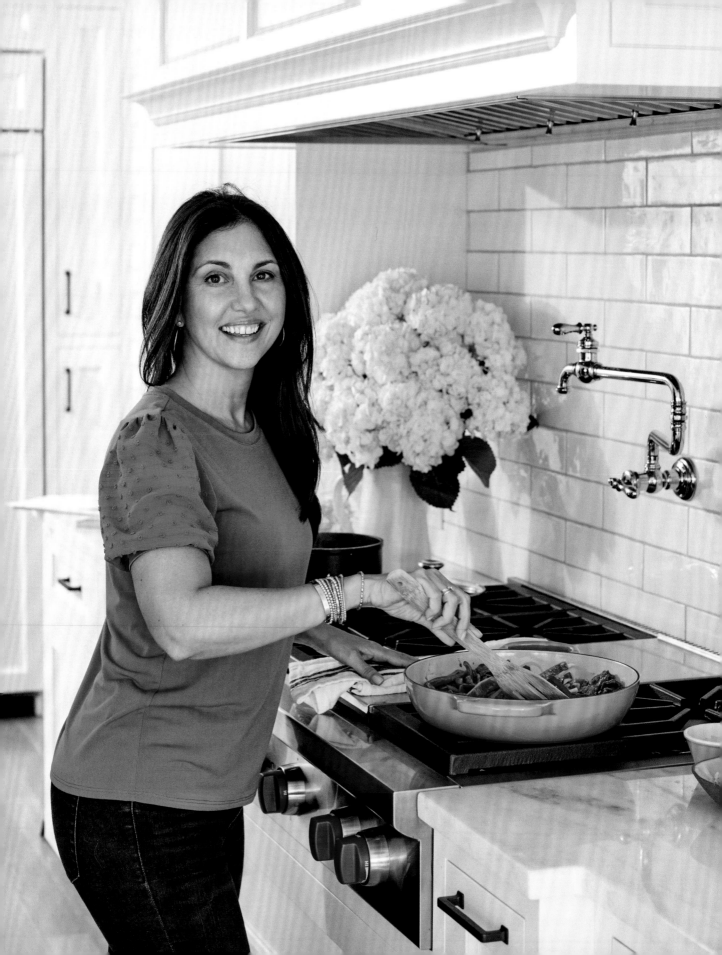

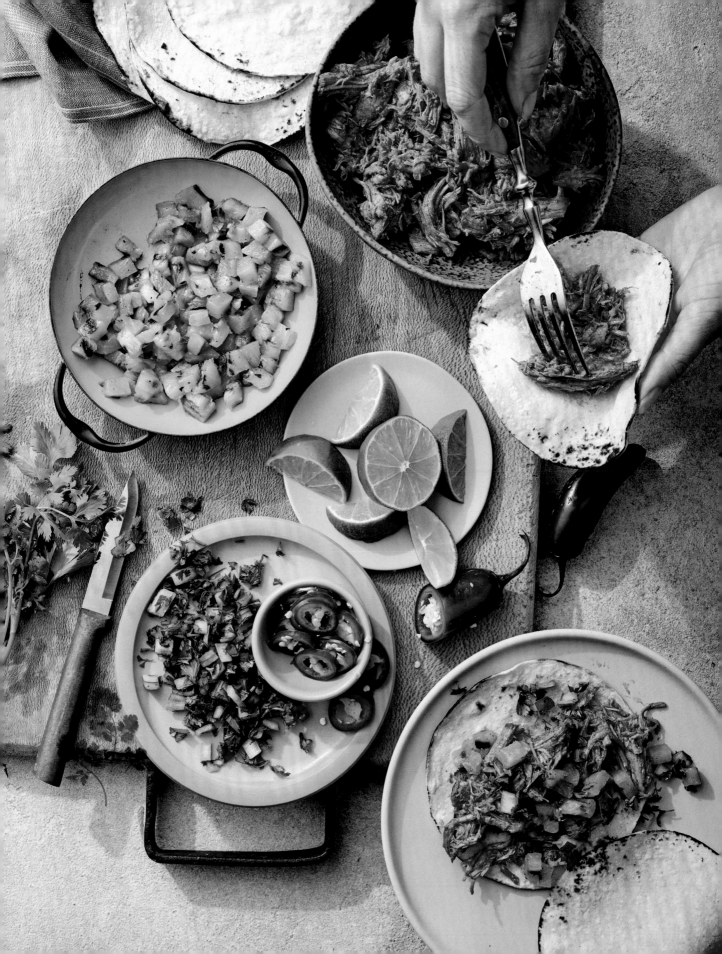

Slow Cooker Tacos al Pastor

SERVES 7

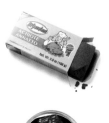

I eat my weight in tacos every time I go to California, and *al pastor* ("shepherd style") tacos are always my favorite. The pork is marinated and cooked on a vertical rotisserie spit with pineapple and carved similarly to a gyro. I re-created them in the slow cooker with a simple marinade inspired by a recipe from Rick Bayless, and my family is obsessed! It makes a lot of pork, so you can freeze the leftovers if you don't have a big crowd to feed. I like to serve this in tortillas with jalapeños, diced grilled pineapple, onion, cilantro, and a wedge of lime.

SKINNY SCOOP: El Yucateco achiote paste can be found in any Mexican market and on Amazon.

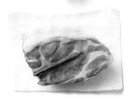

1 (3½-ounce) package El Yucateco achiote paste (see Skinny Scoop)

2 canned chipotle peppers in adobo sauce, minced, plus 2 tablespoons of adobo sauce

4½ pounds trimmed and skinned bone-in pork shoulder

3 (¼-inch-thick) rounds fresh pineapple (about ¼ medium pineapple, peeled)

1 medium red onion, chopped

½ cup chopped fresh cilantro

14 (6-inch) corn tortillas

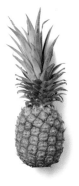

In a blender, combine the achiote paste, chipotle peppers, adobo sauce, ½ tablespoon extra-virgin olive oil, and ¾ cup water. Blend into a smooth marinade.

In a large bowl, season the pork all over with 2 teaspoons kosher salt and rub the marinade all over (use gloves to avoid staining your hands). Cover the bowl and transfer to the refrigerator to marinate overnight, turning it the next morning so the marinade covers all of the pork.

Transfer the pork to a slow cooker, cover, and cook on low for 10 to 12 hours, until tender and falling apart.

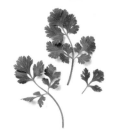

(recipe continues)

Per Serving (2 tacos) ● Calories 524 ● Fat 20 g ● Saturated Fat 6.5 g ● Cholesterol 162 mg
Carbohydrate 33 g ● Fiber 4 g ● Protein 51 g ● Sugars 5 g ● Sodium 975 mg

Transfer the pork to a cutting board, discard the fat and bones, and shred the meat using two forks. Pour the liquid from the slow cooker into a small bowl or liquid measuring cup. Return about 1½ cups of the liquid to the slow cooker along with the shredded pork. Season with additional salt and freshly ground black pepper to taste. Cook on low for 30 minutes to let the flavors meld into the pork.

Heat a grill or broiler on high. Spray both sides of the pineapple with oil (if broiling, place on a sheet pan). Grill or broil 6 inches from the heat, flipping halfway, until browned and softened, 3 to 5 minutes on each side. Cut the core out of the pineapple, then chop the pineapple into small pieces.

In a small bowl, combine the red onion and cilantro.

Heat the tortillas for 30 seconds on each side on the grill (or over an open flame on a gas stove). Transfer to a plate and cover with a clean kitchen towel to keep warm.

To serve, divide the tortillas among plates and place ¼ cup of pork on each tortilla. Top each with 1½ tablespoons of the onion-cilantro mixture and 1 heaping tablespoon of the diced pineapple.

Madison's Steak Tacos
with Cilantro-Lime Rice

SERVES 4

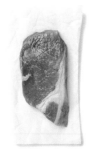

Madison loves steak tacos, and every time she goes to Chipotle, she gets them with cilantro-lime rice inside the taco. If it works in a burrito, why not in a taco? I love how the rice inside the taco keeps the tortilla from getting soggy. You can make the steak on the grill, a grill pan, or even in an air fryer!

1 (1-pound) sirloin steak, 1 to 1¼ inches thick

¼ small red onion, sliced

1 beefsteak tomato, chopped

½ cup chopped fresh cilantro

2 limes, 1 halved, 1 cut into wedges for serving

¾ cup uncooked long-grain rice

12 (6-inch) corn tortillas

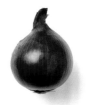

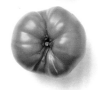

Spray the steak with olive oil and season both sides with 1 teaspoon kosher salt and freshly ground black pepper to taste. Let stand at room temperature while preparing the pico de gallo and rice.

To make a pico de gallo, in a medium bowl, combine the red onion, tomato, ¼ cup of the cilantro, ¼ teaspoon kosher salt, and the juice of one lime half.

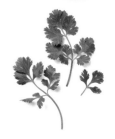

In a small heavy-bottomed pot with a tightly fitting lid, combine the rice, 1½ cups water, 1 teaspoon extra-virgin olive oil, and ½ teaspoon kosher salt. Bring to a boil over high heat. Cook until the water is reduced to just skimming the top of the rice. Reduce the heat to low and cover. Cook for about 15 minutes, then remove from the heat. Keep covered an additional 5 minutes so the rice finishes cooking with the steam. Uncover and fluff the rice with a fork.

In a medium bowl, combine the cooked rice with the remaining ¼ cup chopped cilantro, the juice of the remaining lime half, and 1 teaspoon extra-virgin olive oil and toss until completely mixed.

(recipe continues)

Per Serving (3 tacos) ● Calories 471 ● Fat 11 g ● Saturated Fat 3 g ● Cholesterol 76 mg
Carbohydrate 64 g ● Fiber 6 g ● Protein 31 g ● Sugars 2 g ● Sodium 590 mg

Preheat the grill or grill pan over high heat. Place the steak on the grill or grill pan and cook until slightly charred on one side, 3 to 4 minutes. Flip the steak and continue to grill until browned and the internal temperature reads 135°F for medium-rare, 3 to 4 minutes longer. The time will vary depending on the thickness of your steak. (Alternatively, to cook in an air fryer, preheat the air fryer to 400°F and cook the steak for 4 to 5 minutes per side for medium-rare.) Transfer the steak to a cutting board, tent loosely with foil, and let rest for 5 minutes.

Meanwhile, char the tortillas for 30 seconds on each side on the grill or over a flame on the stove.

Thinly slice the steak across the grain. Assemble the tacos by placing 3 tortillas on each plate, then top each with 3 tablespoons rice, the sliced steak, and pico de gallo. Serve with lime wedges on the side.

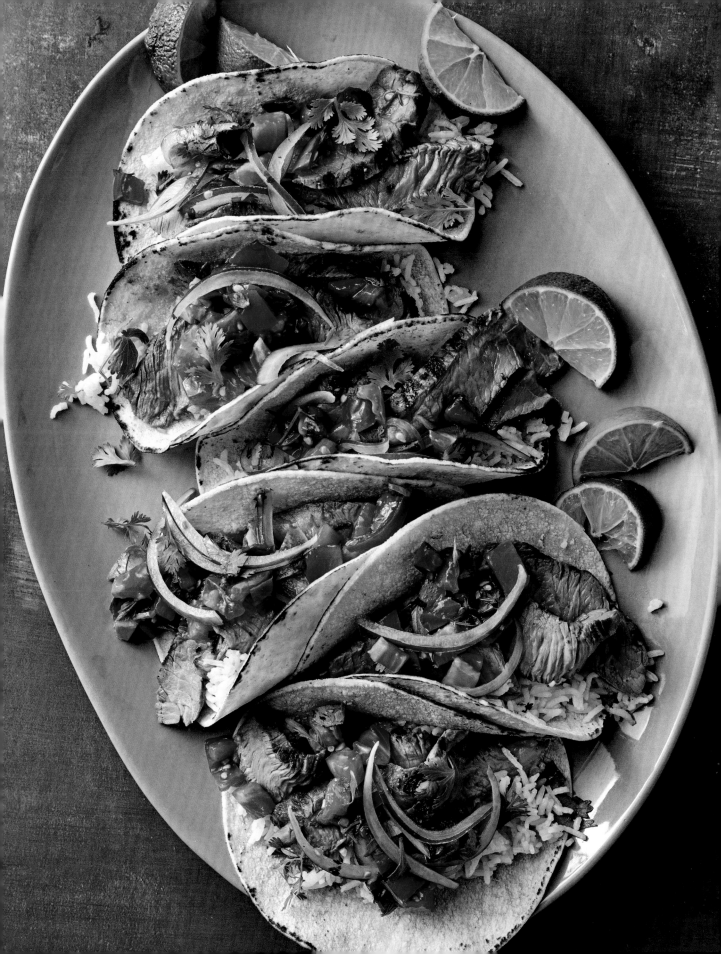

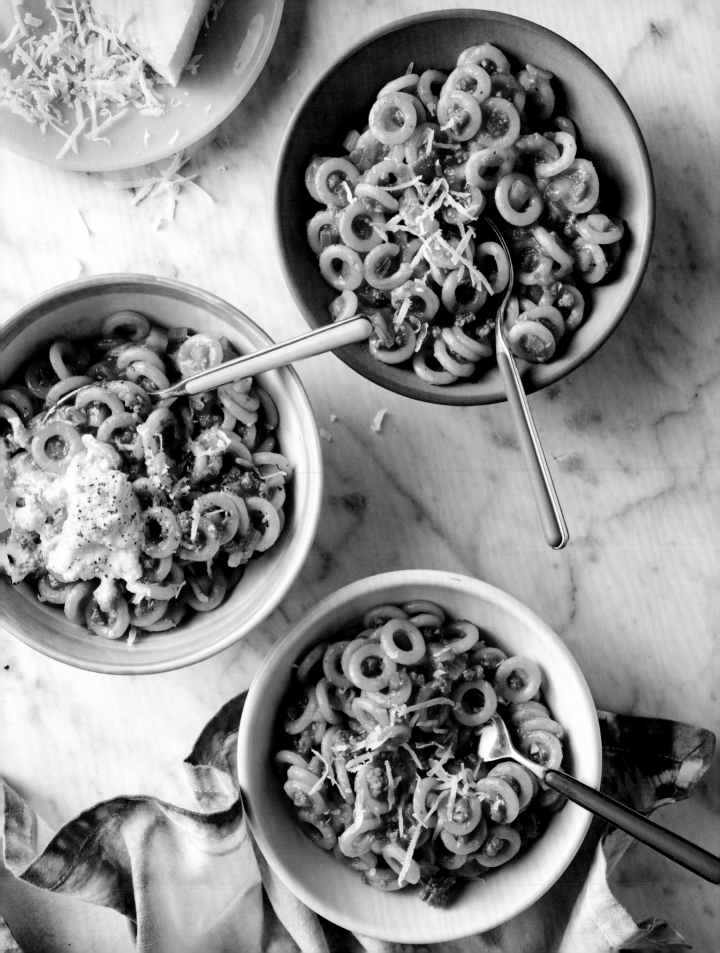

Instant Pot Spaghetti Rings with Beef

SERVES 4

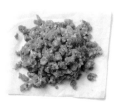

O-shaped pasta is such a fun shape for the kiddos, and this homemade recipe is a thousand percent tastier and healthier than anything you'll get from a can. It's fast and easy, and my family just devours it! Plus, it even has some hidden veggies in the mix. If you have picky kids, use a mini food processor to finely mince the veggies and they won't even notice them. For an extra-cheesy touch, serve with a dollop of ricotta and grated cheese on top.

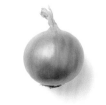

½ pound ground beef (93% lean)

½ cup minced onion

½ cup minced celery

½ cup minced carrots

2 garlic cloves, minced

2½ cups (10 ounces) ring-shaped pasta, such as anelletti, or a gluten-free small pasta shape

2 cups good-quality jarred marinara sauce

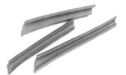

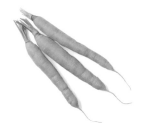

Press the sauté button on an electric pressure cooker. When it's very hot, spray with oil and add the beef and ½ teaspoon kosher salt. Cook, breaking up the meat, until browned, 4 to 5 minutes. Add the onion, celery, carrots, and garlic and sauté until softened, 3 to 4 minutes. Press cancel.

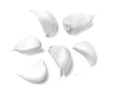

Stir 2 cups water and ¾ teaspoon kosher salt into the pot, scraping the bottom of the pot to deglaze and making sure nothing is stuck to the bottom. Add the pasta and stir well. Pour the marinara sauce evenly over the uncooked pasta, making sure it completely covers it. (Do not stir or you will get a burn message.)

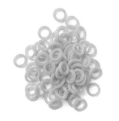

Seal and cook on high pressure for 6 to 8 minutes (the cook time depends on your pasta; use half the time listed on the package). Quick release, then open when the pressure subsides and give everything a big stir. Taste and adjust the salt if needed. Divide among bowls and serve immediately.

NO PRESSURE COOKER? NO PROBLEM! Sauté the meat and vegetables as directed in a large heavy pot or Dutch oven over medium heat. Stir in the water, salt, marinara, and pasta. Bring to a boil over high heat. Reduce the heat to medium-low, cover, and cook, until the pasta is al dente and the liquid is absorbed, 20 to 25 minutes, stirring every 5 minutes.

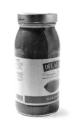

Per Serving (generous 1½ cups) ● Calories 438 ● Fat 9 g ● Saturated Fat 2.5 g
Cholesterol 36 mg ● Carbohydrate 64 g ● Fiber 5.5 g ● Protein 23 g ● Sugars 8 g
Sodium 836 mg

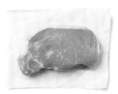

Parmesan Pork Chops

SERVES 4

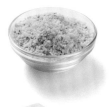

My family devours these pork chops every time I make them! They come out so juicy and delicious, you might want to make a few extra, because my husband, Tommy, always goes for seconds. You can use bone-in or boneless pork chops; they take about the same time to cook. I always serve them with a simple salad and a starch or veggie side, such as Creamed Spinach with Mushrooms (page 259) or Braised Swiss Chard (page 252).

4 boneless center-cut pork chops, ¾ inch thick, fat trimmed (5 ounces each trimmed)

¼ cup seasoned bread crumbs, regular or gluten-free

¼ cup freshly grated Parmesan cheese

½ teaspoon garlic powder

1 large egg, beaten

1 (9-ounce) bag radicchio and romaine salad mix (6 cups)

1 tablespoon red wine vinegar

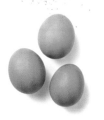

Preheat the oven to 425°F. Spray a sheet pan with olive oil (or use nonstick foil for easy cleanup, if desired).

Season the pork chops all over with ¼ teaspoon kosher salt. In a large shallow bowl, combine the bread crumbs, Parmesan, and garlic powder. Place the beaten egg in another shallow bowl. Dip the pork into the egg, then the crumb mixture, pressing to adhere. Transfer to the prepared sheet pan and spray the top of the chops with oil.

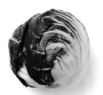

Bake the chops until the internal temperature reaches 145°F, about 20 minutes, or longer if your chops are thicker. (Alternatively, to cook in an air fryer, preheat the air fryer to 400°F. Lightly spray the basket with oil. Cook the pork chops for 12 minutes, flipping halfway.)

While the pork cooks, in a large bowl, toss the salad mix with 1½ tablespoons extra-virgin olive oil, the vinegar, ¼ teaspoon kosher salt, and ⅛ teaspoon freshly ground black pepper.

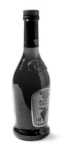

Serve the chops with the salad.

Per Serving (1 chop + 1½ cups salad) ● Calories 286 ● Fat 12 g ● Saturated Fat 3 g Cholesterol 129 mg ● Carbohydrate 7 g ● Fiber 1.5 g ● Protein 38 g ● Sugars 1 g Sodium 468 mg

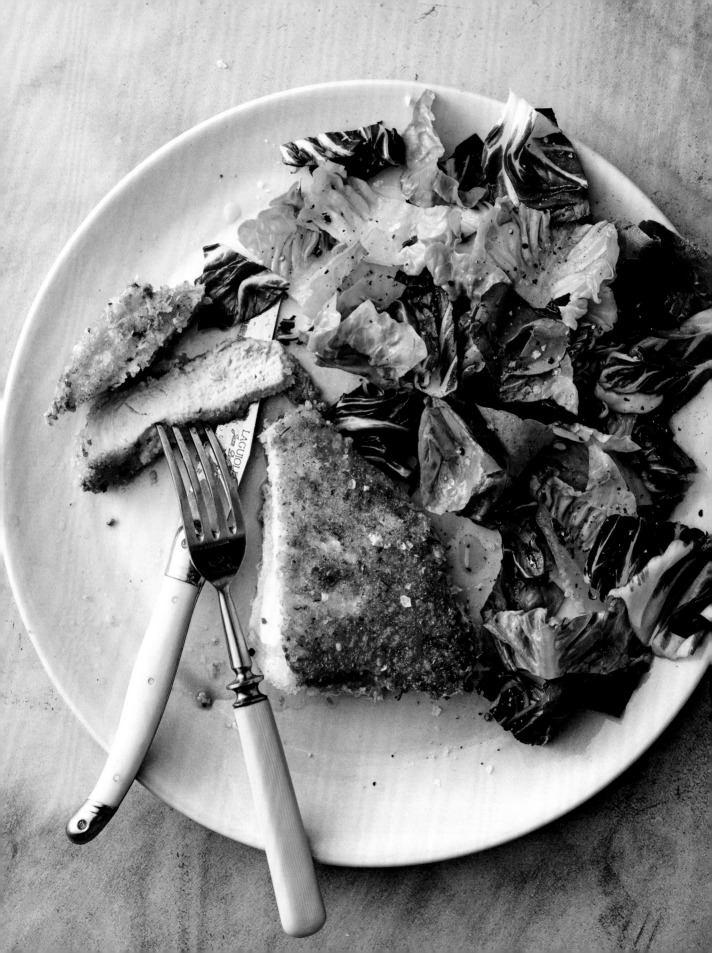

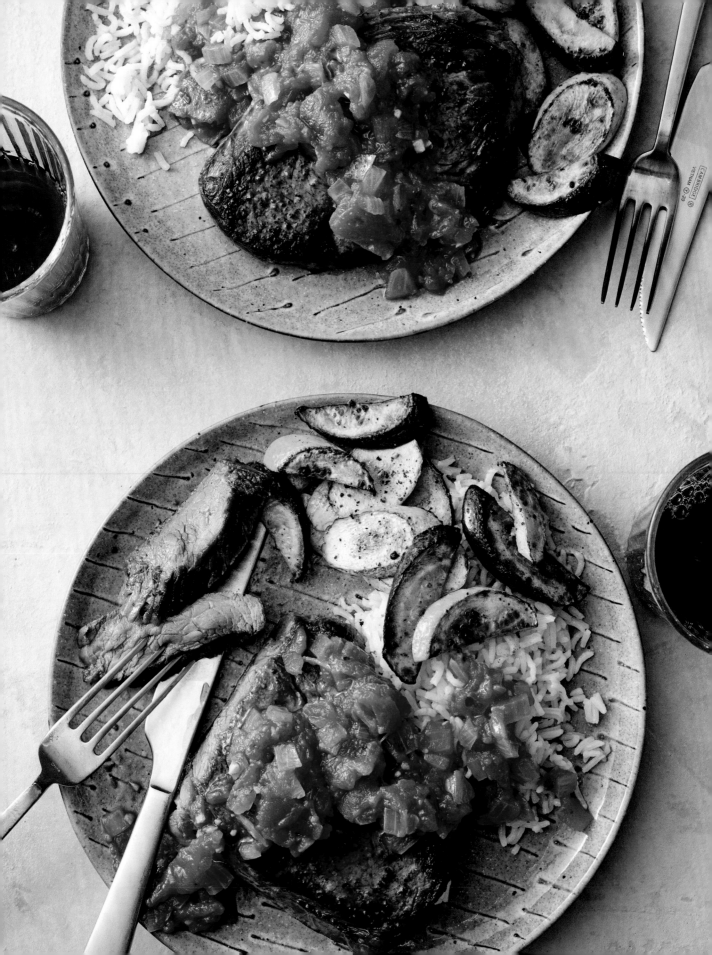

Steak with Pizzaiola Sauce

SERVES 4

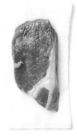

Many moons ago when I worked in New York City, I used to get steak pizzaiola from an Italian restaurant for lunch. Steak pizzaiola does not resemble a modern-day pizza and instead is meat served in a flavorful pizza-style red sauce. The simple tomato sauce in this recipe is also wonderful over pork chops, and for an extra punch of flavor, add capers or olives along with the tomatoes. Serve with potatoes, rice, or roasted vegetables on the side.

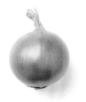

4 sirloin steaks (6 ounces each), about 1 inch thick

1 yellow onion, finely diced

4 garlic cloves, finely minced

¼ teaspoon crushed red pepper flakes

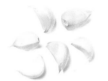

¼ cup dry white wine or broth

½ (28-ounce) can whole peeled San Marzano tomatoes, crushed by hand (about 1½ cups)

1 teaspoon chopped fresh oregano or ½ teaspoon dried

Season the steaks on both sides with ½ teaspoon kosher salt and freshly ground black pepper to taste.

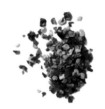

Heat a medium skillet over medium heat and add ½ tablespoon extra-virgin olive oil, the onion, garlic, and pepper flakes. Cook, stirring frequently, until browned, 4 to 5 minutes.

Add the wine to deglaze the skillet, scraping up any browned bits, and cook until most of the wine has reduced, 30 seconds to 1 minute. Add the tomatoes and their juices, the oregano, ¾ teaspoon kosher salt, and ground black pepper to taste. Reduce the heat to medium-low, cover, and cook until the sauce has thickened, 10 to 12 minutes.

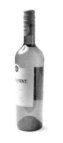

Meanwhile, heat a large skillet or cast-iron skillet over high heat. When the skillet is hot, spray with olive oil. Add the steaks to the skillet in a single layer and cook until browned, about 3 minutes per side for medium-rare, or longer, if desired.

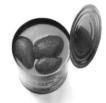

Transfer the steaks to 4 plates. Top the steaks with the pizzaiola sauce (about ⅓ cup sauce for each serving) and serve immediately.

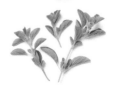

Per Serving (1 steak + ⅓ cup sauce) ● Calories 305 ● Fat 11 g ● Saturated Fat 3.5 g Cholesterol 114 mg ● Carbohydrate 12 g ● Fiber 2 g ● Protein 38 g ● Sugars 7 g Sodium 593 mg

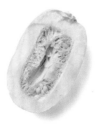

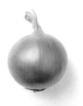

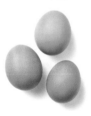

Spaghetti Squash Carbonara

SERVES 4

This dish might have a short ingredient list, but trust me, it's huge on flavor! While the squash roasts, you crisp up the bacon and gently caramelize the onions, then you finish the dish in the same skillet—so easy. Don't be shy with the black pepper or the grated cheese, since they do a lot of the heavy lifting in this simple dish. This is best served with a very lemony arugula salad.

2 small or 1 large spaghetti squash (5 pounds total), halved lengthwise and seeded

8 slices center-cut bacon

1 small yellow onion, diced small

2 large eggs, at room temperature

½ cup freshly grated Parmesan or Pecorino Romano cheese (or a combination), plus more (optional) for serving

Preheat the oven to 400°F. Line a baking sheet with foil.

Season the cut sides of the squash with ½ teaspoon salt and freshly ground black pepper to taste. Place the squash on the prepared baking sheet, cut side down, and roast until very tender, about 1 hour.

Meanwhile, line a plate with paper towels and set a large skillet over medium heat. Add the bacon and cook, stirring occasionally, until crispy, about 10 minutes. Transfer to the paper towels and pour off all but 1 teaspoon of the bacon fat. Crumble the bacon and set aside.

Reduce the heat under the skillet to low. Add the onion and sauté, stirring frequently, until lightly browned, 5 to 8 minutes. Leave the onion in the pan and remove from the heat.

Crack the eggs into a small bowl and add the cheese and ¼ teaspoon freshly ground black pepper. Whisk until combined and set aside.

When the squash is done, carefully flip over each half and rake a fork through the flesh. When it's cool enough to handle (but still warm), use a fork to scrape out all the flesh and add to the skillet with the onion. Cook over low heat for a minute or two to cook off any lingering steam.

Using a wooden spoon or tongs, stir the squash constantly while you pour in the egg and cheese mixture, and continue to stir until fully incorporated. It should look thick but not wet. Fold in the reserved bacon bits. To serve, top with more grated cheese and black pepper as desired.

Per Serving (1⅓ cups) ● Calories 352 ● Fat 14 g ● Saturated Fat 5 g ● Cholesterol 109 mg Carbohydrate 46 g ● Fiber 9.5 g ● Protein 17 g ● Sugars 20 g ● Sodium 710 mg

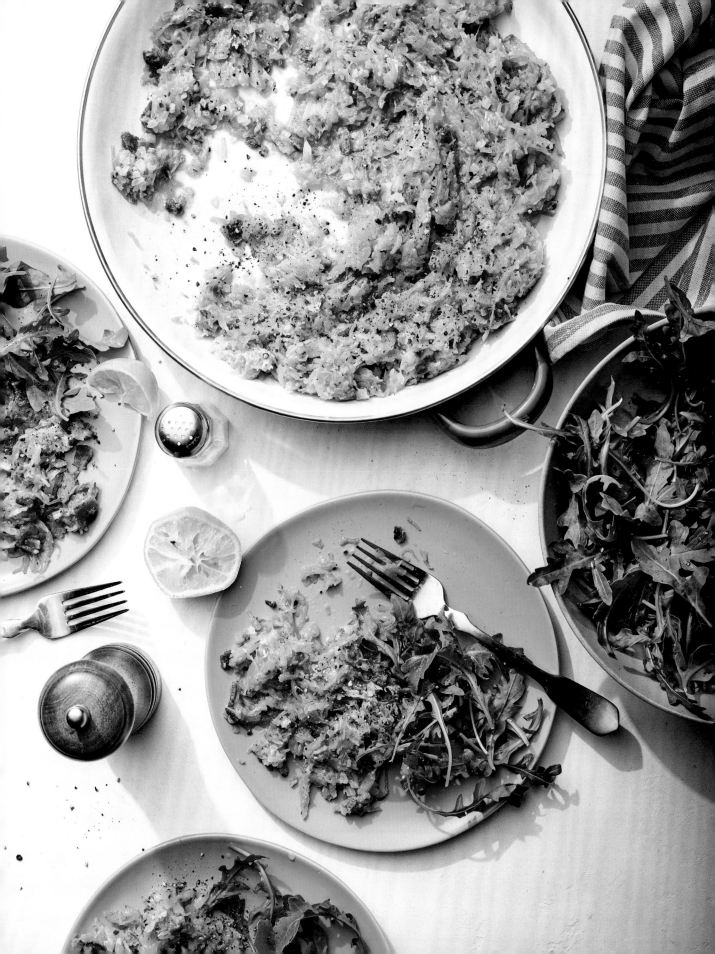

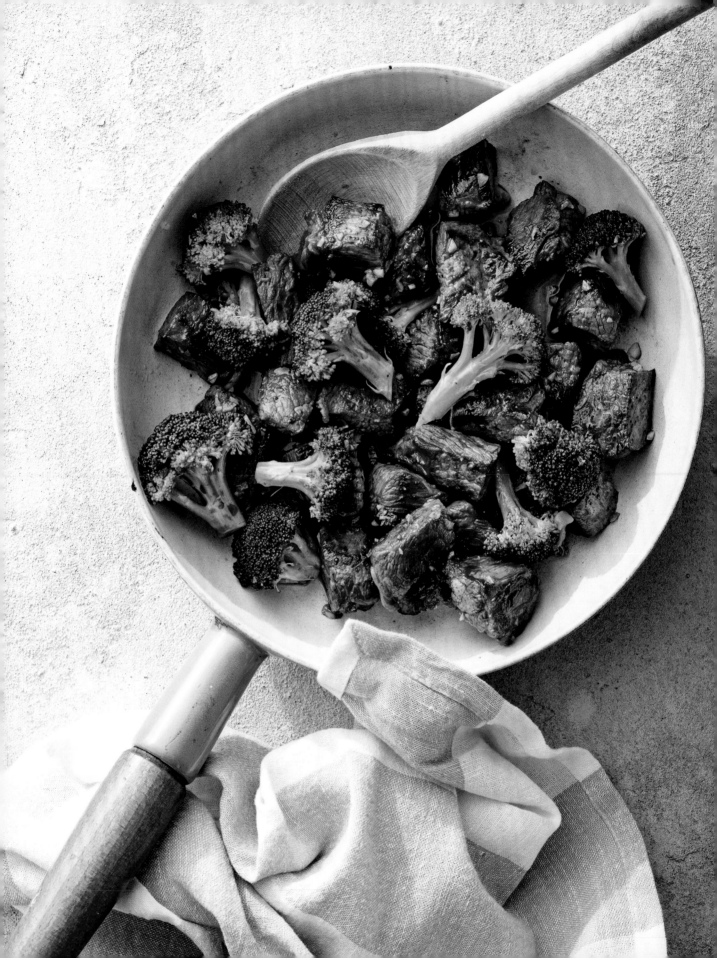

Garlic-Butter Steak Bites with Broccoli

SERVES 4

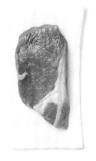

I love a good steak, but I also love steak bites (cubed sirloin steak) because they're so quick and easy to cook! Not to mention, steak smothered in garlic butter is just a perfect combination. Of course, I had to add some veggies to this dish, and you can never go wrong with beef and broccoli. If you want to change things up, though, chopped bell peppers and onions are also a great idea. The best part? The entire meal takes less than 15 minutes from start to finish! Serve over rice, mashed potatoes, cauliflower, or your favorite grain and you're all set.

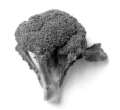

1¼ pounds sirloin steak or filet mignon, cut into 1-inch cubes

4 cups broccoli florets (10 ounces)

2 tablespoons salted butter

4 garlic cloves, minced

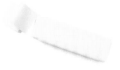

Season the steak with 1 teaspoon kosher salt and freshly ground black pepper to taste.

Heat a large cast-iron or 12-inch heavy skillet over high heat. When hot, spray with olive oil. Add the steak in a single layer. (Don't overcrowd the pan; if your pan is smaller, work in batches.) Let the steak sear undisturbed until the bottom is browned, about 1 minute. Cook, stirring occasionally, until golden brown all over, about 2 minutes more. Set aside on a large plate.

Reduce the heat to low and wipe out the skillet. Spray the pan with oil and add the broccoli, 2 tablespoons water, and ⅛ teaspoon kosher salt. Cover and cook, stirring halfway, until crisp-tender and bright green, about 2 minutes. Scoop out of the skillet and set aside with the steak.

Increase the heat under the skillet to medium-low and add the butter. When melted, add the garlic and cook, stirring, until golden, about 1 minute. Return the broccoli and beef with any juices and stir to coat well. Serve immediately.

Per Serving (1½ cups) ● Calories 269 ● Fat 14 g ● Saturated Fat 6.5 g ● Cholesterol 110 mg
Carbohydrate 6 g ● Fiber 2 g ● Protein 33 g ● Sugars 1 g ● Sodium 463 mg

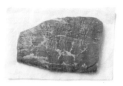

Grilled London Broil
with Tomatoes, Onion, and Basil

SERVES 6

This is one of my favorite ways to prepare grilled steak in the summer when tomatoes are at their peak. Although you can use any steak, London broil is perfect to cook for four to six people because it's inexpensive and you have only one steak to mind and flip instead of several smaller pieces.

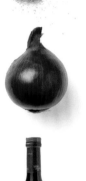

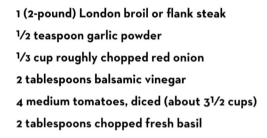

1 (2-pound) London broil or flank steak

1/2 teaspoon garlic powder

1/3 cup roughly chopped red onion

2 tablespoons balsamic vinegar

4 medium tomatoes, diced (about 31/2 cups)

2 tablespoons chopped fresh basil

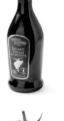

Poke the steak all over with a fork. Season with 1¼ teaspoons kosher salt, freshly ground black pepper to taste, and the garlic powder. Set aside at room temperature for about 30 minutes while you prepare the rest of the dish.

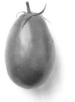

In a large bowl, combine the red onion, 1 tablespoon extra-virgin olive oil, the balsamic vinegar, ¼ teaspoon kosher salt, and freshly ground black pepper to taste. Let the onion sit for 2 to 3 minutes to mellow its sharp taste. Add the tomatoes and basil and toss to combine. Adjust the salt to taste, if needed.

Preheat the grill or broiler on high heat. Cook the steak until it registers 130° to 140°F for medium-rare, about 7 minutes per side, or longer, if desired. Remove the steak from the grill and loosely tent with foil. Let it rest for 10 minutes.

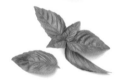

Carve the steak into thin slices across the grain. Transfer to a serving platter, top with the tomato-onion salad, and serve.

Per Serving (4 ounces steak + generous ½ cup salad) ● Calories 269 ● Fat 12 g
Saturated Fat 4.5 g ● Cholesterol 104 mg ● Carbohydrate 5 g ● Fiber 1 g ● Protein 34 g
Sugars 3 g ● Sodium 372 mg

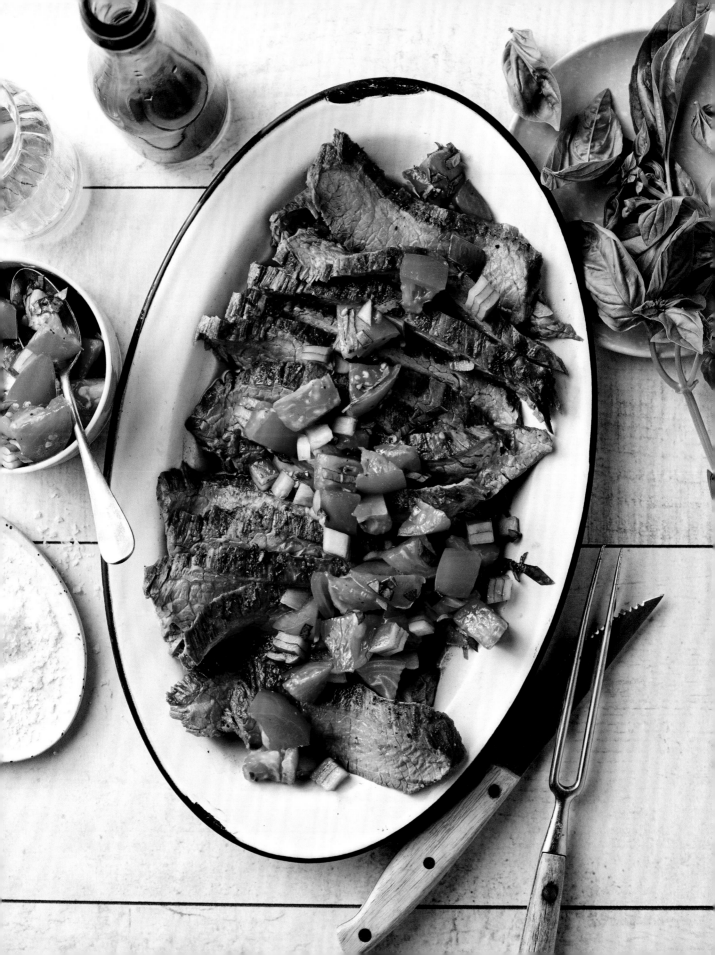

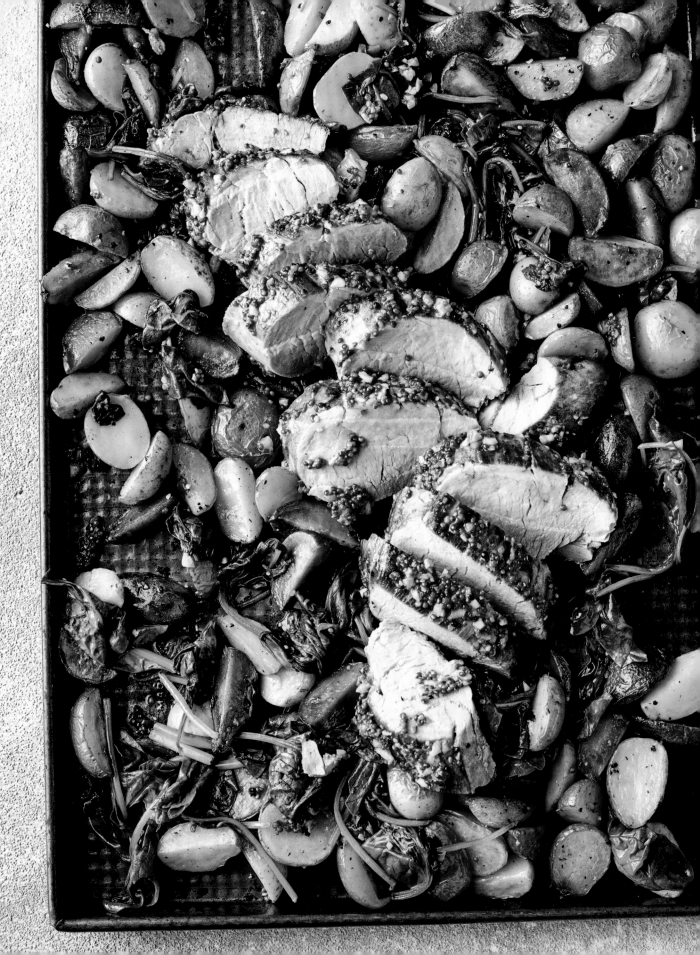

Sheet Pan Pork Tenderloin with Potatoes and Spinach

SERVES 4

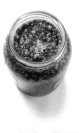

This dish came out better than I even hoped! It has only five ingredients, but it's packed with flavor thanks to one of my favorite refrigerator staples, whole-grain Dijon mustard. I love the grainy texture and tender pop of mustard seeds. It gives a plain piece of pork a whole new dimension. And who knew you could wilt spinach on a sheet pan? This one-pan dish is ready in less than 40 minutes, and if you use foil, cleanup is easy, too.

2 tablespoons whole-grain Dijon mustard (I love Maille Old Style), plus more for serving

4 garlic cloves, minced

1 (1½-pound) pork tenderloin

1½ pounds baby potatoes, quartered

1 (6-ounce) bag baby spinach

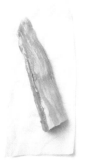

Preheat the oven to 425°F. Spray a sheet pan with oil (or for easy cleanup, line it first with foil and then spray with oil).

In a small bowl, mix the mustard, half of the garlic, ½ teaspoon kosher salt, and freshly ground black pepper to taste. Place the tenderloin on one side of the prepared sheet pan and spread the mustard-garlic mixture all over it.

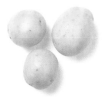

On the other side of the sheet pan, toss the potatoes with 2½ tablespoons extra-virgin olive oil, ½ teaspoon kosher salt, and freshly ground black pepper to taste.

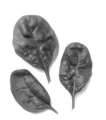

Roast until the pork reaches an internal temperature of 140°F and the potatoes are browned and tender, about 30 minutes, tossing the potatoes halfway.

Transfer the pork to a cutting board and let it rest for 5 minutes before serving (the temperature will climb to 145°F). Meanwhile, stir the spinach and remaining minced garlic into the potatoes. Return the pan to the oven and continue to roast until the spinach wilts, 2 to 3 minutes more.

Slice the pork and serve with the potatoes and spinach, with more mustard for the pork on the side.

Per Serving (4½ ounces pork + generous ½ cup veggies) ● Calories 409 ● Fat 13 g
Saturated Fat 2.5 g ● Cholesterol 111 mg ● Carbohydrate 31 g ● Fiber 4 g ● Protein 40 g
Sugars 2 g ● Sodium 584 mg

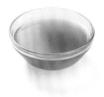

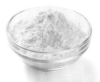

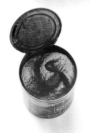

Baked Beef Stew
with Butternut Squash

SERVES 6

Warm and hearty beef stew is the best cold-weather comfort food, and it's even better made with winter squash in place of potatoes for extra flavor and nutrition. Most stew recipes begin and end on the stovetop, but I prefer baking this stew in the oven because it's so much easier! It's completely hands-off cooking—no need to stir or monitor the heat of the stovetop all day. After just a few hours in the oven, you'll have fork-tender beef in a veggie-rich gravy that's perfect served over rice or with crusty bread. You can use acorn squash or pumpkin in place of butternut, if you'd like.

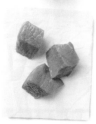

2 cups low-sodium beef broth*

3 tablespoons all-purpose or gluten-free flour

2 tablespoons tomato paste

2¼ pounds lean beef chuck stew meat, trimmed and cut into 1-inch cubes

4 cups 1-inch cubes peeled butternut squash

1 large onion, cut into 1-inch pieces

3 sprigs of fresh thyme

*Read the label to be sure this product is gluten-free.

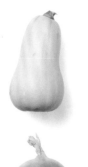

Preheat the oven to 375°F.

In a blender, combine the broth, flour, tomato paste, 1¼ teaspoons kosher salt, and ¼ teaspoon freshly ground black pepper and blend until smooth.

Arrange the beef, squash, onion, and thyme in a 9 × 13-inch baking dish. Pour the broth mixture on top and cover tightly with foil. Bake until the meat and vegetables are tender, about 2 hours.

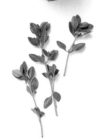

Remove the foil, discard the thyme, and stir. Serve warm.

Per Serving (1⅓ cups) ● Calories 301 ● Fat 8 g ● Saturated Fat 3 g ● Cholesterol 109 mg
Carbohydrate 20 g ● Fiber 2.5 g ● Protein 40 g ● Sugars 5 g ● Sodium 425 mg

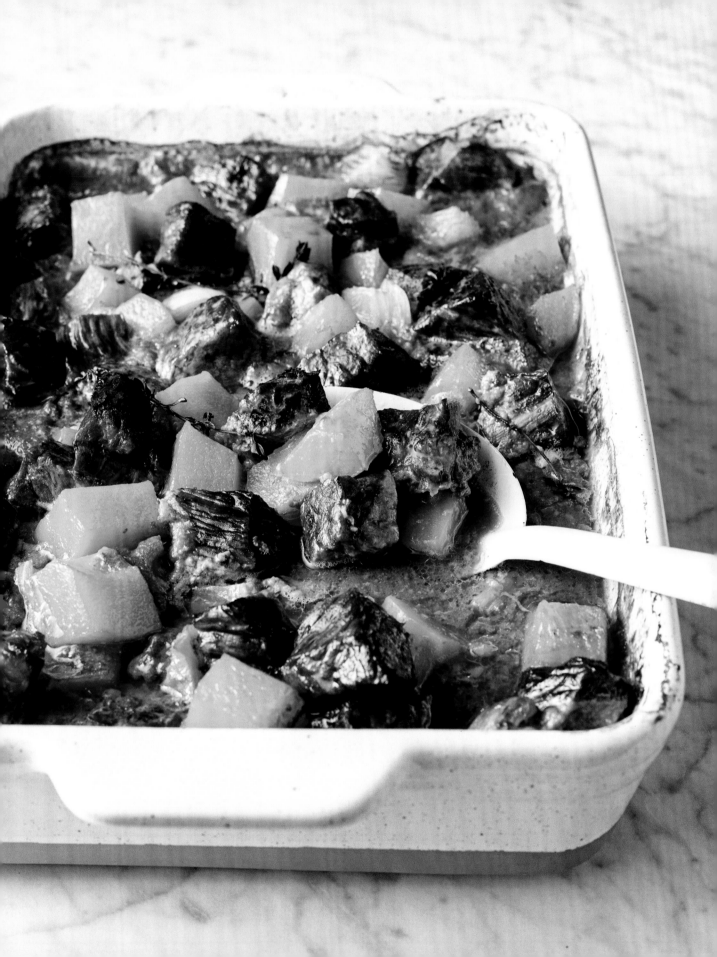

From
the Sea

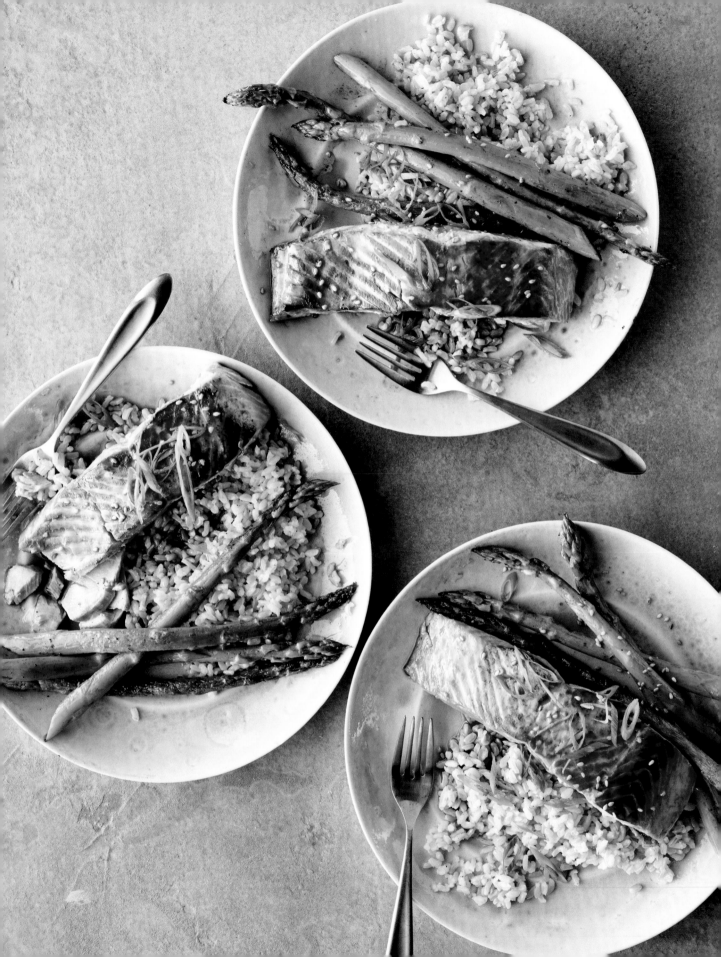

Sheet Pan Teriyaki Salmon with Asparagus

SERVES 4

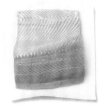

This is the easiest teriyaki salmon! The sauce uses just two ingredients and it caramelizes beautifully in the broiler. The sweetness comes from the mirin (sweetened rice wine), so there's no need to add additional sugar or honey. If asparagus is not in season, green beans can be used instead.

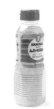

4 skinless salmon fillets (6 ounces each)

¼ cup mirin

¼ cup reduced-sodium soy sauce or gluten-free tamari

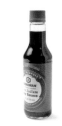

1 pound asparagus, tough ends trimmed

3 cups cooked brown rice, heated

1 teaspoon toasted sesame seeds

1 medium scallion, green tops only, thinly sliced, for garnish

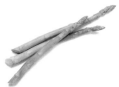

Pat the salmon dry with paper towels. In a large shallow bowl, combine the mirin and soy sauce. Add the salmon to the bowl and marinate for about 10 minutes, flipping halfway.

Adjust an oven rack to 6 inches from the heating element and preheat the broiler to high. Line a sheet pan with foil.

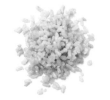

Carefully transfer the salmon to one side of the prepared sheet pan, reserving the teriyaki marinade in the bowl. Add the asparagus to the other side of the sheet pan and spray the asparagus a few times with olive oil and add a pinch of kosher salt. Broil the salmon and asparagus until the fish flakes easily with a fork and the asparagus is slightly charred, flipping both halfway, 3 to 4 minutes on each side.

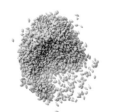

Meanwhile, transfer the reserved marinade to a small skillet. Place over low heat and cook until slightly thickened, 2 to 3 minutes.

To serve, scoop ¾ cup of rice into each of four bowls and top with the salmon and asparagus. Drizzle each serving with the reduced sauce and sprinkle with the sesame seeds and scallion greens.

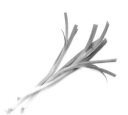

Per Serving (1 salmon fillet + ¼ of the asparagus + ¾ cup rice) ● Calories 458 ● Fat 12 g
Saturated Fat 2 g ● Cholesterol 94 mg ● Carbohydrate 46 g ● Fiber 5 g ● Protein 41 g
Sugars 8 g ● Sodium 767 mg

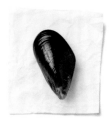

Mussels in Coconut-Tomato Broth

SERVES 4

Eating mussels at home always feels special, but it's such an easy dish to pull off because of how relatively affordable mussels are, their short cooking time, and how it's all done in one pot. This light coconut broth (inspired by Asian and Caribbean flavors) enhances, rather than overwhelms, the delicate taste of the mussels. If you'd like some heat, though, add some crushed red pepper flakes or 1 diced red chile along with the garlic.

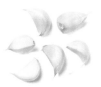

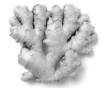

2¹/₂ pounds mussels (about 64), scrubbed and debearded

1 tablespoon minced garlic

1 teaspoon grated fresh ginger

4 tablespoons chopped fresh cilantro

1¹/₂ cups cherry tomatoes, quartered

1 (13.5-ounce) can light coconut milk

8 ounces crusty bread, regular or gluten-free, cut into 4 pieces and toasted

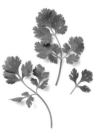

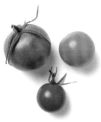

Discard any mussels with broken shells. In a large heavy pot or Dutch oven, heat 1 teaspoon extra-virgin olive oil over medium heat. Add the garlic, ginger, and 2 tablespoons of the cilantro and cook until fragrant, about 1 minute. Add the cherry tomatoes and cook until they start to soften, about 2 minutes.

Add the coconut milk and ¼ teaspoon kosher salt and bring to a simmer. Add the mussels and cover the pot. Reduce the heat to low and cook until the mussels open, 5 to 6 minutes. Discard any mussels that don't open.

Divide the mussels and broth among four bowls and sprinkle with the remaining 2 tablespoons cilantro. Serve with the toasted bread.

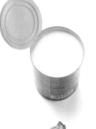

Per Serving (about 16 mussels + ¾ cup broth + 2 ounces bread) ● Calories 456 ● Fat 13 g Saturated Fat 5.5 g ● Cholesterol 72 mg ● Carbohydrate 44 g ● Fiber 2 g ● Protein 38 g Sugars 4 g ● Sodium 1,194 mg

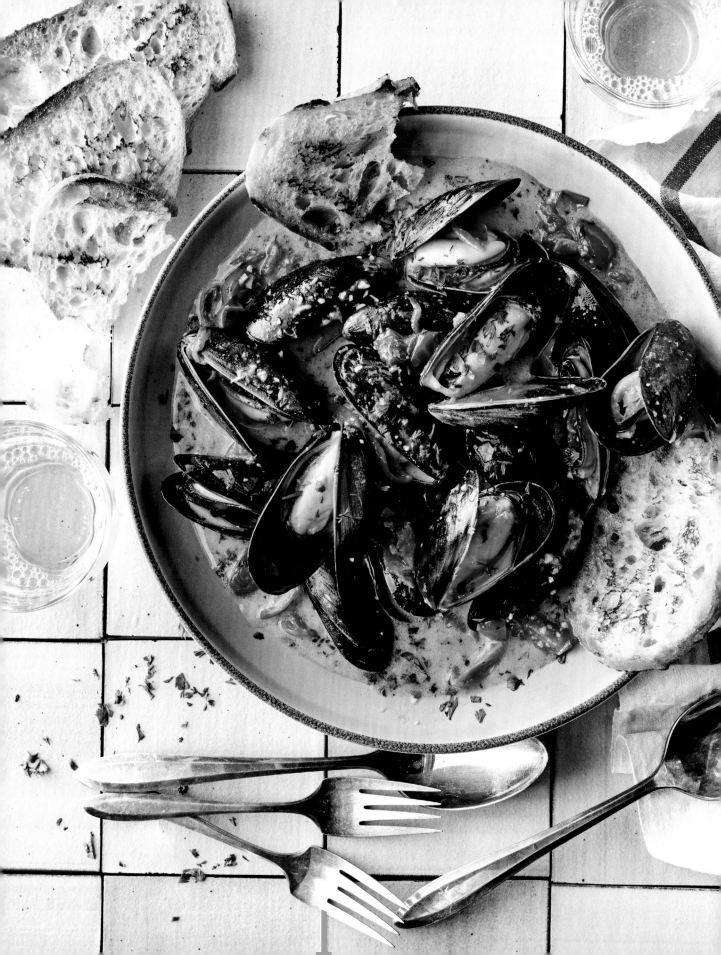

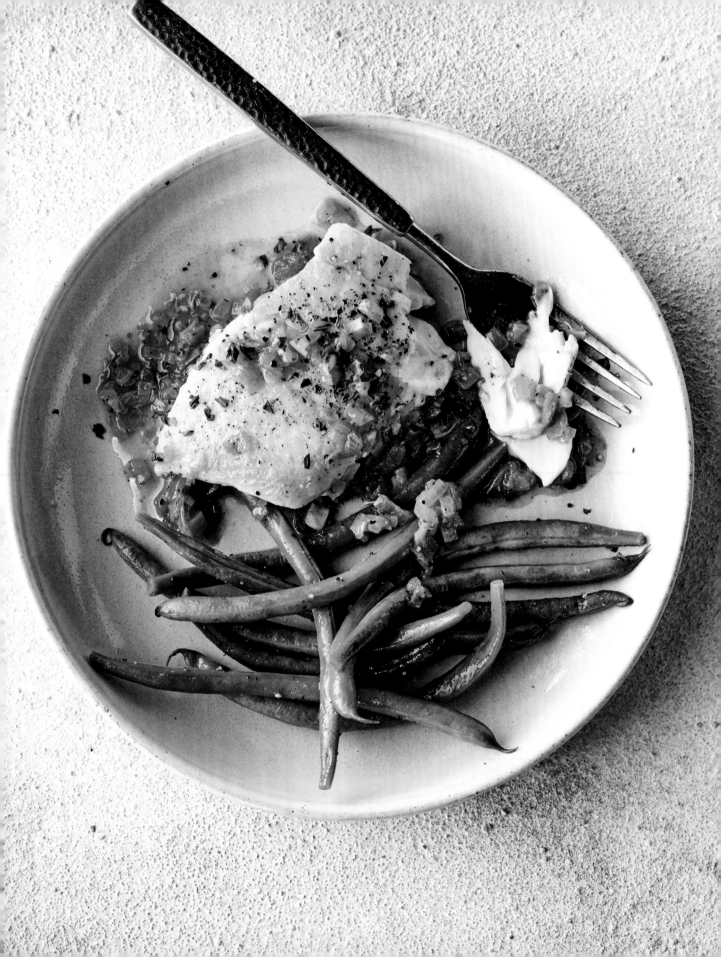

Skillet Fish with Caramelized Shallots and Lemon Brown Butter Sauce

SERVES 4

Butter, lemon, and sweet flaky whitefish are a match made in heaven! Searing the fish and browning the butter make this dish even more divine, and the quick caramelized shallots bring a sweet bite. You need only a little butter to create a rich sauce worthy of a fancy restaurant. Any fresh whitefish can be used in this dish; I love it with halibut, but I usually buy local or whatever my fishmonger tells me is freshest. Serve the fish with green beans or asparagus.

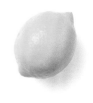

4 halibut fillets (6 ounces each) or striped bass, haddock, flounder, or fluke

1 lemon, halved

3 tablespoons salted butter

2 small shallots, finely chopped

Finely chopped fresh flat-leaf parsley, for garnish

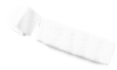

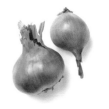

Pat the fish dry with paper towels and season with ¼ teaspoon kosher salt and freshly ground black pepper to taste. Place a large skillet over medium-high heat and spray with olive oil. Add the fish and cook until browned on the outside and opaque halfway through, 3 to 4 minutes, depending on the thickness. Gently flip the fish and cook until it flakes easily with a fork, 2 to 3 minutes more. Remove from the skillet and set aside on a plate.

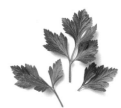

Meanwhile, juice half of the lemon. Cut the other lemon half into 4 wedges for serving. Set both aside.

Reduce the heat under the skillet to medium and add the butter to the pan, swirling to coat. Once melted, the butter will begin to foam; continue to cook, stirring, until it just turns golden brown, 2 to 3 minutes. Add the shallots and cook, scraping the browned bits from the pan with a wooden spoon, until softened and caramelized, about 1 minute.

Reduce the heat to low and quickly add the lemon juice, 2 tablespoons water, ⅛ teaspoon salt, and black pepper to taste and whisk to combine. Return the fish to the pan to warm through, spooning the sauce over the fish, about 30 seconds.

Divide the fish and the pan sauce among four plates (or transfer all of it to a serving platter) and top with the parsley. Serve with the lemon wedges.

Per Serving (1 fillet) ● Calories 242 ● Fat 11 g ● Saturated Fat 6 g ● Cholesterol 106 mg
Carbohydrate 3 g ● Fiber 0.5 g ● Protein 32 g ● Sugars 1 g ● Sodium 292 mg

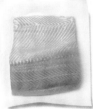

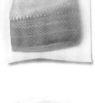

Air Fryer Crispy Salmon Nuggets

SERVES 2

These bite-size panko-crusted salmon nuggets just explode with flavor. You get the crunch from the crispy coating and a juicy center with every bite! This recipe would also work with cod or any other whitefish.

SKINNY SCOOP: If you don't have lemon pepper on hand, use a mixture of freshly ground black pepper and grated lemon zest. Also, if you want to make a simple tartar sauce, combine ¼ cup fat-free Greek yogurt, ¼ cup light mayonnaise, 2 tablespoons chopped dill pickles, juice of ½ lemon, and chopped fresh dill. Mix and serve with the salmon.

12 ounces skinless wild salmon fillet, 1½ inches thick, or arctic char or steelhead trout

2 tablespoons light mayonnaise

½ teaspoon lemon pepper or garlic pepper seasoning (see Skinny Scoop)

¼ teaspoon sweet paprika

½ cup seasoned panko bread crumbs, regular or gluten-free

Lemon wedges, for serving (optional)

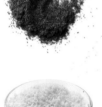

Cut the salmon into sixteen 1½-inch cubes and season with ¼ teaspoon kosher salt.

In a medium bowl, combine the mayonnaise, lemon pepper, and paprika. Place the panko in a separate shallow bowl. Add the salmon to the mayonnaise mixture and toss to coat, then transfer to the panko and toss again to coat.

Place the salmon on a work surface and spray the top sides with olive oil.

Spray an air fryer basket with olive oil. Add the salmon to the basket in a single layer, oiled side down. Spray the other side of the salmon with more oil and cook at 400°F until golden and crisp, 6 to 7 minutes, flipping halfway through.

Transfer the salmon nuggets to a plate and serve with lemon wedges, if desired.

NO AIR FRYER? NO PROBLEM! Preheat the oven to 425°F. Arrange the breaded salmon nuggets on a baking sheet and spray with oil. Bake until the salmon nuggets are golden and crisp, 8 to 10 minutes; no need to flip.

Per Serving (8 nuggets) ● Calories 322 ● Fat 15 g ● Saturated Fat 2 g ● Cholesterol 96 mg Carbohydrate 10 g ● Fiber 0.5 g ● Protein 35 g ● Sugars 1 g ● Sodium 545 mg

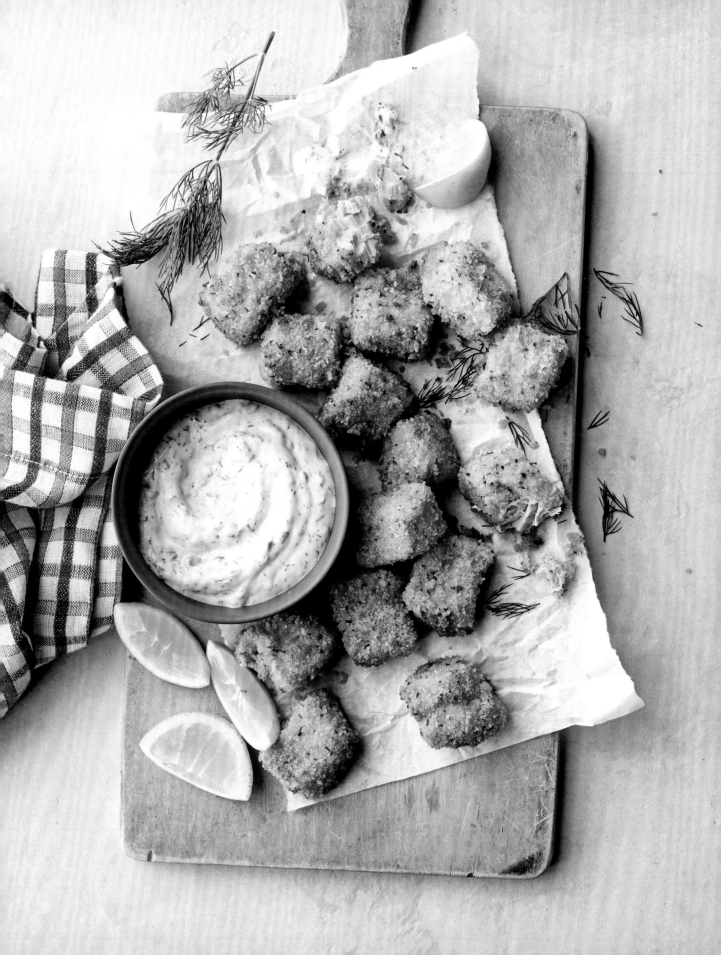

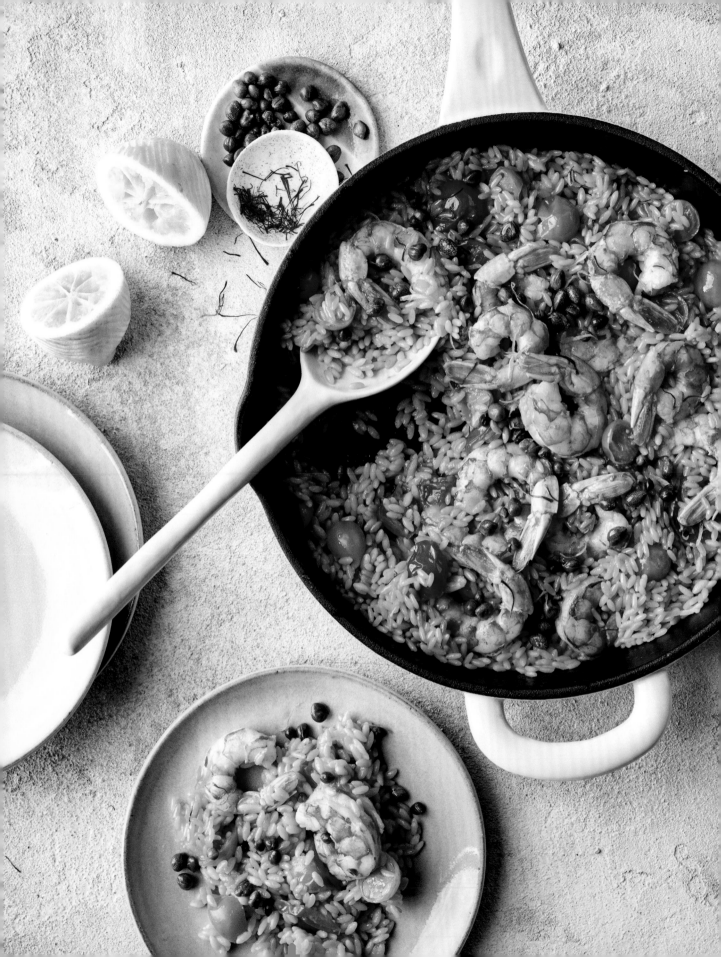

One-Pan Shrimp and Saffron Orzo

SERVES 4

This one-pan pasta dish gives me paella vibes! Paella is a classic Spanish rice dish made with rice, saffron, veggies, and protein cooked in one pan, but here I've swapped out the rice for rice-shaped orzo pasta. It's a really versatile dish, so you can make it with any seafood you like. I used just shrimp for this version, but you can do half shrimp and half littleneck clams, or add some fish or even lobster meat.

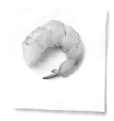

1 pound peeled and deveined large shrimp

8 ounces orzo pasta (1¹/₃ cups)

2 cups chicken or vegetable broth

1 teaspoon saffron threads

1 cup halved mixed color cherry tomatoes

Grated zest and juice of ¹/₂ lemon

2 tablespoons capers, drained

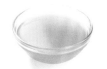

In a large bowl, season the shrimp with ¼ teaspoon kosher salt and freshly ground black pepper to taste.

In a large deep skillet, heat 1 tablespoon extra-virgin olive oil over medium heat. Add the orzo and cook, stirring frequently, until toasted, 3 to 4 minutes.

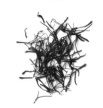

Add the broth and saffron and bring to a boil over high heat. Stir in the tomatoes and season with ½ teaspoon kosher salt. Reduce the heat to low, cover, and cook until the orzo is partially cooked, about 8 minutes.

Stir in the shrimp, cover, and cook until the liquid is absorbed, the pasta is tender, and the shrimp are opaque, 4 to 5 minutes more. Uncover, and if there's still some liquid, cook uncovered for 1 more minute. Remove from the heat.

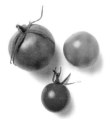

Squeeze the lemon over the pasta and top with the zest and capers before serving.

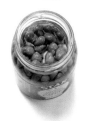

Per Serving (1½ cups) ● Calories 359 ● Fat 7 g ● Saturated Fat 1.5 g ● Cholesterol 168 mg
Carbohydrate 43 g ● Fiber 2.5 g ● Protein 30 g ● Sugars 3 g ● Sodium 709 mg

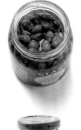

Broiled Fish with Salsa Verde

SERVES 4

This herby, garlicky green sauce, made with capers and anchovies, is a perfect complement to any whitefish. It's similar to an Argentinian chimichurri, but don't confuse it with a Mexican salsa verde, which is made with tomatillos. The sauce can be made up to 4 days ahead, although the color will dull after a day or two.

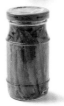

2 tablespoons capers, drained, plus 1 tablespoon of the brine

2 oil-packed anchovy fillets

2 garlic cloves, coarsely chopped

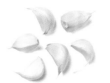

2/3 cup fresh flat-leaf parsley

1/8 teaspoon crushed red pepper flakes

4 white-fleshed fish fillets (6 ounces each), such as cod, halibut, or striped bass

Lemon wedges, for serving

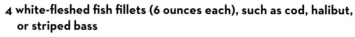

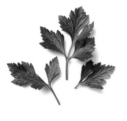

In a small food processor, combine the capers, anchovies, and garlic and pulse until finely chopped. Add the parsley and pulse a few times. Add ¼ cup extra-virgin olive oil, the caper brine, and pepper flakes and pulse until chopped and coarse. If too thick, add a tablespoon of water to loosen. Set the salsa verde aside.

Adjust an oven rack to 6 inches from the heating element and preheat the broiler to high.

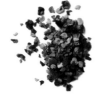

Spray a large baking sheet with olive oil and arrange the fish fillets in a single layer on top. Season both sides of the fish with ¾ teaspoon salt and freshly ground black pepper to taste. Broil until opaque and cooked through, 5 to 8 minutes depending on the thickness. (No need to flip.)

Serve the fish topped with the salsa verde and with lemon wedges on the side.

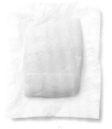

Per Serving (1 fillet + 2 tablespoons salsa verde) ● Calories 249 ● Fat 15 g ● Saturated Fat 2 g Cholesterol 82 mg ● Carbohydrate 2 g ● Fiber 0.5 g ● Protein 27 g ● Sugars 0 g ● Sodium 906 mg

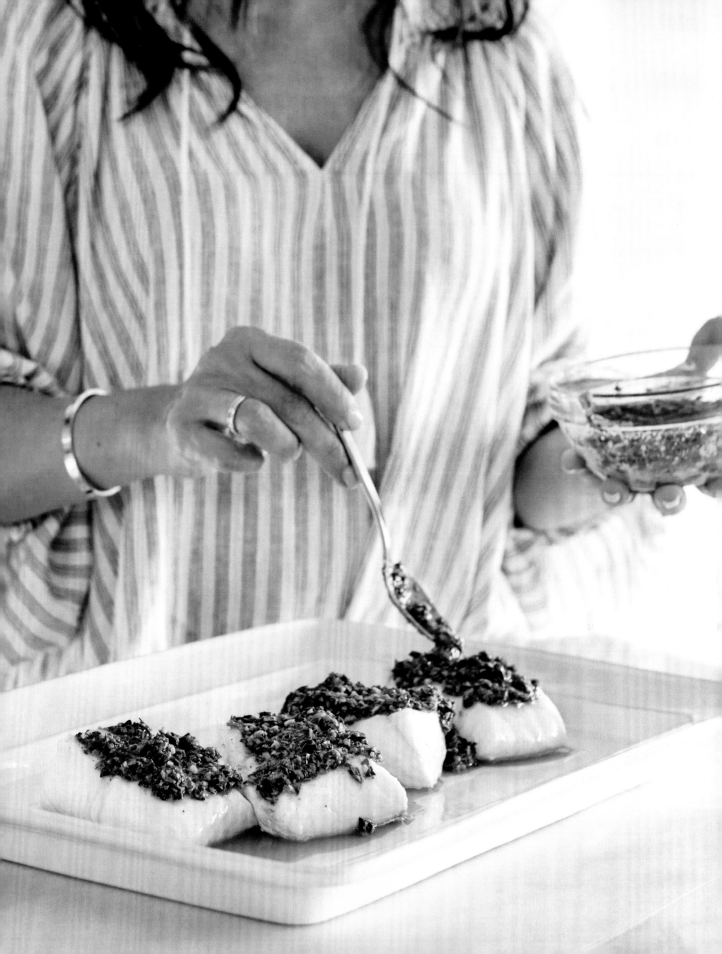

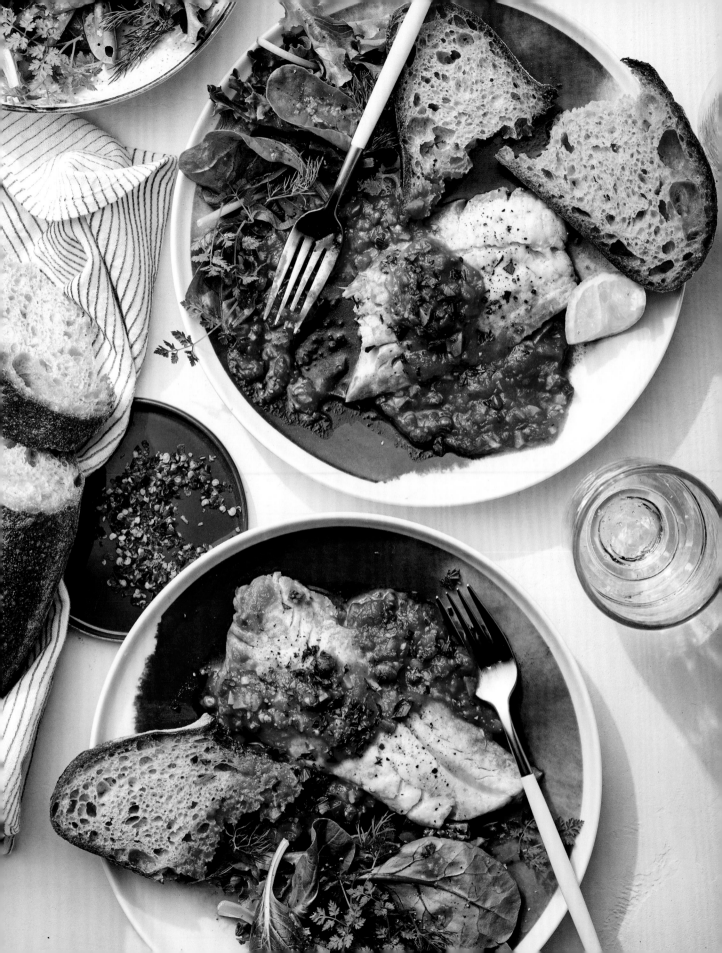

Red Snapper
with Tomatoes and Olives

SERVES 2

Seafood cooked in this style is called Livornese, meaning it originated from the Italian port town of Livorno in Tuscany. Made with tomatoes, capers, olives, white wine, and garlic, this is my brother's favorite way to eat fish. He eats it over pasta, but you can also serve it as is, or with a salad and some bread. I used red snapper here, but any whitefish fillet will work. Garnish with chopped fresh parsley if you have it on hand.

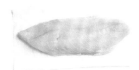

2 skinless fish fillets (6 ounces each), such as red snapper, cod, or flounder

8 mixed pitted oil-marinated olives, drained and chopped, plus 1 teaspoon of the oil

2 garlic cloves, minced

1 cup good-quality marinara sauce

¼ cup dry white wine

1 tablespoon capers, drained, plus 1 teaspoon of the brine

⅛ teaspoon crushed red pepper flakes, or more to taste

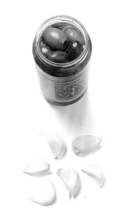

Season the fish with ¼ teaspoon kosher salt and freshly ground black pepper to taste.

In a skillet large enough to hold both fish fillets, heat the oil from the olives over medium heat. Add the garlic and cook, stirring, until golden, about 1 minute. Add the marinara sauce and the wine and simmer for 1 minute to let the alcohol cook out. Reduce the heat to low, then add the olives, capers, caper brine, and pepper flakes. Simmer for 2 to 3 minutes to let the flavors meld.

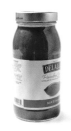

Nestle the fish in the sauce, cover, and cook until the fish flakes easily with a fork, 6 to 8 minutes (depending on the thickness). Using a wide spatula, carefully transfer the fish to a serving plate (it will be delicate). Spoon the sauce over the fish and serve immediately.

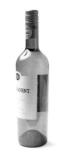

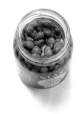

Per Serving (1 fillet + ½ cup sauce) • Calories 277 • Fat 7 g • Saturated Fat 1 g • Cholesterol 82 mg
Carbohydrate 13 g • Fiber 1 g • Protein 33 g • Sugars 5 g • Sodium 791 mg

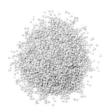

Gingery Shrimp and Quinoa "Fried Rice"

SERVES 4

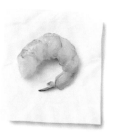

This ginger-infused "fried rice" dish swaps out the rice for quinoa, and that's a really good thing for your body! Quinoa is a complete protein, meaning it contains all nine essential amino acids your body needs. It's also a good source of the minerals magnesium and copper, which play important roles in energy metabolism and bone health. Plus, it offers more dietary fiber and protein than brown rice. I really loved this with sesame oil, so if you have any in your pantry, use it in place of the vegetable oil called for!

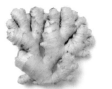

1 cup white quinoa,* rinsed well

1 pound peeled and deveined shrimp, cut into 1-inch pieces

1 tablespoon grated fresh ginger and/or minced garlic

1 cup frozen peas and carrots (no need to thaw)

6 scallions, white and green parts kept separate, chopped

2 large eggs, beaten

3 tablespoons reduced-sodium soy sauce or gluten-free tamari

*Read the label to be sure this product is gluten-free.

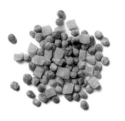

Cook the quinoa according to the package directions.

Meanwhile, in a medium bowl, toss the shrimp with ½ tablespoon of the ginger. Heat a large nonstick wok or deep skillet over high heat. Spray with oil, add the shrimp, and cook until pink and cooked through in the center, about 1 minute per side. Remove the shrimp from the wok and set aside.

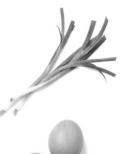

Add 2 teaspoons vegetable oil, the remaining ½ tablespoon ginger, the frozen vegetables, and scallion whites to the wok. Cook until browned, stirring, about 2 minutes. Push the vegetable mixture to one side of the pan. Add the eggs to the cleared space and scramble.

Add the cooked quinoa and shrimp along with the soy sauce and mix well until thoroughly combined, another 30 seconds. Top with the scallion greens and serve.

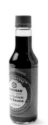

Per Serving (1½ generous cups) ● Calories 366 ● Fat 9 g ● Saturated Fat 2.5 g
Cholesterol 261 mg ● Carbohydrate 34 g ● Fiber 5 g ● Protein 35 g ● Sugars 1 g
Sodium 600 mg

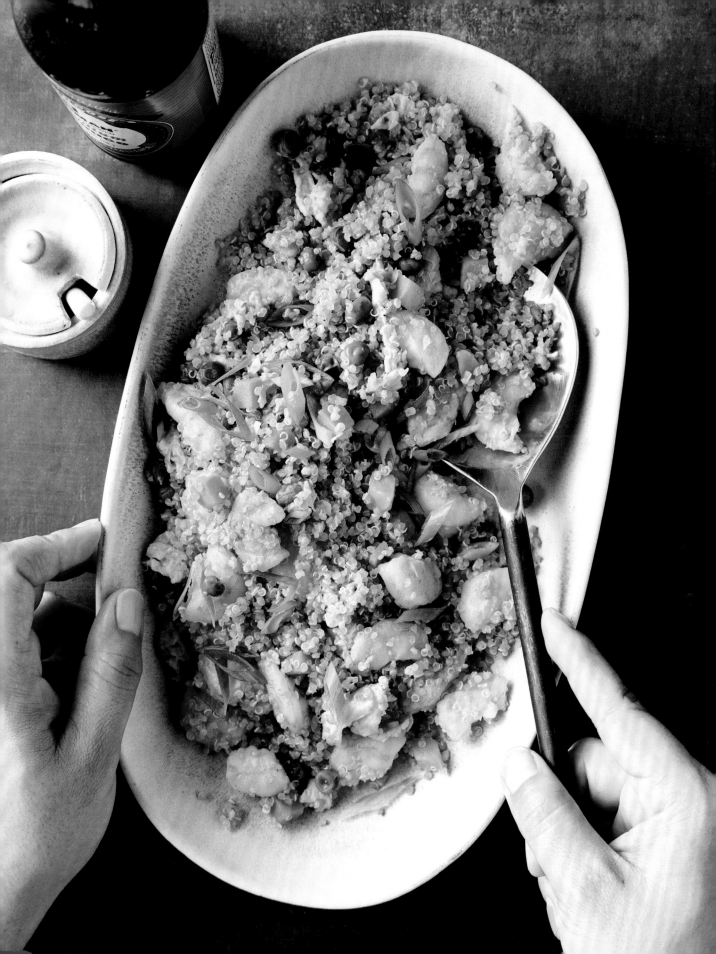

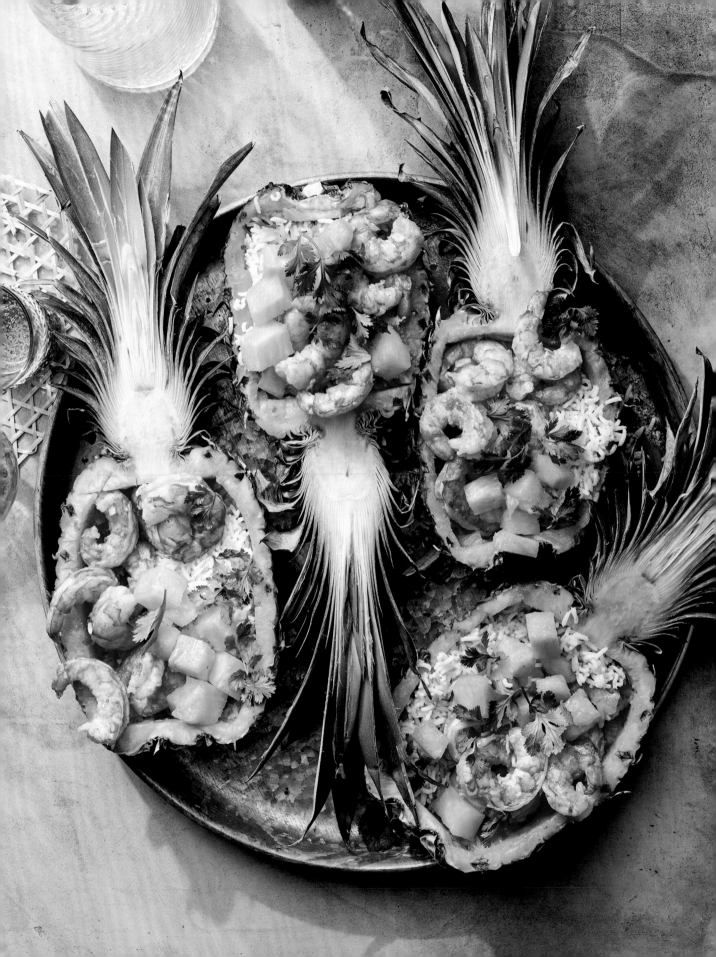

Sweet and Spicy Shrimp Pineapple Boats

SERVES 4

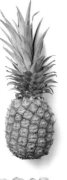

I really love the combination of pineapple and shrimp. They're great together in stir-fries and on skewers, but I especially love the duo in these spicy rice boats. It's not just delicious—using the pineapple as a serving dish makes it pretty to look at, too!

SKINNY SCOOP: If you prefer to skip the whole pineapples, you can use 3 cups diced fresh pineapple and simply serve in bowls. I also recommend using half garlic and half ginger, if you have them both on hand for the best flavor.

2 whole medium pineapples (see Skinny Scoop)

1 tablespoon minced fresh ginger and/or garlic

1¼ pounds peeled and deveined extra-large shrimp

¼ cup Thai sweet chili sauce

1 tablespoon Sriracha sauce

3 cups cooked basmati rice, warmed

¼ cup chopped fresh cilantro or scallions, for garnish

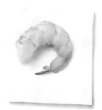

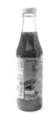

Cut each pineapple in half lengthwise. Cut out and discard the core, then slice the pineapple flesh into chunks by making a 1-inch grid pattern, being careful not to cut through the outer skin. Use a large serving spoon to scoop out the pieces and hollow out both halves to make four bowls. Cut a piece off the underside of the pineapple halves to create a flat base. Cut the pineapple flesh into 1-inch chunks until you have 3 cups. (Save the remainder for another meal or snack.)

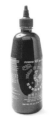

In a large nonstick skillet or wok, heat ½ tablespoon extra-virgin olive or vegetable oil over medium-high heat. Add the ginger and/or garlic and stir-fry until fragrant, about 30 seconds. Add the shrimp and cook until opaque, 2 to 3 minutes. Add the Thai sweet chili sauce and Sriracha and stir until heated through, about 30 seconds.

Fill each pineapple boat with ¾ cup rice and top each with the shrimp mixture. Arrange the pineapple cubes alongside the shrimp. Garnish with cilantro or scallions and serve.

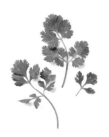

Per Serving (1 boat) ● Calories 422 ● Fat 5 g ● Saturated Fat 1.5 g ● Cholesterol 210 mg
Carbohydrate 60 g ● Fiber 2.5 g ● Protein 33 g ● Sugars 20 g ● Sodium 475 mg

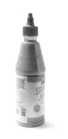

Spicy Crab Sushi Stacks

SERVES 2

 Q GF DF

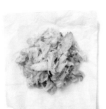

Here's a way to get your sushi fix in just minutes! Grab some crabmeat (imitation will also work), cucumbers, and frozen brown rice and whip up this easy dish that looks like you put in a lot of effort. If you've tried the popular shrimp stacks on Skinnytaste.com, you'll love this variation. You can swap the crab for cooked salmon, sushi-grade tuna, or cooked diced shrimp, and swap out half the cucumber for avocado if you like.

SKINNY SCOOP: You can make your own spicy mayo by combining mayo and Sriracha. You can use equal parts or less Sriracha to make it milder. I like it spicy so I usually top my stack with even more Sriracha!

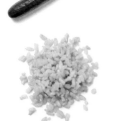

2 tablespoons spicy Sriracha mayo, plus more (optional) for topping (see Skinny Scoop)

8 ounces (1½ cups) lump crabmeat (canned or imitation is also fine)

2 cups diced peeled cucumber (about 1 medium)

1⅓ cups cooked or frozen brown rice, warmed

4 teaspoons reduced-sodium soy sauce or gluten-free tamari

2 teaspoons furikake or black and white sesame seeds

¼ cup chopped fresh chives

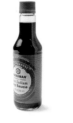

In a medium bowl, combine the Sriracha mayo and crab.

Spray the inside of a 1-cup dry measuring cup with oil, then, in this order, layer in ½ cup cucumber, then one-quarter (2 ounces) of the spicy crab, and ⅓ cup rice, gently packing as you go.

Carefully turn the cup upside down onto a plate to turn the stack out, lightly tapping the bottom of the cup if necessary. Repeat to make 4 stacks. Drizzle each stack with 1 teaspoon soy sauce plus more spicy mayo (optional) on top. Sprinkle with the furikake and chives.

Serve immediately.

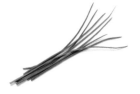

Per Serving (2 stacks) • Calories 369 • Fat 12 g • Saturated Fat 1.5 g • Cholesterol 116 mg
Carbohydrate 34 g • Fiber 3 g • Protein 28 g • Sugars 2 g • Sodium 924 mg

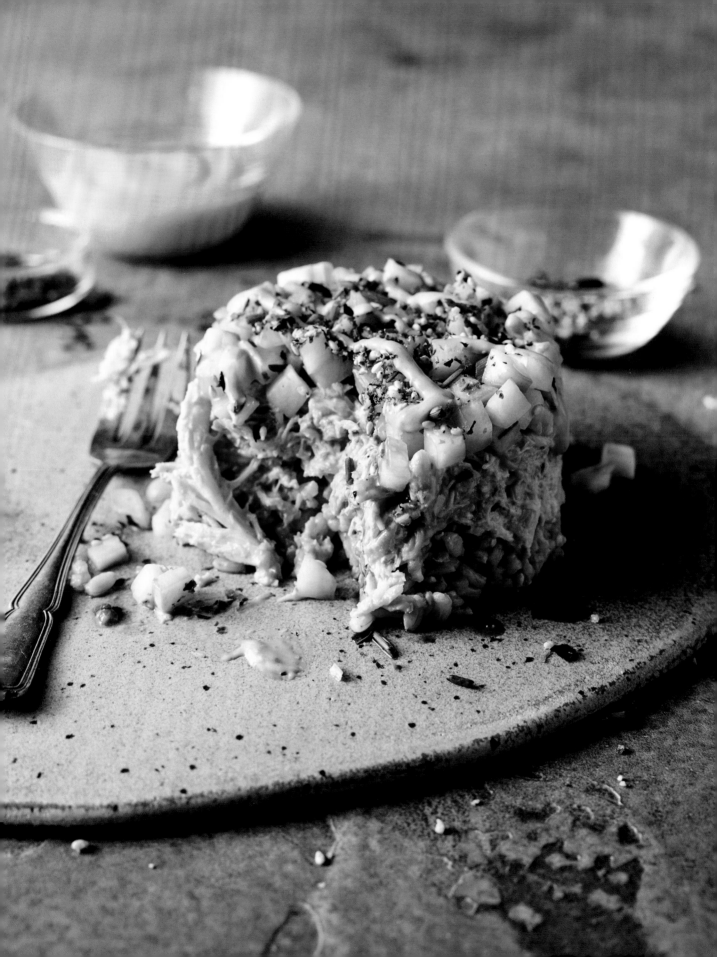

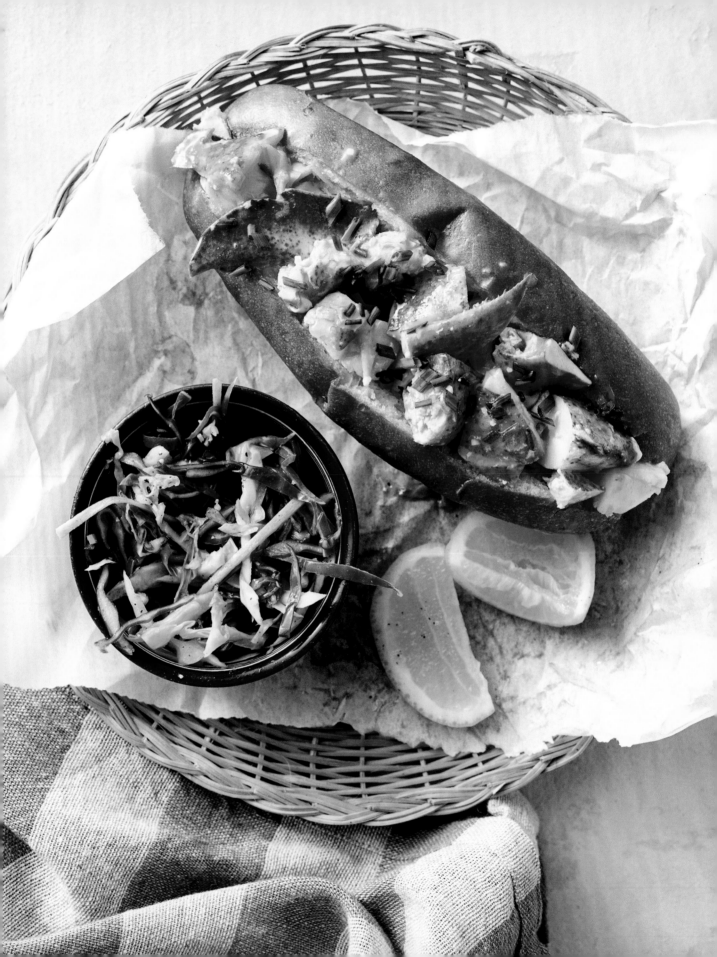

Butter-Poached Lobster Rolls

SERVES 4

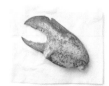

Lobster rolls just scream summer! A quarter pound of lobster poached in butter served on a toasted bun, end of story. When I get a lobster roll, I always prefer a warm, buttery Connecticut-style lobster roll rather than a cold New England–style one with mayo. Frozen lobster tails or claws work great here if you can't get fresh. Serve with a side of coleslaw, corn on the cob, or baked fries for the perfect summer meal.

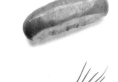

2 tablespoons salted butter

16 ounces fresh or thawed frozen lobster meat, claws or tails, cut into 1-inch pieces

1 large garlic clove, chopped

4 split-top buns, warmed, grilled, or lightly toasted

¼ cup minced fresh chives

1 lemon, cut into wedges

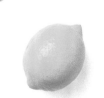

Heat a medium skillet over medium-low heat and add the butter. When the butter is almost melted, stir in the lobster meat. Reduce the heat to low, cover, and gently cook for 1 minute. Add the garlic and cook until the lobster is opaque and firm, 3 to 5 minutes.

Remove from the heat and divide the lobster among the rolls. Garnish with the chives and serve with lemon wedges.

Per Serving (1 roll) ● Calories 280 ● Fat 9 g ● Saturated Fat 4.5 g ● Cholesterol 95 mg Carbohydrate 21 g ● Fiber 1 g ● Protein 27 g ● Sugars 2 g ● Sodium 419 mg

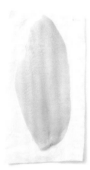

Flounder Milanese

SERVES 4

The flounder for this Milanese is lightly pan-fried using just a spray of olive oil (look for propellant-free varieties such as Bertolli) and topped with a simple arugula salad dressed in lots of fresh lemon. It's one of my favorite fish recipes, and trust me, even non-fish eaters will love this dish! I love the crunchy exterior without the oily coating you would normally get from frying. You can use any whitefish fillets—it's great with grouper or whatever's available fresh in your area.

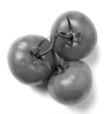

4 skinless flounder fillets (6 ounces each)

6 cups baby arugula

1 medium vine tomato, finely diced

1½ lemons

1 large egg

¾ cup seasoned bread crumbs, regular or gluten-free

Season the fish with ¼ teaspoon kosher salt and freshly ground black pepper to taste.

In a medium bowl, combine the arugula, tomato, the juice from the half lemon, and ½ tablespoon extra-virgin olive oil. Season with ¼ teaspoon each kosher salt and ground black pepper, toss, and set aside.

Slice the remaining lemon into 4 wedges and set aside for serving.

In a shallow bowl, beat the egg with 1 tablespoon water. Place the bread crumbs in another shallow bowl. Dip each fillet into the egg, then the bread crumbs, pressing gently to adhere. Set aside on a plate.

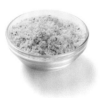

Heat a large nonstick skillet over medium heat. Spray one side of the fish with a generous amount of olive oil, then lay it in the pan oil side down. Spray the top side of the fish generously to coat. Cook until the crumbs are golden on both sides and the fish is opaque and cooked through, 4 to 5 minutes per side.

To serve, place a fillet on each of four plates and top each with one-quarter of the arugula salad. Serve immediately with the lemon wedges on the side.

Per Serving (1 fillet + 1½ cups salad) ● Calories 270 ● Fat 6 g ● Saturated Fat 1.5 g
Cholesterol 128 mg ● Carbohydrate 15 g ● Fiber 2 g ● Protein 37 g ● Sugars 3 g
Sodium 682 mg

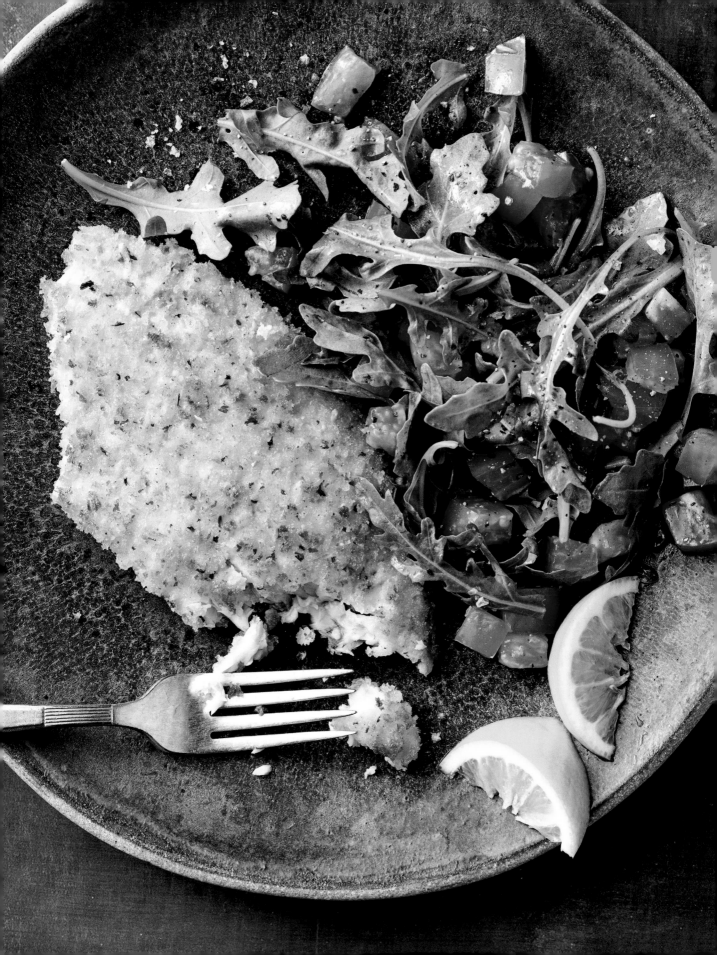

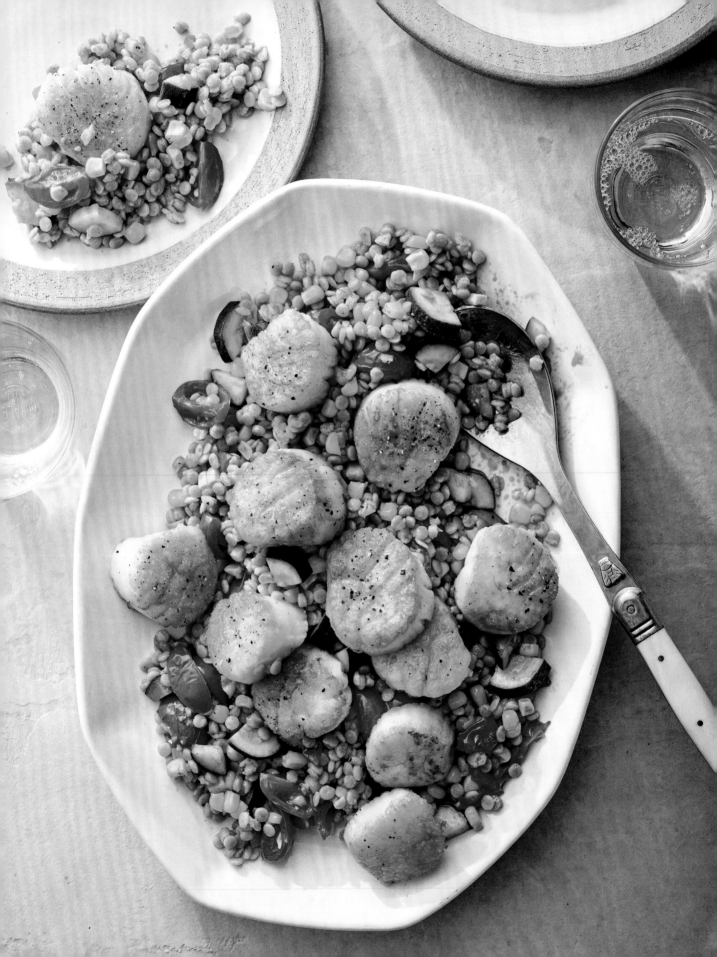

Seared Scallops with Summer Couscous

SERVES 4

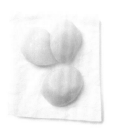

Q

This seafood dish is loaded with summer corn, tomatoes, and zucchini, but you can certainly make this anytime of the year. My daughter Madison fell in love with scallops when she tried this recipe. If you want to level this up, you can finish it with a squeeze of basil oil on top. To make basil oil, blanch a bunch of basil in boiling water for 20 to 30 seconds and cold-shock in an ice bath. Dry well, then puree it in the blender with extra-virgin olive oil.

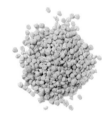

16 large scallops (1 to 1¼ pounds)

5 ounces (1 cup) whole wheat pearl couscous

3 garlic cloves, minced

1 cup corn kernels, fresh (from 1 large ear) or frozen

1 small zucchini (about 7 ounces), cut into ¼-inch pieces

1 cup cherry tomatoes, quartered

2 tablespoons freshly grated Pecorino Romano cheese

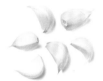

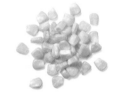

Rinse the scallops and pat dry with a paper towel. Season with ½ teaspoon kosher salt and freshly ground black pepper to taste.

In a medium pot, combine 1¼ cups water with ½ teaspoon kosher salt and bring to a boil over high heat. Add the couscous, stir, and cook until the water is absorbed and the couscous is tender, 8 to 12 minutes, or according to the package directions.

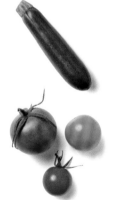

Meanwhile, heat a large skillet over high heat. When hot, add ½ tablespoon extra-virgin olive oil and place the scallops in the pan. Cook, undisturbed, until the bottom forms a nice caramel-colored crust, 2 to 3 minutes. Flip the scallops over and cook until the center is slightly translucent (you can check this by viewing them from the side; be careful not to overcook) and the bottom is seared, 2 to 3 minutes more. Remove from the pan and set aside on a warm plate.

Reduce the heat under the skillet to medium-low. Add ½ tablespoon extra-virgin olive oil and the garlic and cook until golden, 20 to 30 seconds. Add the corn, zucchini, and tomatoes and season with ¼ teaspoon kosher salt and ground black pepper to taste. Cook until the vegetables are tender, about 2 minutes (be careful not to overcook the zucchini or it will become mushy). Add the couscous and Pecorino to the skillet and cook for 1 minute to combine.

Divide the couscous among four plates, top with the scallops, and serve.

Per Serving (4 scallops + 1 generous cup couscous) ● Calories 311 ● Fat 6 g ● Saturated Fat 1 g
Cholesterol 29 mg ● Carbohydrate 42 g ● Fiber 7 g ● Protein 23 g ● Sugars 4 g ● Sodium 705 mg

On the
Side

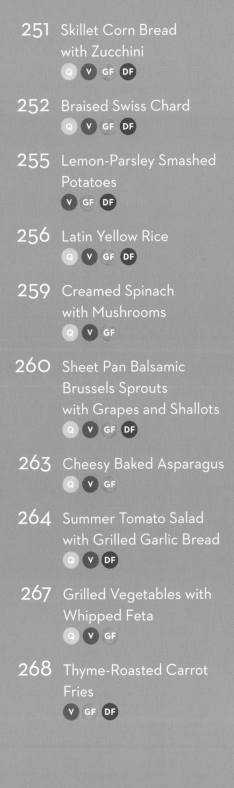

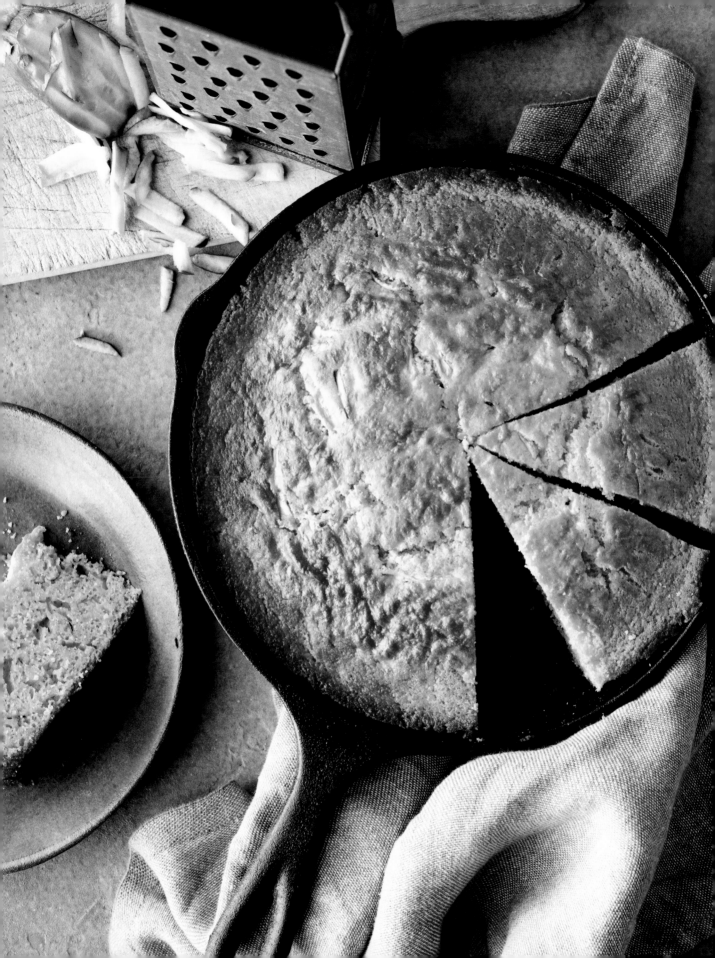

Skillet Corn Bread with Zucchini

SERVES 12

The secret to making this corn bread moist and delicious is grated zucchini! If it works for quick bread, why not corn bread? You can't even taste it, and if you don't want to see speckles of green for picky kids, you can peel the zucchini before grating it. It's quick, slightly sweet, and ready in just 30 minutes! Perfect right out of the oven topped with a little butter or serve it with soup, stews, chili, or your favorite BBQ dishes. Make a spicy, cheesy variation by adding one or two chopped jalapeños along with some shredded cheddar to the batter along with the milk.

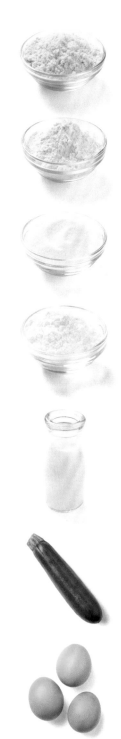

1 cup coarse yellow cornmeal

1 cup all-purpose or gluten-free flour, such as Cup4Cup

½ cup sugar

3½ teaspoons baking powder

1 cup fat-free milk or nondairy milk

1 cup (4 ounces) grated zucchini (no need to squeeze)

3 large eggs

Preheat the oven to 400°F. Spray a 9-inch cast-iron skillet or round cake pan generously with oil.

In a medium bowl, whisk together the cornmeal, flour, sugar, baking powder, and 1 teaspoon kosher salt.

Make a well in the center of the dry ingredients and add the milk, zucchini, eggs, and 3 tablespoons neutral oil, such as canola or grapeseed. Stir just until the mixture comes together and only a few lumps remain.

Pour the batter into the prepared pan and bake until the top is lightly browned, the sides have pulled away from the pan, and a toothpick inserted into the center comes out clean, 22 to 25 minutes.

Cut into 12 wedges and serve hot or warm.

Per Serving (1 wedge) ● Calories 165 ● Fat 5 g ● Saturated Fat 1 g ● Cholesterol 47 mg
Carbohydrate 26 g ● Fiber 1 g ● Protein 4 g ● Sugars 10 g ● Sodium 267 mg

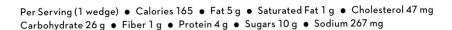

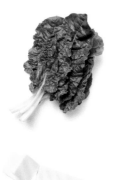

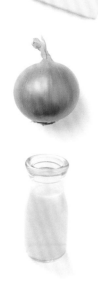

Braised Swiss Chard

SERVES 4

This is my favorite way to eat Swiss chard, which is known as *acelgas* in Colombia. My mom and aunt make these tasty, braised greens all the time. The leaves and stems are separated and then sautéed in butter and simmered in milk. They come out creamy and delicious and are perfect as a side with steak or other meats. To make it dairy-free, rice milk and vegan butter would work fine here.

2 large bunches Swiss chard (24 ounces total), rinsed well

2 tablespoons unsalted butter or vegan butter

1 cup chopped yellow onion

1 cup 2% milk or rice milk

Separate the Swiss chard leaves from the stems and cut the leaves into ½-inch-wide strips. Finely chop the stems, keeping them separate.

In a medium pot or deep skillet, heat the butter over medium heat. When the butter has melted, add the onion and sauté until softened, 2 to 3 minutes. Add the Swiss chard stems and cook, stirring, until just tender, about 3 minutes. Stir in the leaves, cover, and cook until they start to wilt, 2 to 3 minutes. Season with ½ teaspoon kosher salt and a pinch of freshly ground black pepper. Stir in the milk, reduce the heat to low, cover, and cook until the leaves are very tender, 5 to 6 minutes. Serve immediately.

Per Serving (¾ cup) ● Calories 130 ● Fat 7 g ● Saturated Fat 4.5 g ● Cholesterol 20 mg
Carbohydrate 13 g ● Fiber 3.5 g ● Protein 6 g ● Sugars 7 g ● Sodium 530 mg

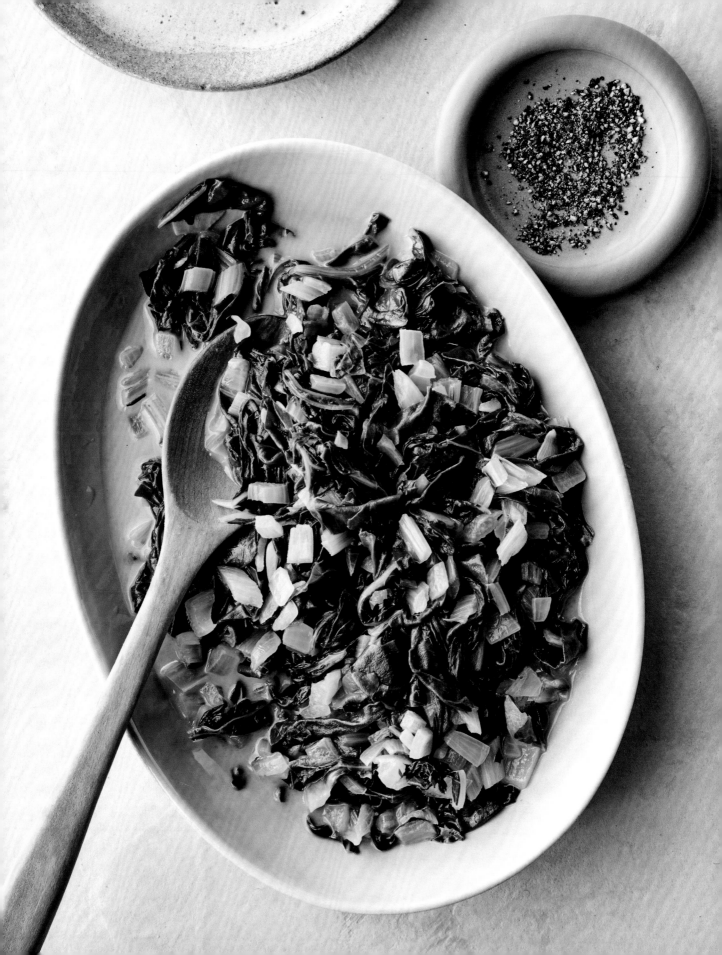

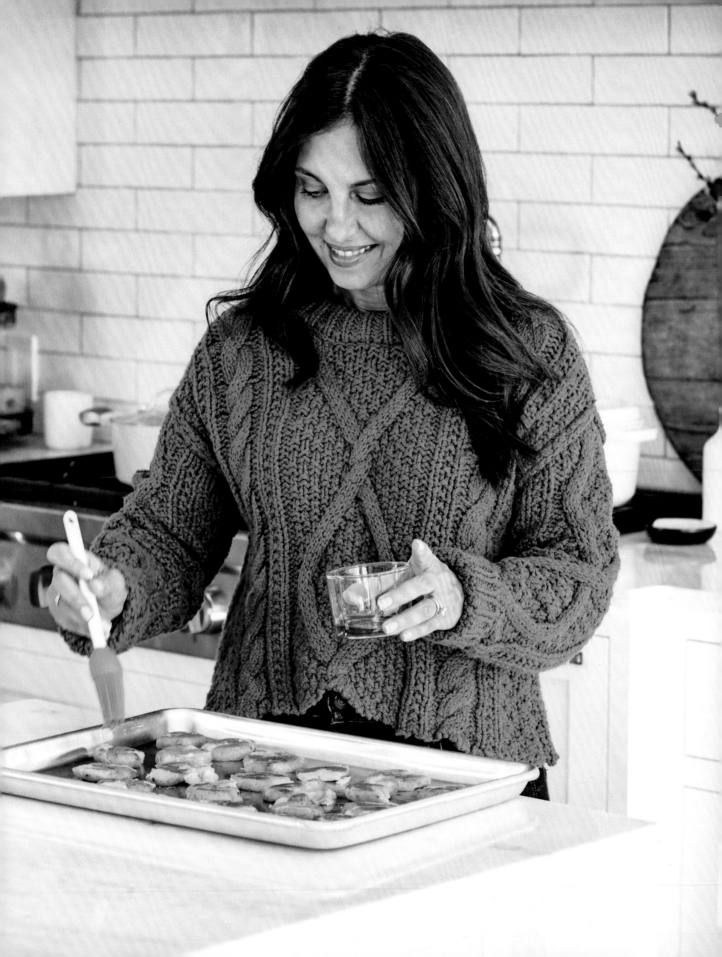

Lemon-Parsley Smashed Potatoes

SERVES 4

Crispy smashed potatoes are my go-to when I need an easy side dish to pair with steak, lamb, or any type of roast. You can season these potatoes with a variety of spices and herbs, but this simple combo with lemon zest and parsley is one of my favorites. If you boil and then bake the potatoes, they always come out delicious, perfectly crisp and tender on the inside. Try them with Air Fryer Chicken Drumsticks (page 175) or Sheet Pan Spatchcock Chicken with Brussels Sprouts (page 154).

16 baby gold potatoes (about 1 pound total)

½ teaspoon garlic powder

½ teaspoon sweet paprika

1 teaspoon grated lemon zest, plus lemon wedges (optional) for serving

1 tablespoon finely chopped fresh parsley

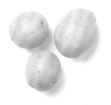

Preheat the oven to 425°F. Spray a sheet pan with oil.

In a medium pot, combine the potatoes with cold water to cover and 1 teaspoon kosher salt. Bring to a boil over high heat and cook until a knife easily pierces to the center of each potato, about 20 minutes.

Meanwhile, in a small bowl, combine the garlic powder, paprika, ½ teaspoon kosher salt, and ⅛ teaspoon freshly ground black pepper.

Drain the potatoes and place on a clean work surface. Use the bottom of a glass to gently press and squash the potato.

Place the smashed potatoes in a single layer on the prepared sheet pan. Lightly brush with ½ tablespoon extra-virgin olive oil and sprinkle both sides of each potato with the spice mix.

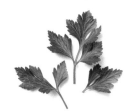

Roast until crisp and golden, about 20 minutes, flipping halfway.

In a small bowl, combine the lemon zest, parsley, and ⅛ teaspoon kosher salt. Top the potatoes with the lemon zest and parsley mixture. Serve with lemon wedges, if desired.

Per Serving (4 potatoes) ● Calories 96 ● Fat 2 g ● Saturated Fat 0.5 g ● Cholesterol 0 mg
Carbohydrate 18 g ● Fiber 3 g ● Protein 2 g ● Sugars 1 g ● Sodium 194 mg

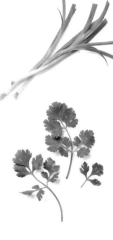

Latin Yellow Rice

SERVES 8

I love all kinds of rice—fried rice, rice and beans, sushi rice, you name it. But my homemade yellow rice is definitely at the top of the list! Every time I make it, everyone asks me for the recipe. My method will give you perfect rice every single time. It pairs wonderfully with any protein, from steaks and pork chops to grilled chicken, fish, or beans.

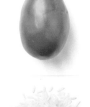

5 medium scallions, chopped

½ cup chopped fresh cilantro

2 garlic cloves, minced

1 medium tomato, diced

2 cups uncooked long-grain rice (I use Canilla extra-long grain)

1 large (about 12 grams) chicken or veggie bouillon cube*

1 (5-gram) packet sazón seasoning with achiote (about ½ tablespoon)

*Read the label to be sure this product is gluten-free.

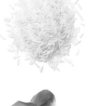

In a heavy-bottomed medium pot with a tight-fitting lid, heat 4 teaspoons extra-virgin olive oil over medium heat. Add the scallions, cilantro, and garlic and cook until tender, about 2 minutes. Add the tomato and cook until softened, about 1 minute. Add the rice and slightly toast, stirring frequently, about 2 minutes.

Add 4 cups water, the bouillon cube, sazón seasoning, and 1 teaspoon kosher salt. Taste the water for salt; it should be flavorful. If not, adjust as needed.

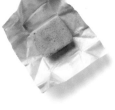

Bring the mixture to a boil over high heat, stirring only once. Once most of the water evaporates and just barely skims the top of the rice, reduce the heat to very low, cover, and cook for 15 minutes. Remove from the heat and let sit at least 5 more minutes without removing the lid. (The steam will finish cooking the rice.)

Fluff with a fork and serve.

Per Serving (¾ cup) ● Calories 200 ● Fat 3 g ● Saturated Fat 0.5 g ● Cholesterol 0 mg
Carbohydrate 39 g ● Fiber 1 g ● Protein 4 g ● Sugars 1 g ● Sodium 460 mg

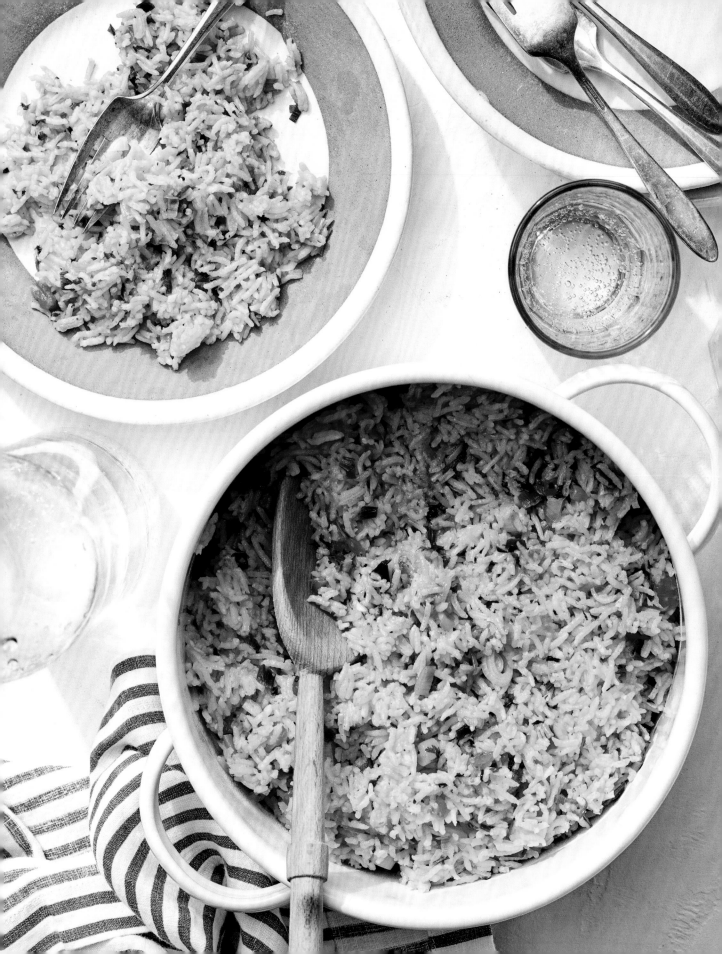

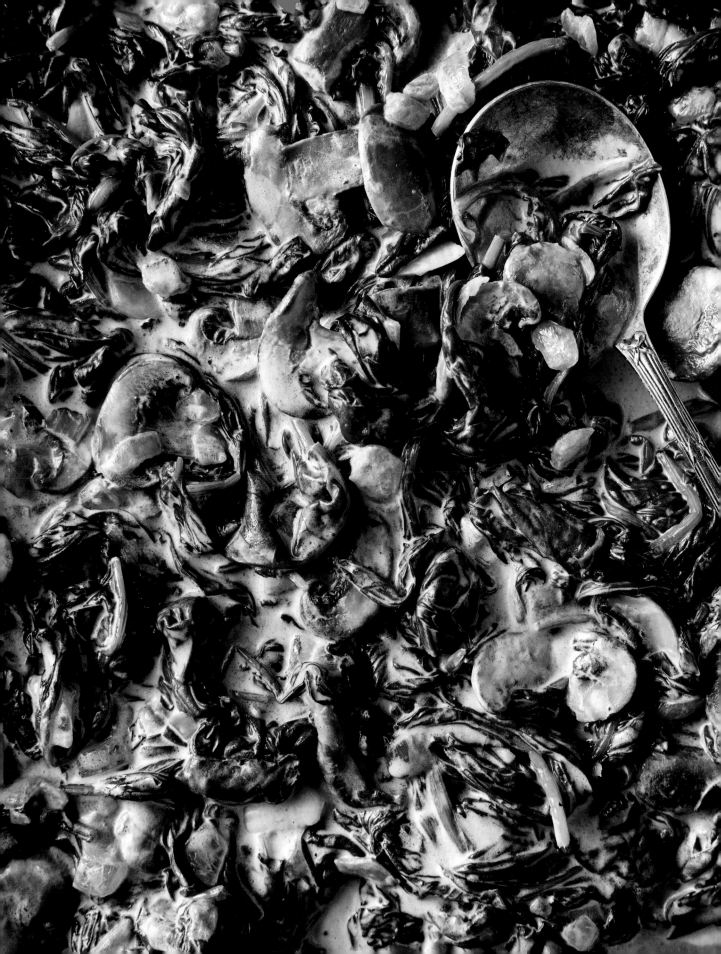

Creamed Spinach with Mushrooms

SERVES 4

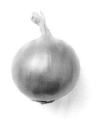

Creamed spinach is one of my family's favorite steakhouse sides, but when I make it at home, I love using Greek yogurt in place of cream to make it a bit lighter. No one knows the difference!

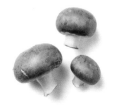

½ small onion, finely diced

4 ounces sliced cremini or white mushrooms

2 garlic cloves, thinly sliced

Pinch of freshly grated nutmeg

10 ounces baby spinach

⅓ cup whole-milk plain Greek yogurt

In a large skillet, heat 2 teaspoons extra-virgin olive oil over medium heat until shimmering. Add the onion and sauté until translucent, about 3 minutes. Stir in the mushrooms and ¼ teaspoon kosher salt and cook until the mushrooms start to brown, 3 to 4 minutes. Add the garlic and cook until fragrant, about 30 seconds more. Stir in the nutmeg.

Gradually add the spinach, stirring each addition until it wilts. Season with ⅛ teaspoon kosher salt and continue to cook until the spinach is wilted and tender, but not overcooked, 3 to 5 minutes. Remove from the heat.

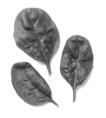

Add the yogurt to a large bowl and fold in a spoonful of the spinach mixture until incorporated. Add the remaining spinach and toss to coat completely. Serve immediately.

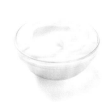

Per Serving (½ cup) ● Calories 75 ● Fat 3 g ● Saturated Fat 0.5 g ● Cholesterol 2 mg
Carbohydrate 8 g ● Fiber 2.5 g ● Protein 5 g ● Sugars 3 g ● Sodium 170 mg

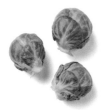

Sheet Pan Balsamic Brussels Sprouts with Grapes and Shallots

SERVES 4

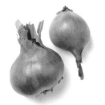

Roasting grapes in the oven concentrates their sweetness and makes them a lovely addition to Brussels sprouts. If you want to make this a one-pan meal, season a pork loin with salt and pepper and add it to the sheet pan. It should take the same time to cook, about 20 minutes or until a thermometer inserted in the center of the loin registers 145°F.

12 ounces Brussels sprouts, trimmed and quartered

4 large or 5 small shallots, peeled and quartered lengthwise

1 cup seedless red grapes

2 tablespoons balsamic vinegar, plus more (optional) for serving

4 sprigs of fresh rosemary or thyme

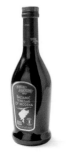

Preheat the oven to 400°F.

In a large bowl, combine the Brussels sprouts, shallots, grapes, vinegar, 2 teaspoons extra-virgin olive oil, ½ teaspoon kosher salt, and freshly ground black pepper to taste and toss well.

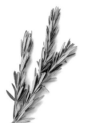

Spread the mixture in an even layer on a sheet pan and nestle in the fresh herb sprigs. Roast until the Brussels sprouts are tender and the grapes burst, about 20 minutes.

Serve warm with more balsamic for drizzling, if desired.

Per Serving (1 cup) ● Calories 135 ● Fat 3 g ● Saturated Fat 0.5 g ● Cholesterol 0 mg
Carbohydrate 26 g ● Fiber 5.5 g ● Protein 5 g ● Sugars 14 g ● Sodium 172 mg

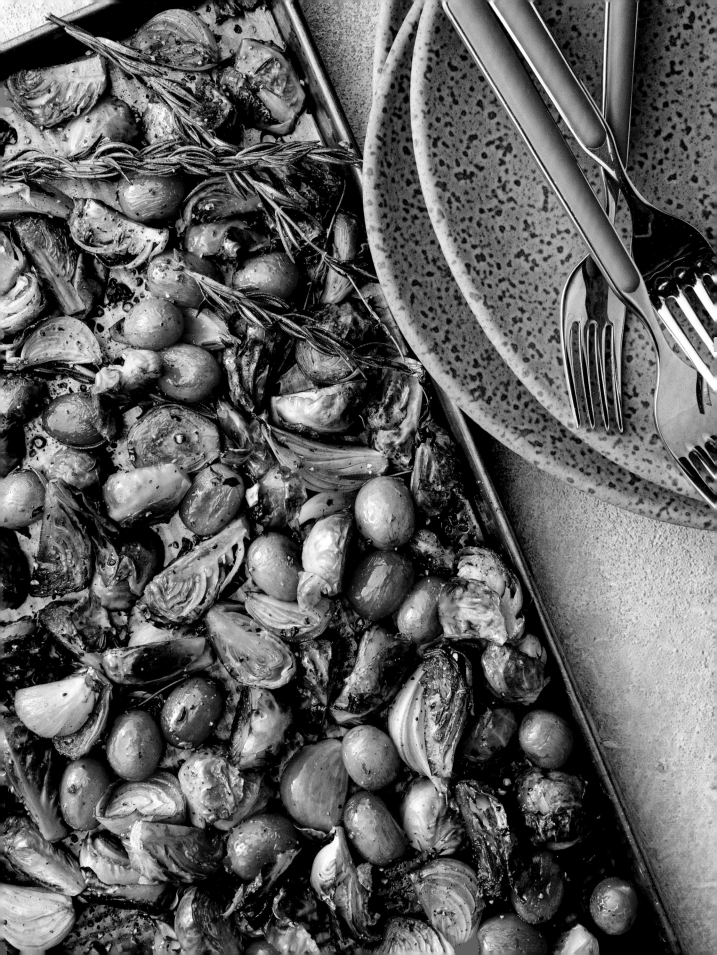

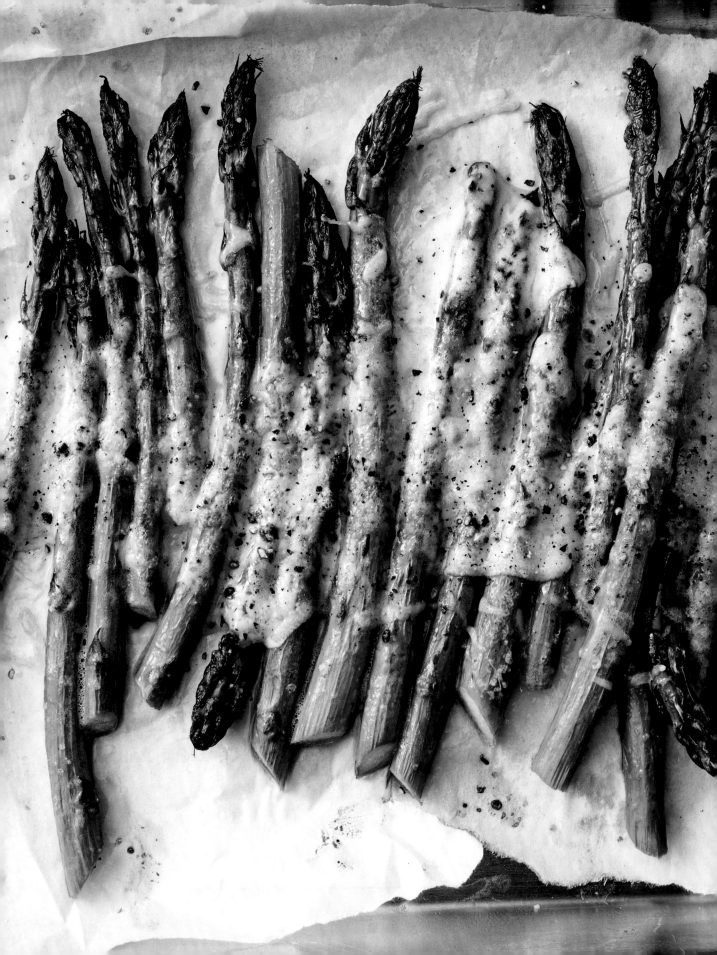

Cheesy Baked Asparagus

SERVES 4

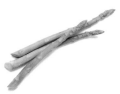

I love roasted asparagus, and I also love Fontina cheese, so combining the two just seemed natural. The pairing makes a really simple side dish that's worthy of being the star of the show. Although the melted Fontina works beautifully with asparagus, you can also try this with a different cheese, such as mozzarella. It makes a great side to go with salmon, shrimp, or chicken.

1 pound asparagus, tough ends trimmed

3 tablespoons freshly grated Parmesan cheese

3 ounces fontina cheese, thinly sliced

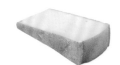

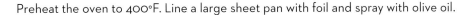

Preheat the oven to 400°F. Line a large sheet pan with foil and spray with olive oil.

Arrange the asparagus on the prepared sheet pan in a single layer and spray with olive oil. Sprinkle with the Parmesan, ¼ teaspoon kosher salt, and freshly ground black pepper to taste. Roast until crisp-tender, 12 to 14 minutes.

Remove the pan from oven and push the asparagus spears together so they are close to each other and touching. Arrange the fontina slices over the center and bake until the cheese melts, 2 to 4 minutes. Top with more black pepper and serve.

Per Serving (¼ of the asparagus) ● Calories 121 ● Fat 8 g ● Saturated Fat 4.5 g
Cholesterol 28 mg ● Carbohydrate 5 g ● Fiber 2.5 g ● Protein 9 g ● Sugars 2 g
Sodium 240 mg

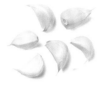

Summer Tomato Salad with Grilled Garlic Bread

SERVES 4

I had to include this recipe because it's a staple in our house every summer! Tommy eats this salad all season long as a main dish with some grilled bread, but we also serve it as a side dish or an appetizer. It's always a hit. Just be sure to use the highest quality ingredients here for the best results.

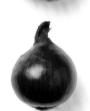

3 garlic cloves, 2 minced, 1 halved crosswise

5 large heirloom or beefsteak tomatoes, cut into 1-inch cubes (about 7 cups)

½ cup chopped red onion

8 to 10 fresh basil leaves, chopped

4 slices sourdough or other rustic bread (about 1 ounce each)

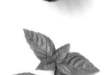

In a large bowl, combine the minced garlic, tomatoes and their juices, red onion, basil, and 1 tablespoon extra-virgin olive oil. Season with 1½ teaspoons kosher salt and freshly ground black pepper to taste and gently toss to combine. Let the tomato mixture sit at room temperature, stirring occasionally, for about 20 minutes to let the flavors meld (the juices from the tomatoes will release and make the best liquid for dipping that bread in).

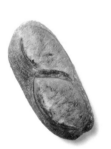

Preheat the grill to medium-high and clean the grates. Spray both sides of the bread slices with olive oil and sprinkle with a pinch of kosher salt. Grill the bread until toasted and grill marks appear, 1 to 2 minutes per side. When cool enough to handle, rub the cut side of the halved garlic all over both sides of the bread.

Divide the tomatoes among four bowls and serve with the bread. (If serving as an appetizer, grill extra bread and place the tomatoes in a large bowl and provide a spoon for topping the bread.)

Per Serving (1¼ cups tomatoes + 1 ounce bread) ● Calories 160 ● Fat 5 g ● Saturated Fat 0.5 g
Cholesterol 0 mg ● Carbohydrate 26 g ● Fiber 4 g ● Protein 5 g ● Sugars 8 g ● Sodium 621 mg

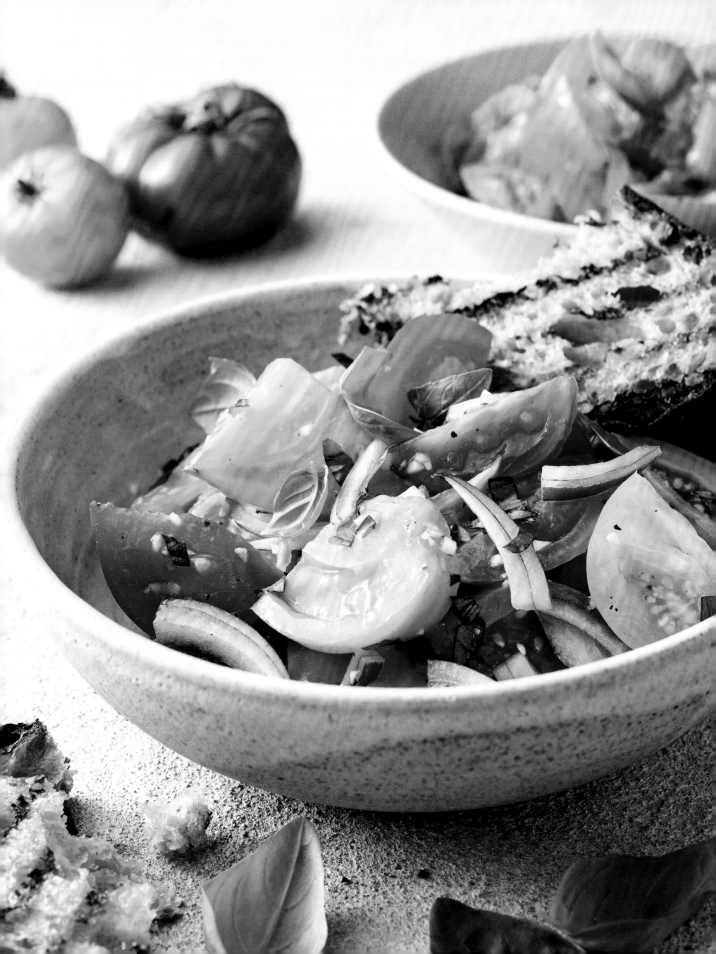

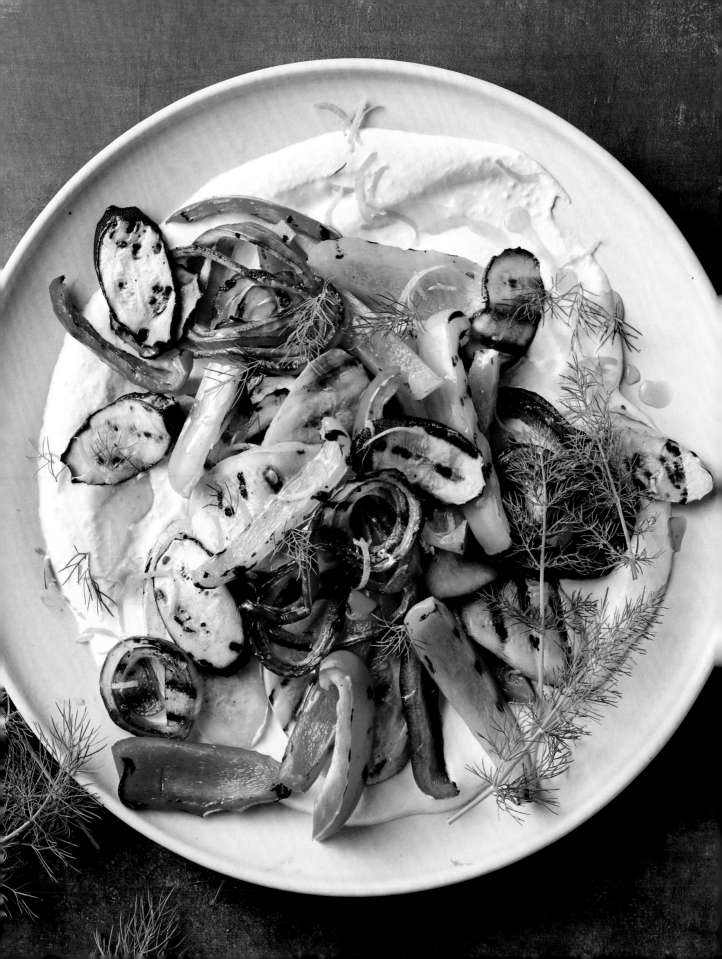

Grilled Vegetables with Whipped Feta

SERVES 6

Dining alfresco with lots of grilled veggies and a glass of rosé … this is how I like to eat all summer long! Made with only a handful of ingredients and in only a few minutes, this is a greater-than-the-sum-of-its-parts dish, perfect to have up your sleeve for an easy dinner or a last-minute hosting or potluck. Look for feta that comes in a block and packed in brine, rather than precrumbled in a carton. The feta whips up light and airy in the food processor, and it goes great with grilled veggies or even as a refreshing dip or a sandwich spread. Make this a light meal with wedges of grilled pita bread.

Grated zest and juice of ½ lemon

1 (8-ounce) block feta cheese in brine, drained and crumbled (2 cups)

½ cup plain 2% Greek yogurt

1 large red onion, sliced into ¼-inch-thick rounds

4 medium multicolor bell peppers, cut into ½-inch-wide strips

3 medium summer squash (8 ounces each), a mix of yellow squash and green zucchini, cut on an angle into slices ¼ inch thick

Chopped fresh dill, for garnish

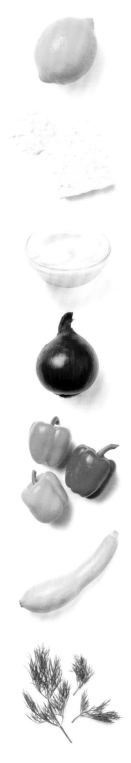

In a food processor, combine the lemon juice, feta, yogurt, and 2 tablespoons extra-virgin olive oil. Process until smooth and airy. You may need to pause and scrape down the sides once or twice. (The whipped feta can be served at room temperature or chilled; it will keep in the fridge for up to 1 week.)

Heat the grill or grill pan over medium-high heat.

Spray the onion slices, bell peppers, squash, and zucchini all over with extra-virgin olive oil. Season with ½ teaspoon kosher salt and freshly ground black pepper to taste. Grill the vegetables, turning occasionally, until nicely charred, 10 to 12 minutes.

Smear the whipped feta on a large platter, then drizzle with a little olive oil and sprinkle with the lemon zest. Top with the grilled veggies, garnish everything with dill, and serve.

Per Serving (1½ cups vegetables + ¼ cup sauce) ● Calories 214 ● Fat 14 g ● Saturated Fat 7 g
Cholesterol 36 mg ● Carbohydrate 13 g ● Fiber 3 g ● Protein 10 g ● Sugars 9 g ● Sodium 457 mg

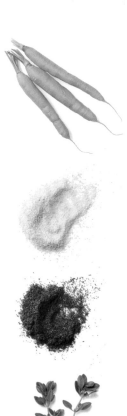

Thyme-Roasted Carrot Fries

SERVES 4

These carrots are so tender and irresistible! I'm not the biggest fan of cooked carrots, but when I make these roasted carrot fries, I just can't stop eating them. These are great to meal prep, too—I make a batch and keep them refrigerated for up to 4 days to serve with a quick protein and some grains for an easy lunch.

8 large carrots (about 8 inches each), peeled

1 teaspoon garlic powder

1 teaspoon sweet paprika

3 tablespoons chopped fresh thyme

Preheat the oven to 425°F.

Cut the carrots into even sticks by first cutting them into 4-inch lengths, then quartering the thicker ends and cutting the thinner ends into thirds. Place in a large bowl and combine with 3 tablespoons extra-virgin olive oil, the garlic powder, paprika, 1 teaspoon kosher salt, and ¼ teaspoon freshly ground black pepper. Toss well to evenly coat the sticks.

Line a large baking sheet with parchment paper. Transfer the carrot sticks to the prepared baking sheet and arrange in a single layer. Bake for 20 minutes.

Remove the pan from the oven and add the thyme, stirring so the carrots are coated on all sides. Return to the oven and bake until the carrots are tender, 20 to 25 minutes more. Season with ¼ teaspoon salt and serve.

Per Serving (about ¾ cup) ● Calories 155 ● Fat 11 g ● Saturated Fat 1.5 g ● Cholesterol 0 mg Carbohydrate 15 g ● Fiber 4.5 g ● Protein 2 g ● Sugars 7 g ● Sodium 451 mg

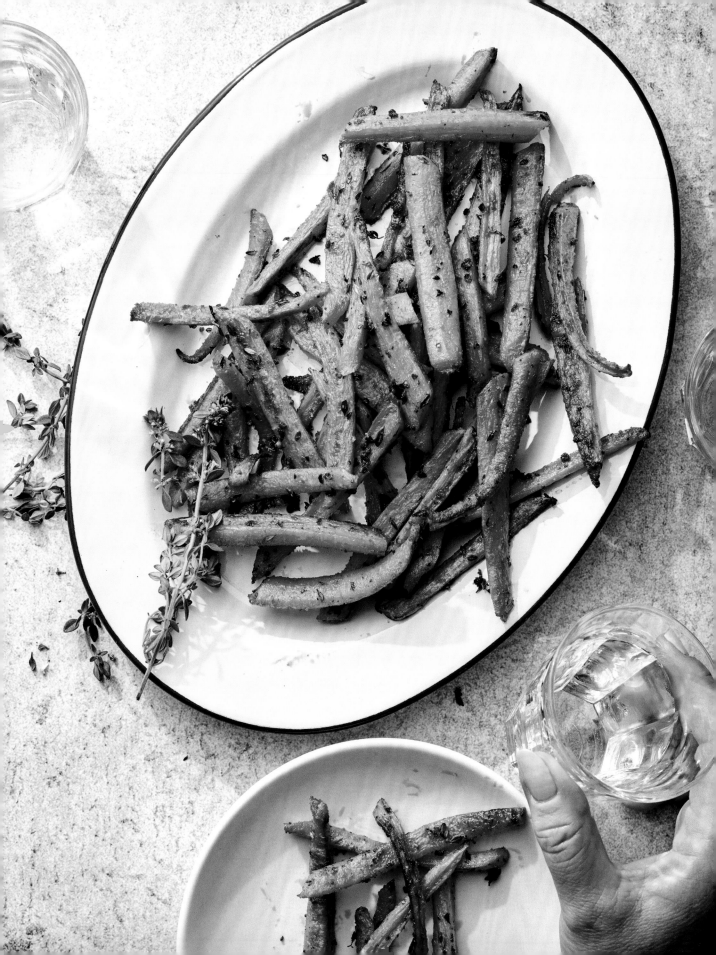

Sweet
Tooth

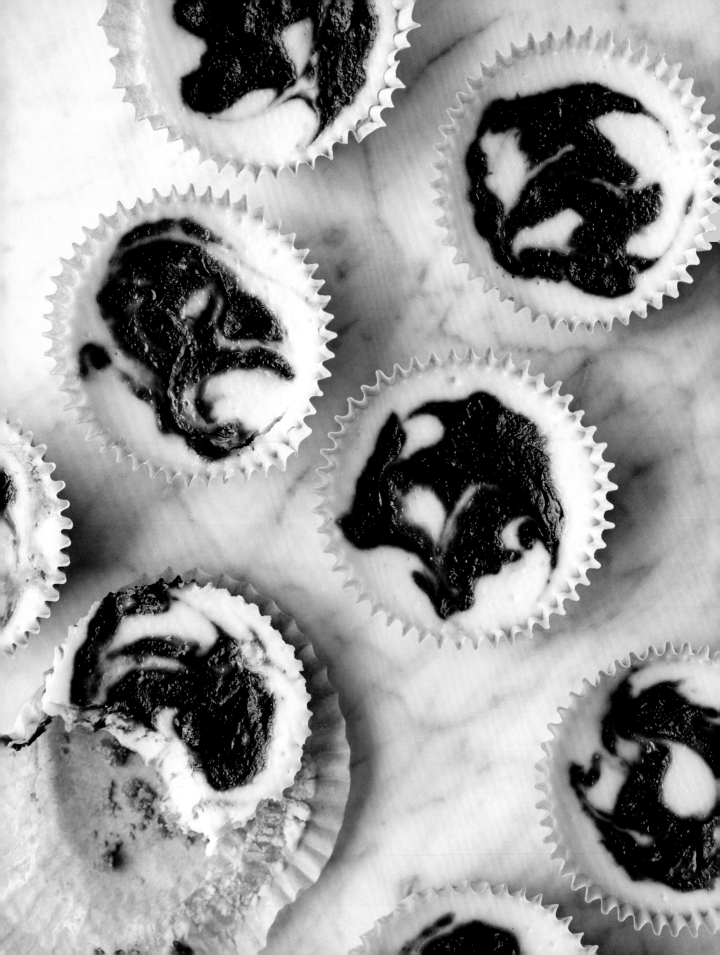

Mini Blueberry Swirl Cheesecakes

MAKES 8 MINI CHEESECAKES

These individual cheesecakes are so creamy, and since they're made in muffin tins, they're also an easy way to control your portions. Instead of blueberries, try them with fresh strawberries or raspberries. For extra flavor, stir in ½ teaspoon vanilla extract along with the cream cheese.

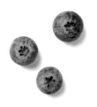

½ cup blueberries

4 tablespoons sugar

1 (8-ounce) block ⅓-less-fat cream cheese, at room temperature

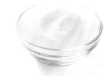

¼ cup light sour cream or plain low-fat yogurt, at room temperature

1 large egg, at room temperature

4 whole graham crackers (about 2 ounces total)

2 tablespoons unsalted butter, melted

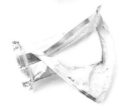

Preheat the oven to 350°F. Line 8 cups of a muffin tin with paper liners and spray evenly with cooking spray.

In a small saucepan, combine the blueberries and 1 tablespoon of the sugar. Cook over medium heat, stirring constantly and gently smashing the berries, until slightly reduced and thickened, 4 to 5 minutes. Remove from the heat and set aside.

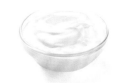

In a large bowl, with an electric mixer, beat together the cream cheese, sour cream, egg, and remaining 3 tablespoons sugar on medium-high speed until thoroughly combined and smooth, about 30 seconds.

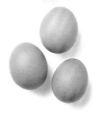

Place the graham crackers in a zip-top plastic bag and seal. Use a rolling pin to crush into fine crumbs. Transfer to a small bowl, add the melted butter, and stir to combine.

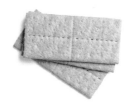

Scoop 1½ tablespoons of the crumb mixture into each muffin cup, pressing down to create a layer of crust. Divide the cheesecake batter evenly among the cups, dolloping slightly less than 3 tablespoons in each, then smooth the tops with a spoon. Top each with a heaping teaspoon of the blueberry sauce, and using a toothpick or skewer, swirl the blueberry topping into the batter.

Bake the cheesecakes until they are set but still slightly jiggly, 20 to 24 minutes, rotating the pan front to back halfway through. Place the pan on a wire rack to cool for about 1 hour, then refrigerate for 2 hours before serving.

Per Serving (1 mini cheesecake) ● Calories 175 ● Fat 11 g ● Saturated Fat 6.5 g
Cholesterol 54 mg ● Carbohydrate 14 g ● Fiber 0.5 g ● Protein 3.5 g ● Sugars 9 g ● Sodium 179 mg

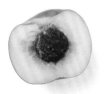

Juicy Peach Cobbler

SERVES 8

Cobbler is one of my favorite desserts to make in the summer. Be sure to let your peaches get extra ripe, so they're at their sweetest and juiciest. Serve with a dollop of vanilla yogurt, whipped cream, or ice cream on top.

SKINNY SCOOP: If you can't find self-rising flour, use 1 cup all-purpose flour and 1½ teaspoons baking powder instead.

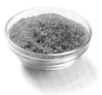

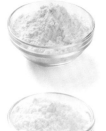

8 peaches, peeled, pitted, and sliced (about 8 cups)

⅓ cup plus 2 tablespoons raw or granulated sugar

1 cup self-rising flour (see Skinny Scoop)

¼ teaspoon baking soda

3 tablespoons cold salted butter, cut into cubes

⅔ cup low-fat buttermilk

¼ teaspoon ground cinnamon

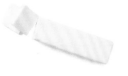

Preheat the oven to 350°F. Spray a 9 × 9-inch baking dish with oil.

In a large saucepan, combine the peaches, ⅓ cup of the sugar, and ⅛ teaspoon kosher salt and stir to mix thoroughly. Cover and cook over medium heat, stirring occasionally, until the peaches are juicy, 5 to 10 minutes. Remove from the heat and set aside.

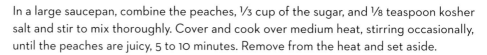

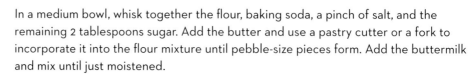

In a medium bowl, whisk together the flour, baking soda, a pinch of salt, and the remaining 2 tablespoons sugar. Add the butter and use a pastry cutter or a fork to incorporate it into the flour mixture until pebble-size pieces form. Add the buttermilk and mix until just moistened.

Transfer the peaches and their juices to the prepared baking dish. Dollop the batter over the peaches and sprinkle the top with the cinnamon.

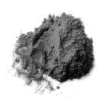

Place the dish on a sheet pan and bake until the peaches are bubbling and the top is golden, 40 to 45 minutes. Serve warm.

Per Serving (generous ¾ cup) • Calories 197 • Fat 5 g • Saturated Fat 3 g • Cholesterol 12 mg
Carbohydrate 37 g • Fiber 2.5 g • Protein 3.5 g • Sugars 24 g • Sodium 304 mg

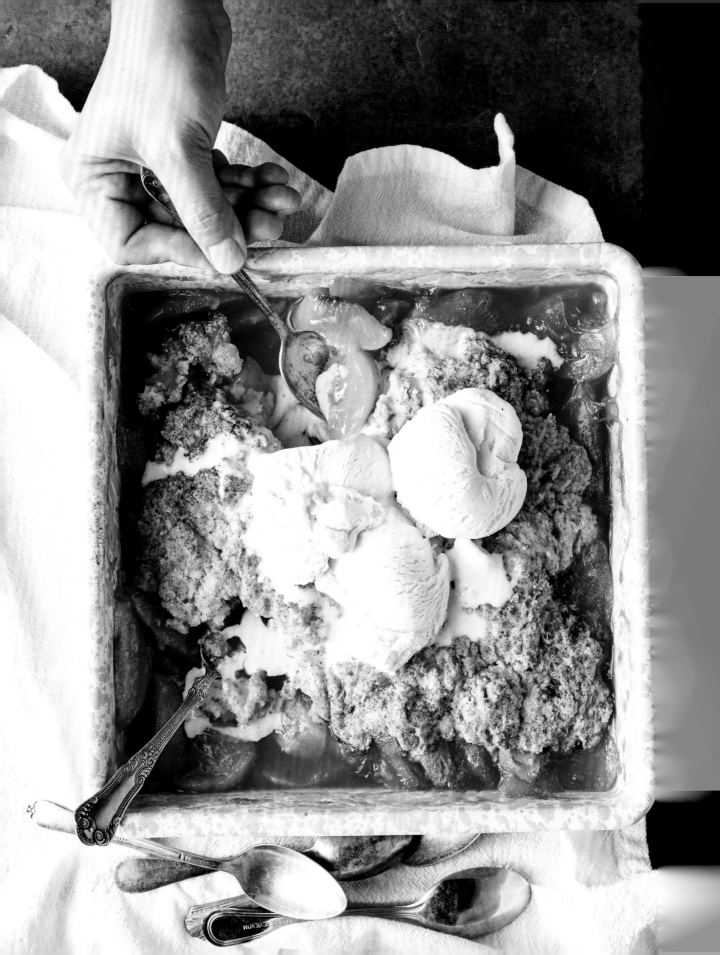

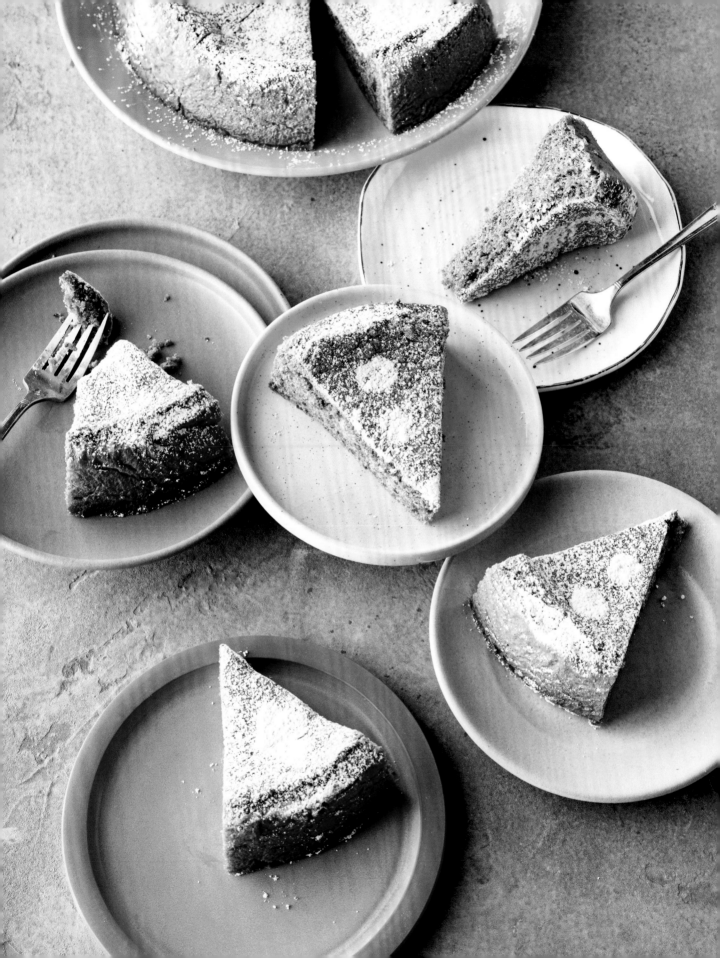

Flourless Pistachio Cake

SERVES 12

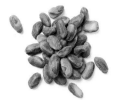

I love this incredibly moist pistachio cake made with a few ingredients—just pistachios, eggs, and sugar, plus some almond extract and a pinch of salt. Dorie Greenspan has a Simple Almond Cake in her cookbook, *Baking Chez Moi*, that my aunt has been making for years, and every time I eat it with her, I say I am going to re-create it with pistachios. I am so glad I finally did, because it's even better than I imagined! I made my own pistachio flour by toasting the raw nuts and throwing them into a food processor. Surprisingly, almond extract really brings out the flavor of the pistachios here.

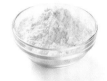

2 cups raw shelled pistachios

Flour or gluten-free flour, for dusting

6 large eggs, separated, at room temperature

2/3 cup raw sugar

1¼ teaspoons almond extract

Powdered sugar (optional), for dusting

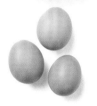

Adjust a rack to the center of the oven and preheat to 325°F.

Spread the pistachios on a sheet pan and bake until the pistachios smell nutty and are lightly toasted, 6 to 8 minutes. Set the pistachios aside to cool completely.

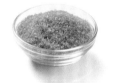

Leave the oven on but increase the temperature to 350°F. Spray a 9-inch springform pan with cooking spray, then line with a round of parchment paper and dust with flour (use gluten-free all-purpose flour blend to keep the cake gluten-free).

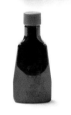

Transfer the cooled pistachios to a food processor and pulse until finely ground to a texture of coarse sugar or cornmeal, which will take about 1 minute total. If you see any pistachio bits starting to clump together around the bottom edge of the processor bowl, stop pulsing and scrape and stir the nuts to evenly distribute them before continuing. Don't overprocess or you will make nut butter.

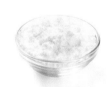

In a large bowl, whisk together the egg yolks and all but 2 tablespoons of the raw sugar until the yolks become thick and pale in color, about 1 minute. Whisk in the almond extract and a pinch of kosher salt and set aside.

(recipe continues)

Per Serving (1 slice) ● Calories 179 ● Fat 11 g ● Saturated Fat 2 g ● Cholesterol 93 mg
Carbohydrate 16 g ● Fiber 2 g ● Protein 7 g ● Sugars 12 g ● Sodium 45 mg

In a stand mixer fitted with the whisk (or in a bowl with a hand mixer), beat the egg whites on medium speed until they become opaque, about 1 minute. Sprinkle in the remaining 2 tablespoons raw sugar, increase the speed to medium-high, and continue to beat the egg whites until they hold medium peaks, about 2 minutes.

With a flexible rubber spatula, mix the egg yolks so the sugar that has settled on the bottom is mixed well, then stir in about one-quarter of the beaten egg whites. Scrape the remaining egg whites over the yolks and add half of the pistachio flour. Partially fold into the yolks, gently. While the mixture still has a few streaks of white left, add the remaining pistachio flour and gently fold in until you have a uniform batter.

Scrape the batter into the prepared springform pan and smooth the top with the rubber spatula.

Bake the cake until the top is golden and springy to the touch, about 30 minutes. Let cool on a wire rack for 5 minutes, then run a butter knife along the edges of the cake pan.

Invert the cake pan onto the rack, remove the sides and bottom, and peel away the parchment paper. Turn the cake right side up and allow to cool completely.

Dust with powdered sugar, if desired, and cut into 12 slices.

Cinnamon-Apple Tarte Tatin

SERVES 8

Tarte Tatin is basically a French apple pie ... that happened by accident! It is named for the Tatin sisters, who attempted to save a failed apple pie by serving it to their guests upside down. The tart is fruit (usually apples) caramelized in butter and sugar that is baked underneath a pastry top but is inverted before serving. This recipe uses a lot less butter than the Tatin sisters' version, but it's still wonderful. If you want to make this recipe even easier, feel free to use store-bought piecrust. Serve with ice cream or whipped topping.

4½ tablespoons cold unsalted butter

¾ cup plus 2 tablespoons all-purpose flour, plus more for dusting

2 teaspoons plus ⅓ cup packed dark brown sugar

3 to 4 tablespoons ice water, as needed

6 sweet medium apples, such as Honeycrisp or Gala, peeled and cored

½ teaspoon ground cinnamon

Cut 3 tablespoons of the butter into ½-inch cubes.

In a medium bowl, combine the flour, ¼ teaspoon kosher salt, and 2 teaspoons of the brown sugar. Add the cubes of butter and mix with a fork until the butter is in pea-size pieces. Add 3 tablespoons ice water and mix just until the dough holds together. If it feels dry, add more ice water 1 teaspoon at a time, until it's malleable. Shape into a disc and wrap in plastic wrap or your favorite eco-friendly alternative and transfer to the refrigerator to chill while preparing the filling. (The dough can be refrigerated for up to 2 days in advance.)

Slice each apple into 8 wedges and toss with the cinnamon in a large bowl.

In a 10-inch cast-iron or other ovenproof skillet, melt the remaining 1½ tablespoons butter over medium heat. Stir in the remaining ⅓ cup brown sugar until thoroughly combined, then remove from the heat and spread the sugar so it coats the bottom of the pan.

(recipe continues)

Per Serving (1 slice) ● Calories 214 ● Fat 7 g ● Saturated Fat 4 g ● Cholesterol 17 mg
Carbohydrate 38 g ● Fiber 2 g ● ● Protein 2 g ● Sugars 22 g ● Sodium 39 mg

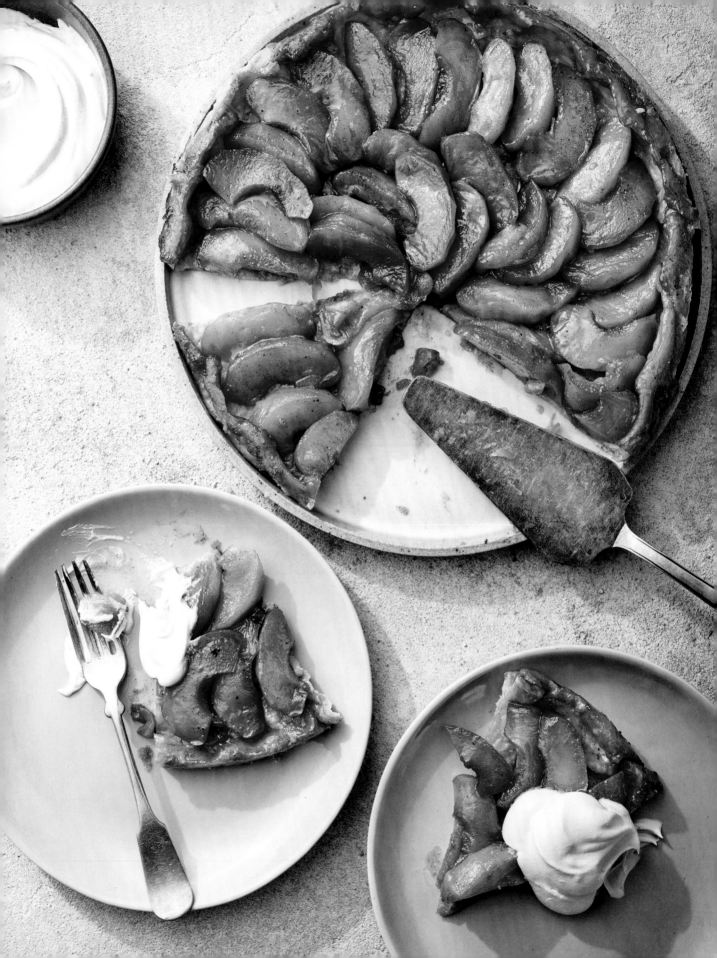

Carefully arrange the apple wedges in a circular pattern over the brown sugar mixture (it's okay if they overlap). Return the pan to medium-low heat and cook until the apples have lightly softened, 12 to 15 minutes. Remove from the heat and let cool.

Preheat the oven to 400°F.

On a lightly floured surface, roll out the dough into a 12-inch round. Drape the dough over the apples and carefully tuck the overhang between the apples and the inside of the pan as best you can, creating a rimmed crust. Bake until the crust is golden, 25 to 30 minutes.

Remove the tart from the oven and let it cool a bit. Place a large rimmed platter or baking sheet over the top of the skillet. Hold the skillet in place (make sure you are wearing oven mitts) and flip both the skillet and the platter simultaneously to invert the tart, being careful with any pan juices that may leak out. (It's smart to do this over the sink.) Carefully lift the skillet away from the platter and rearrange any apples that may have moved.

Slice the tart into 8 slices. Serve warm.

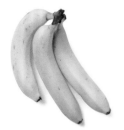

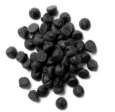

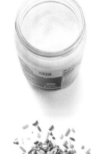

Chocolate Shell Nice Cream

SERVES 4

Ripe bananas transform into a healthy soft-serve ice cream when you freeze then pulse them in a food processor! Top with a homemade magic shell using whatever chocolate that works for you—it works with dairy-free or sugar-free chocolate chips, too. Look for bananas with lots of brown spots, but not yet brown all over, for best results!

4 very ripe medium bananas

½ cup plus 1 tablespoon sugar-free semisweet chocolate chips, such as Lily's

1 tablespoon coconut oil

Sprinkles and/or chopped nuts (optional), for topping

Line a plate or baking sheet (one that will fit in your freezer) with parchment paper. Slice the bananas into 1-inch pieces and arrange them in an even layer on the plate. Cover with another sheet of parchment paper and freeze until firm, at least 6 hours.

Place the frozen banana slices into a food processor. Blend until the mixture is smooth and some air has been whipped in, stopping often to move the pieces to help them catch on the blades, 5 to 10 minutes, depending on your machine. Spread the "nice cream" into a loaf pan in an even layer and freeze again until firm, about 2 hours, for a soft-serve consistency. Cover with plastic wrap if freezing for longer, for up to 3 months.

When ready to serve, put the chocolate chips and coconut oil in a small microwave-safe bowl and heat in 30-second intervals, stirring with a spatula after each, until the chocolate is just melted.

To serve, use an ice cream scoop and divide the nice cream into each bowl. Drizzle 1½ tablespoons of the chocolate mixture over each serving. If desired, sprinkle with toppings. Let the shell set until it hardens, about 2 minutes. Serve immediately.

Per Serving (scant ⅔ cup) ● Calories 223 ● Fat 11 g ● Saturated Fat 7.5 g ● Cholesterol 0 mg Carbohydrate 41 g ● Fiber 12 g ● Protein 3 g ● Sugars 14 g ● Sodium 1 mg

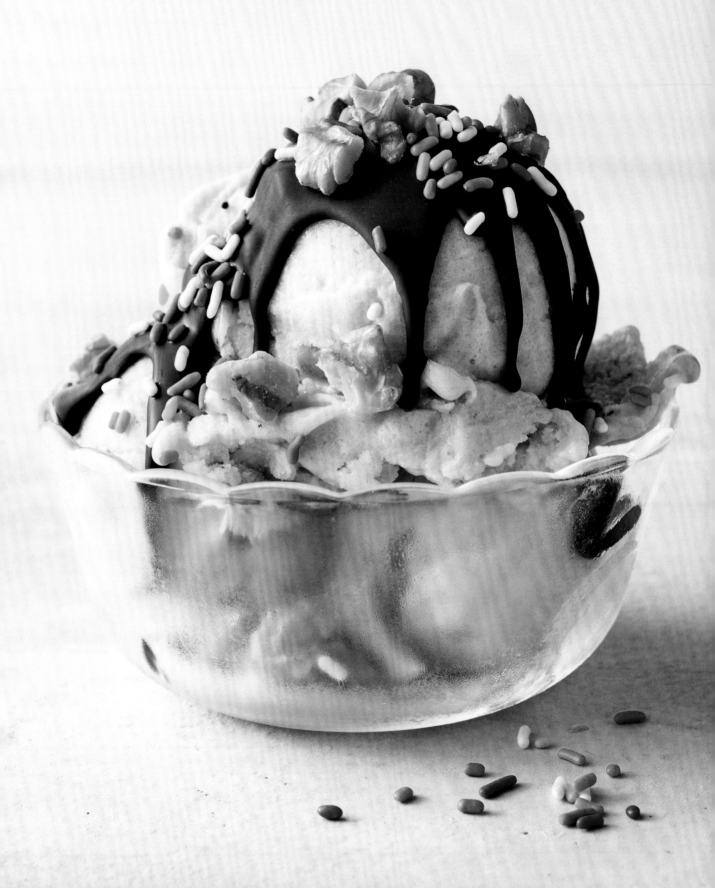

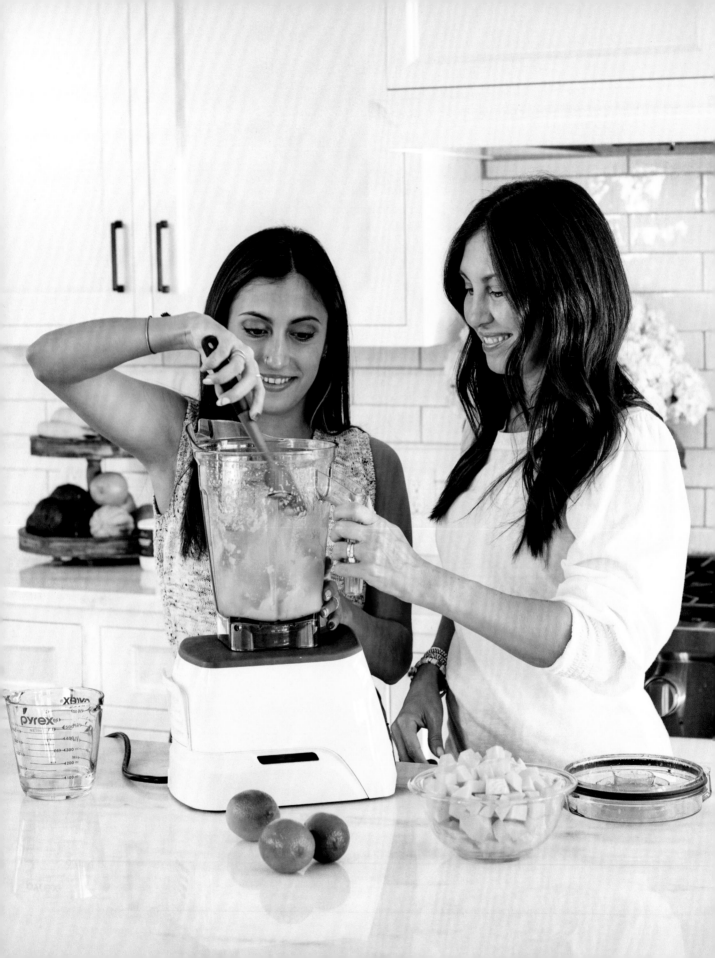

Blender Mango Sorbet

SERVES 4

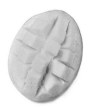

Ripe mango, a touch of sugar, and a little lime juice are all you need to make a refreshing dessert to cool you off on hot summer days. You don't need a fancy ice cream machine to make this sorbet, just a good high-powered blender. Since sorbets have very little fat, they freeze much firmer than ice cream, so I usually make this to be eaten right away. If you plan on freezing it, take it out 10 minutes before eating to soften.

2 large mangoes, peeled, pitted, and diced (about 2½ cups)

2 tablespoons sugar

1 teaspoon fresh lime juice

Place the diced mangoes on a small sheet pan and freeze until solid, 2 to 3 hours.

In a small pot, combine the sugar and ½ cup water and cook over medium heat, whisking until the sugar dissolves, about 1 minute. Let cool completely.

When the mango is frozen solid, transfer the sugar syrup to a blender. Add the lime juice and the frozen mango and blend until smooth, adding a little more water if it's too thick.

Divide the sorbet among bowls and eat right away.

Per Serving (generous ½ cup) ● Calories 92 ● Fat 0.5 g ● Saturated Fat 0 g ● Cholesterol 0 mg Carbohydrate 24 g ● Fiber 2 g ● Protein 0.5 g ● Sugars 22 g ● Sodium 2 mg

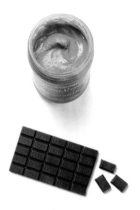

Frozen Peanut Butter Cups

MAKES 12 PEANUT BUTTER CUPS

Tommy has a sweet tooth and he just loves peanut butter cups. I re-created a simplified version of his favorite treat with sugar-free chocolate and they passed the Tommy test with flying colors! We store them in the freezer, so the peanut butter holds its shape.

6 tablespoons smooth peanut butter

3 ounces sugar-free dark chocolate bar (I love Lily's chocolate), chopped

Coarse sea salt

Line 12 cups of a mini-muffin tin with mini paper liners. (If you don't have a mini-muffin tin, for each peanut butter cup, stack 2 or 3 mini liners together so they hold their shape. Arrange them on a small sheet pan.)

In a small microwave-safe bowl, melt the peanut butter in the microwave until it's easy to pour, 30 to 45 seconds.

In another small microwave-safe bowl, melt the chocolate in the microwave in 30-second intervals, stirring after each interval, until completely melted.

Pour about ½ tablespoon of the chocolate into the prepared muffin cups (or carefully pour into the freestanding mini liners on the sheet pan). Top each with ½ tablespoon of the peanut butter. Freeze for 10 minutes, then sprinkle the top with a pinch of sea salt.

Return to the freezer until the peanut butter cups have hardened, 20 to 30 minutes. Serve immediately. Store the peanut butter cups in an airtight container in the freezer for up to 2 months.

Per Serving (2 peanut butter cups) ● Calories 157 ● Fat 13 g ● Saturated Fat 4.5 g
Cholesterol 0 mg ● Carbohydrate 12 g ● Fiber 5.5 g ● Protein 4 g ● Sugars 2 g ● Sodium 89 mg

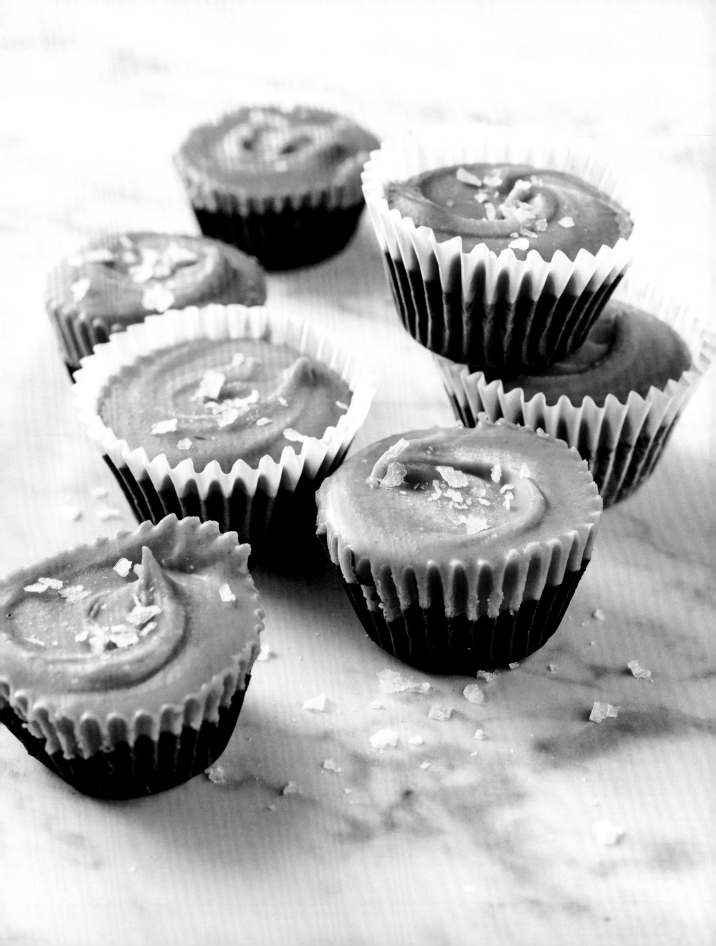

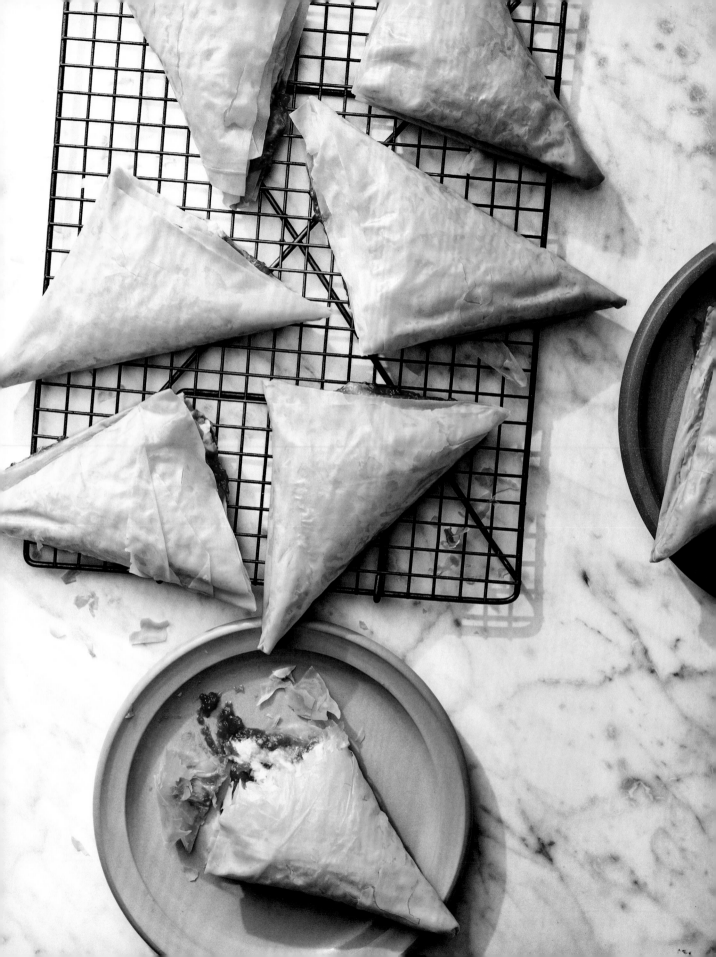

Freezer Strawberry and Cream Cheese Turnovers

MAKES 16 TURNOVERS

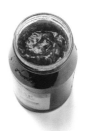

Assemble these turnovers ahead and keep them in your freezer! Then heat them up just like your own homemade toaster strudel. Although you can fill turnovers with just about any type of fruit, I love the combination of cream cheese and jam. Not only is it simple to make (and I almost always have the ingredients on hand), but it's also so delicious. I used strawberry preserves, but feel free to try them with another flavor such as raspberry or apricot.

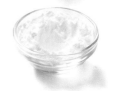

1½ cups low-sugar strawberry preserves

2 teaspoons cornstarch

32 (13 × 9-inch) sheets frozen phyllo dough, thawed

1 cup whipped cream cheese

Powdered sugar, for serving

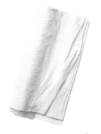

If baking right away, preheat the oven to 350°F. Line a baking sheet with parchment paper.

In a small bowl, stir together the strawberry preserves and cornstarch.

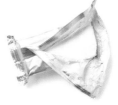

Remove the phyllo dough from the packaging and keep covered with a damp kitchen towel. Stack 2 sheets of phyllo dough on a cutting board and spray lightly with oil. Fold in half lengthwise so you have a long rectangle measuring 4½ × 13 inches.

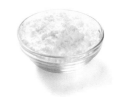

Spread 1 tablespoon of the cream cheese and 1½ tablespoons of the jam at one end of the rectangle. Fold one corner up and over the filling to enclose it in a triangle. Continue folding the triangle over itself (like how you fold a flag) until you reach the other end. Spray the top lightly with oil, then transfer the turnover to the prepared baking sheet, with the seam side down. Repeat with the remaining phyllo and fillings to make 16 turnovers. (At this point, if not baking right away, you can freeze them unbaked for up to 3 months.)

Bake from fresh or frozen until the turnovers are golden and crisp on the outside, 18 to 22 minutes.

Let cool for at least 10 minutes on the baking sheet, then dust with powdered sugar before serving. Refrigerate for up to 3 days.

Per Serving (1 turnover) ● Calories 180 ● Fat 4 g ● Saturated Fat 2 g ● Cholesterol 8 mg
Carbohydrate 31 g ● Fiber 1 g ● Protein 3 g ● Sugars 9 g ● Sodium 226 mg

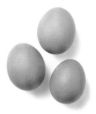

Flourless Sea Salt Brownies

MAKES 12 BROWNIES

Using almond meal in place of wheat flour makes these brownies so incredibly rich and fudgy, it's hard to believe there's absolutely no oil or butter in them! They are lightly sweetened with honey and I use sugar-free chocolate chips. The sea salt accentuates the chocolaty sweetness; I recommend a flaky sea salt like Maldon.

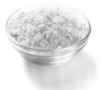

2 large egg whites

1 cup finely ground almond meal, such as Bob's Red Mill

1/2 cup unsweetened cocoa powder

1 teaspoon baking soda

1/2 cup honey

41/2 ounces (3/4 cup) sugar-free chocolate chips (I like Lily's)

1/4 teaspoon flaky sea salt

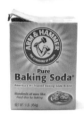

Preheat the oven to 325°F. Spray an 8 × 8-inch pan with oil. Cut a sheet of parchment paper about 8 inches wide and long enough to hang over two sides of the pan (to form a sling so you can easily remove the brownies once baked). Place into the baking pan.

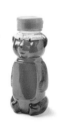

In a medium bowl, whisk the egg whites until fluffy.

In a large bowl, whisk together the almond meal, cocoa powder, baking soda, and 1/4 teaspoon kosher salt. Add the egg whites and stir with a spatula until combined. Add 6 tablespoons water and the honey and stir with the spatula until combined. Fold in the chocolate chips. Scrape the batter into the prepared baking pan.

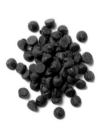

Bake until a toothpick inserted into the center comes out clean, 30 to 35 minutes. Immediately sprinkle the brownies with the flaky sea salt while still warm. Let cool, then refrigerate for about 30 minutes until chilled and firm (this will make it easier to cut cleaner slices).

Cut into 12 brownies and serve. Store in an airtight container in the refrigerator for up to 4 days.

Per Serving (1 brownie) ● Calories 145 ● Fat 8 g ● Saturated Fat 2.5 g ● Cholesterol 0 mg Carbohydrate 22 g ● Fiber 6 g ● Protein 4 g ● Sugars 12 g ● Sodium 180 mg

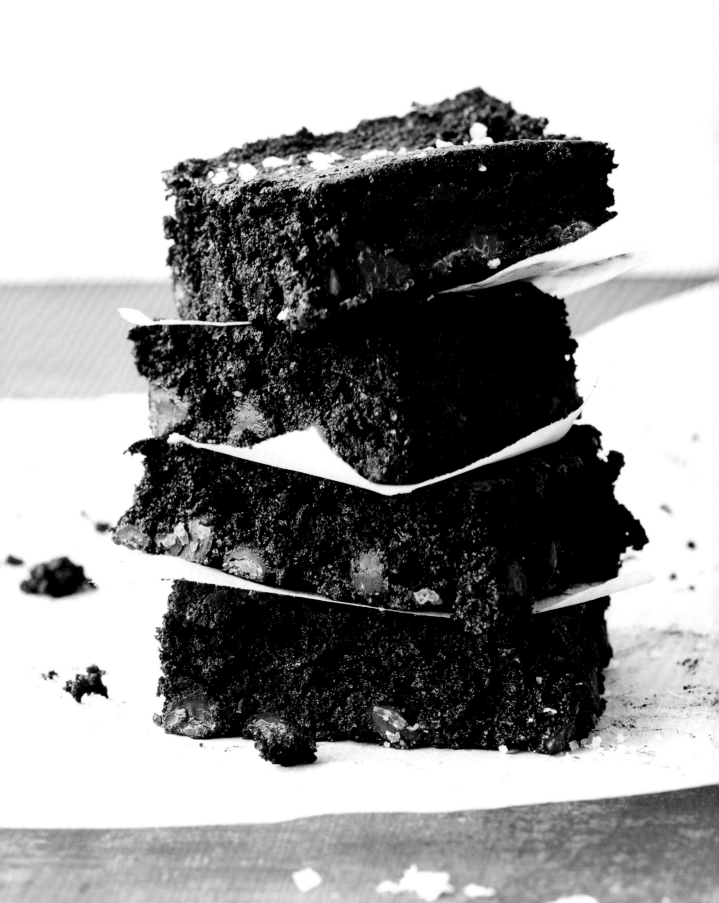

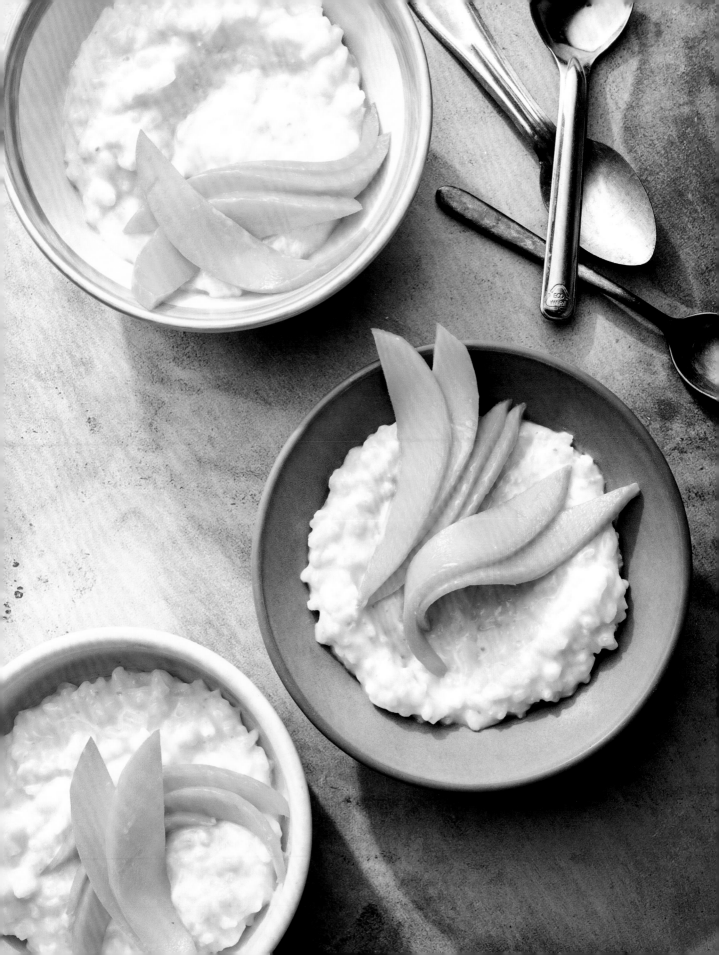

Coconut Rice Pudding with Mango

SERVES 4

The inspiration for this rice pudding came from one of my favorite desserts ever: Thai sticky rice with mango. But instead of using sticky rice in this recipe, I used sushi rice, and the results are creamy and delicious. It's lightly sweetened, letting the flavor of the mangoes shine.

½ cup uncooked sushi rice or short-grain rice, not rinsed

1 cup 2% milk or nondairy milk

½ cup canned light coconut milk

3 tablespoons monk fruit sweetener or sugar

2 mangoes, cut into ½-inch thin slices

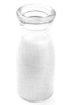

In a heavy-bottomed nonstick medium pot, combine the rice and 1½ cups water. Bring to a boil over medium-high heat and cook uncovered until most of the water is evaporated and just barely skims the top of the rice, 5 to 8 minutes. Cover, reduce the heat to low, and simmer until the rice is tender, about 15 minutes. Remove from the heat and let it sit, covered, for 5 minutes.

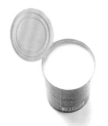

To the rice, add the milk, coconut milk, sweetener, and ⅛ teaspoon kosher salt and stir to combine. Bring to a boil over medium-low heat, then reduce the heat to low and simmer, stirring often, until the rice pudding is thick and creamy, about 15 minutes.

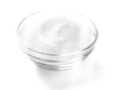

Remove from the heat and spoon into four shallow bowls. Serve warm or chilled, topped with mango.

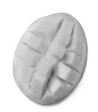

Per Serving (scant ⅔ cup pudding + ½ mango) ● Calories 206 ● Fat 3 g ● Saturated Fat 2.5 g
Cholesterol 5 mg ● Carbohydrate 58 g ● Fiber 2.5 g ● Protein 4 g ● Sugars 19 g ● Sodium 70 mg

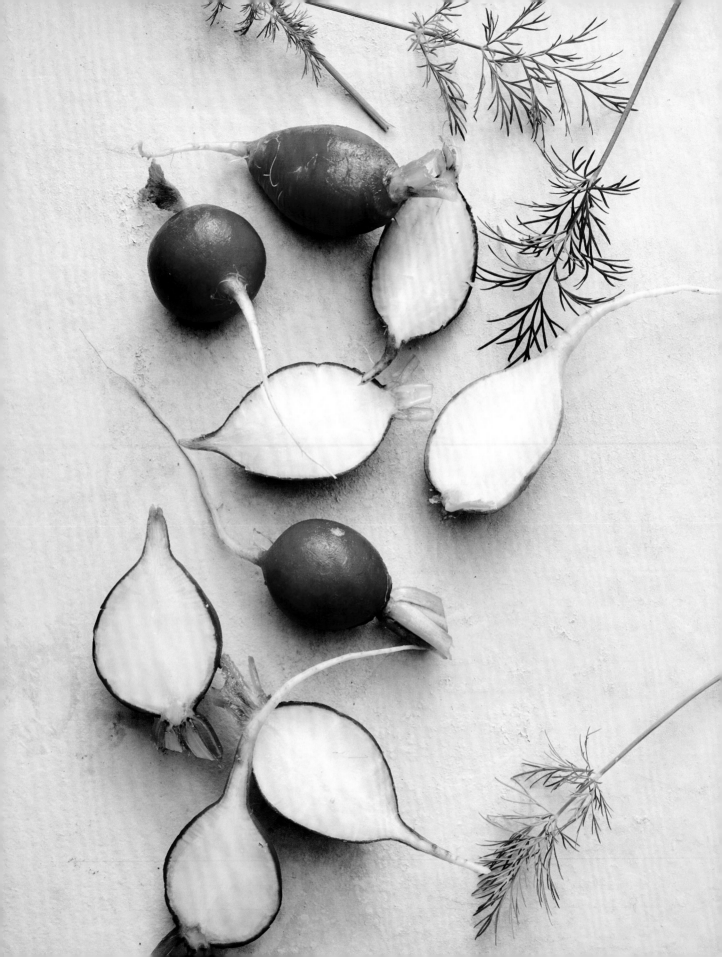

Acknowledgments

I'm forever grateful for the wonderful team who helped put this book together. In addition to the many people who contributed to the creation of this cookbook, I also appreciate the community of readers and fans who have supported me and my work over the years. Your enthusiasm and encouragement are a constant source of inspiration and motivation, and I'm so grateful to have you all in my life. I also want to thank my husband, Tommy, and my kids, Karina and Madison, who always support me and taste-test my recipes. I'm so appreciative for their love and support. And to my parents, for teaching me the joys of cooking.

I'm also grateful to my friend and collaborator Heather K. Jones, R.D., who helped bring this book to life and whose energy, spirit, and positive vibes made the process so much easier. And to the rest of her team, including Danielle Hazard and Jackie Price, who helped make this book the best it could be.

I'm also thankful for my aunt Ligia Caldas, who has been by my side through all of my books and who has been an indispensable source of support and guidance. And to my agent, Janis Donnaud, who has always believed in me and my work.

Finally, a giant thank-you to the terrific team at Clarkson Potter, including Jenn Sit, Ian Dingman, Patricia Shaw, Heather Williamson, Erica Gelbard, Stephanie Davis, Bianca Cruz, and Stephanie Huntwork, who are a pleasure to work with. And to my photographer Eva Kolenko and her fabulous team, including food stylist Emily Caneer, who created such beautiful photos and brought my recipes to life in a way that I never could have imagined. And for the lifestyle photos, Johnny Miller and Susan Spungen, who made the day go effortlessly smooth. Thank you all for your hard work and dedication. This book would not have been possible without you!

Index

Note: Page references in *italics* indicate photographs.

Published in the United States by Clarkson Potter/ Publishers, an imprint of Random House, a division of Penguin Random House LLC, New York.
ClarksonPotter.com
RandomHouseBooks.com

CLARKSON POTTER is a trademark and POTTER with colophon is a registered trademark of Penguin Random House LLC.

Library of Congress Cataloging-in-Publication Data
Names: Homolka, Gina, author. | Jones, Heather K, author. | Kolenko, Eva, photographer. Title: Skinnytaste simple : easy, healthy recipes with 7 ingredients or fewer/ by Gina Homolka with Heather K. Jones, R.D. ; photographs by Eva Kolenko. Description: New York : Clarkson Potter/ Publishers, [2023] | Includes index. | Identifiers: LCCN 2022047835 (print) | LCCN 2022047836 (ebook) | ISBN 9780593235614 (hardcover) | ISBN 9780593235621 (ebook) Subjects: LCSH: Quick and easy cooking. | LCGFT: Cookbooks. Classification: LCC TX833.5 .H665 2023 (print) | LCC TX833.5 (ebook) | DDC 641.5/12—dc23/eng/20221116
LC record available at https://lccn.loc.gov /2022047835
LC ebook record available at https://lccn.loc.gov /2022047836

ISBN 978-0-593-23561-4
eBook ISBN 978-0-593-23562-1
Barnes & Noble ISBN 978-0-593-79664-1

Printed in China

Photographer: Eva Kolenko
Food Stylist: Emily Caneer
Editor: Jennifer Sit
Editorial Assistant: Bianca Cruz
Designer: Ian Dingman
Production Editor: Patricia Shaw
Production Manager: Heather Williamson
Compositor: Merri Ann Morrell and Nick Patton
Copy Editor: Kate Slate
Indexer: Elizabeth T. Parson
Marketer: Stephanie Davis
Publicist: Erica Gelbard
Cover design: Ian Dingman
Cover photographs: Eva Kolenko

10 9 8 7 6 5 4 3 2 1

First Edition

Clarkson Potter/Publishers
New York
clarksonpotter.com

Cover design by Ian Dingman
Cover photographs by Eva Kolenko